Pace Rhythm -

Pace Rhythm -

Echocardiography:
The Normal Examination and
Echocardiographic Measurements

Bonita Anderson

Diploma in Medical Ultrasonography (Cardiac),
Master of Applied Science (Medical Ultrasound),
Accredited Medical Sonographer.

Typesetting, illustrations, layout and design by
MGA Graphics,
PO Box 5443,
Manly, Queensland, 4179.
AUSTRALIA.

First Edition, 2000.
Third Printing: March, 2004.

Printed in Australia by Fergies, Brisbane.

For updates, information and availability visit: http://**www.echotext.info**

ISBN: 0-646-39139-9

Table of Contents

Table of Contents (continued)

Table of Contents (continued)

Preface

The routine echocardiographic examination is a non-invasive investigation that consists of a comprehensive two-dimensional (2-D) examination complemented by additional M-mode (motion-mode), spectral and colour flow Doppler modalities. The 2-D examination provides important and detailed information regarding anatomic structures and relationships as well as allowing the assessment of cardiac function. The M-mode examination provides valuable and superior temporal information while the Doppler examination contributes vital haemodynamic data including the assessment of pressure gradients, volumetric flow, and intracardiac pressures.

Due to the diagnostic potential of echocardiography, the echocardiographic examination has become widely employed as a common cardiac investigative tool which has revolutionised the assessment of gross cardiac pathology and has, therefore, become an integral component in the routine clinical assessment of the cardiac patient.

The primary objective of this text is to provide an educational guide for the cardiac sonographer, which incorporates all aspects of the echocardiographic examination from the routine examination to the more complex haemodynamic calculations. This text is divided into two parts. The first part encompasses the basic principles of two-dimensional imaging, M-mode and Doppler echocardiography as well as the routine echocardiographic examination. Part two covers two-dimensional, M-mode and Doppler measurements and calculations, including basic principles of the techniques, advantages, limitations, and significance of the values obtained. "Step by step" instructions have also been included as a guide for the performance of certain measurements, especially for haemodynamic calculations.

While every attempt has been made to address the techniques currently employed in echocardiography, it is the responsibility of the cardiac sonographer to remain abreast of new echocardiographic developments and techniques. These new techniques should be adopted in order to provide the most relevant and diagnostic information for the cardiologist or physician. Achievement of these goals will ultimately aid in the improved management and treatment of the cardiac patient. Furthermore, it is important to note that this text should not be used in isolation and that readers should seek alternative sources, such as those listed in the reference sections of this text, for a more comprehensive review of the principles and practice of each echocardiographic modality.

Finally, although not covered within the scope of this text, it is important to recognise that all cardiac sonographers must have a comprehensive knowledge of the following:

- normal cardiac anatomy and normal variants,
- the pathological changes in cardiac anatomy which occur due to acquired and congenital heart disease,
- fluid dynamics of normal blood flow and the pathological changes in cardiac blood flow which occur due to acquired or congenital disease, and
- the pathophysiolgly of cardiac disease processes.

A basic knowledge of cardiac auscultation and electrocardiography for correlation of results of the echocardiogram is also important.

Acknowledgments

The primary incentive for writing this book developed as I began training others in echocardiography. At the time there were many excellent references available on the subject, though few were aimed at the novice sonographer. This made the task of teaching quite difficult. I thought that a book was required which concentrated on the basics of echocardiography, addressing the training sonographer in particular. I hope this book has achieved that goal.

As anyone who has ever undertaken a project of this magnitude will know, it takes a lot longer to complete than first anticipated. In fact I am not sure that I would have taken on this task had I realised exactly how long it would take. However, now that the book is finally finished, I would like to take the opportunity to acknowledge those who have supported and encouraged me along the way.

First and foremost, I must acknowledge the enormous support I have received from my family and my husband, Murray. Not only did Murray offer his support during this time, but he is responsible for the production of the finished article. His background as a graphic artist also allowed him to produce many of the illustrations appearing within this text. Without Murray I doubt that this project would ever have gotten off the ground.

I would also like to thank my "boss", Dr Darryl J. Burstow (Senior Staff Cardiologist and Clinical Director of the Echocardiographic Laboratory at the Prince Charles Hospital). Darryl has, by far, been the greatest influence on my career as a cardiac sonographer. He has advised me, taught me, and always encouraged me to do my very best. Darryl also provided expert advise on the content of this book.

I would also like to extend my thanks to Margo Harkness (Senior Lecturer, Queensland University of Technology) who has had an enormous influence on my academic accomplishments. Margo has taught me many valuable lessons, including teaching me how to teach! It is to her credit that I have advanced as far as I have today. I also thank Margo for an exceptional effort in proof-reading this entire text. Margo's attention to detail is beyond compare!

Last but certainly not least, I would like to thank the people with whom I work with on a daily basis at the Prince Charles Hospital. Without their stamina, support and enthusiasm behind me, I would not have been able to find the inspiration necessary to write this book at all. In particular, I wish to thank Cathy Hegerty and Belinda Shearer. Belinda also proof-read this book and provided valuable input from the cardiac sonographer's perspective.

BA

Abbreviations and Symbols

Echocardiographic and Medical:

AR	: aortic regurgitation
ASE	: American Society of Echocardiography
AVA	: aortic valve area
bpm	: beats per minute
BSA	: body surface area
CI	: cardiac index
CO	: cardiac output
CSA	: cross-sectional area
CW	: continuous-wave
D	: diameter
ECG	: electrocardiogram
EF	: ejection fraction
EOA	: effective orifice area
EPSS	: E point-septal-separation
EROA	: effective regurgitant orifice area
FS	: fractional shortening
HOCM	: hypertrophic obstructive cardiomyopathy
IVC	: inferior vena cava
IVRT	: isovolumic relaxation time
LVEDP	: left ventricular end-diastolic pressure
LVOT	: left ventricular outflow tract
MACS	: maximal aortic cusp separation
MPA	: main pulmonary artery
M-mode	: motion mode
MR	: mitral regurgitation
MVA	: mitral valve area
PASP	: pulmonary artery systolic pressure
PDA	: patent ductus arteriosus
PR	: pulmonary regurgitation
PRF	: pulse repetition frequency
PISA	: proximal isovelocity surface area
PW	: pulsed-wave
Q	: flow rate
RAP	: mean right atrial pressure
RBCs	: red blood cells
RVACT	: right ventricular acceleration time
RVOT	: right ventricular outflow tract
RVSP	: right ventricular systolic pressure
SAM	: systolic anterior motion
2-D	: two-dimensional
SV	: stroke volume
TR	: tricuspid regurgitation
VSD	: ventricular septal defect
VTI	: velocity time integral

Statistical:

r	: correlation coefficient
Pt. No.	: patient number
SEE	: standard error of the estimate
vs	: versus

Symbols and Signs:

%	: percentage
<	: less than
>	: greater than
$\leq$	: less than or equal to
$\geq$	: greater than or equal to
π	: pi
Δ	: delta (difference)
θ	: theta
λ	: lambda

Units of Measure:

circ/s	: circumferences per second
cm	: centimetres
cm^2	: centimetres squared
cm/s	: centimetres per second
dB	: decibels
g	: grams
g/m^2	: grams per metre squared
Hz	: Hertz
kHz	: kilohertz
kg	: kilogram
L/min	: litres per minute
$L/min/m^2$	: litres per minute per metre squared
MHz	: megahertz
ms	: milliseconds
m/s	: metres per second
mm	: millimetres
mm/s	: millimetres per second
mm Hg	: millimetres of mercury
mm/s	: millimetres/second
c	: speed of sound (m/s)

A Brief History of Echocardiography

The use of ultrasound in the diagnosis of cardiac disease has been available for more than four decades with the diagnostic potential of this modality first recognised in 1954 when the first continuous recordings of the heart walls were recorded [1].

The term "Echocardiography" was adopted to describe the utility of ultrasound in cardiology in which returning echoes are reflected from the boundaries of cardiac structures. Since this initial application, and through the development of M-mode and two-dimensional "real-time" imaging as well as the evolution of Doppler technology, the diagnostic role of this modality has increased enormously.

In the years that followed, M-mode echocardiography began to play an important role as a diagnostic tool in the evaluation of the cardiac patient. However, the one-dimensional, "ice-pick" information offered by M-mode echocardiography obviously had significant limitations in the examination of the three-dimensional heart. B-mode (brightness-mode) or two-dimensional ultrasound imaging for stationary (non-dynamic) body structures, such as the abdominal organs, had been available for many years. This technique, however, was not practical in the examination of the dynamic heart. Around the mid 1970's, two-dimensional echocardiography became available for clinical practice allowing "real-time", high resolution ultrasonic imaging of the dynamic heart, thus, providing tomographic spatial information in the assessment of cardiac morphology and cardiac function. The additional ability of this technique to allow two-dimensional spatial orientation also facilitated the M-mode evaluation of the heart by overcoming many of the one-dimensional pitfalls of the M-mode technique, such as oblique transection of cardiac chambers.

Despite the advances of M-mode and two-dimensional echocardiography, and much research into the value and ability of these methods to aid in the quantitation of cardiac valvular lesions, there were still many problems that inhibited the sole use of echocardiography as a definitive diagnostic tool. Therefore, these patients ultimately required further definitive invasive investigations such as cardiac catheterisation.

With the advent of spectral Doppler technology in the late 1970's and the validation of Doppler-derived pressure gradients with simultaneous invasive measurements, accurate haemodynamic evaluation of pressure gradients within the heart was possible. This contributed enormously to the diagnostic capability of echocardiography. Further developments in Doppler technology led to the evolution of colour flow Doppler imaging in the mid 1980's. Colour flow Doppler imaging provides immediate and precise spatial information regarding blood flow within the heart and has reduced the Doppler examination time considerably. In the past, colour flow imaging offered only semiquantitative information about blood flow, particularly with respect to regurgitant lesions. Now due to extensive research, colour flow mapping has the ability to yield quantitative information about the severity of such lesions.

The term "Echocardiography" is a collective expression, which has come to include all modalities of ultrasound utilised in the investigation of cardiac anatomy and function. "Echocardiography" refers to the use of (1) two-dimensional, real-time imaging, (2) M-mode traces obtained in conjunction with two-dimensional guidance, (3) spectral Doppler blood flow velocity information, and (4) colour-encoded Doppler maps overlaid on the two-dimensional image.

An additional advantage of echocardiography is the fact that it is a safe, noninvasive technique with no known risk to the patient or the operator at the ultrasonic power levels used [2].

Due to this important factor, as well as the proven value of the haemodynamic and diagnostic data that can be provided by this technique, echocardiography has become widely employed as a common cardiac investigative tool. It has revolutionised the investigation of gross cardiac pathology and has become an integral component in the routine clinical assessment of the cardiac patient. In fact, echocardiography is the most frequently used imaging procedure in the diagnosis of heart disease and rivals or exceeds the more traditional techniques such as chest radiography and electrocardiography [3].

1: Edler, I and Hertz, C.H.: Kungliga Fysuigrafiska Sallskapets I Lund Forhanlinger Bd 24: 1-19,1954; 2: Bioeffects Committee, American Institute of Ultrasound in Medicine: Journal of Ultrasound in Medicine 7 (suppl): S1-S38, 1988; 3: American Society of Echocardiography: Journal of the American Society of Echocardiography 8: S1-S28, 1995.

Chapter 1
Basic Principles of Two-Dimensional Ultrasound Imaging

Basic Principles of Two-Dimensional Imaging

Two-dimensional (2-D) images are produced using ultrasound; thus, it is important that the sonographer is aware of some of the basic principles of ultrasound physics. This chapter covers only the basic principles of 2-D imaging. Readers should seek alternative sources such as those listed in the reference section at the end of this chapter for a more comprehensive review of the principles of 2-D imaging and instrumentation.

Nature of Ultrasound:

Ultrasound or sound is mechanical energy that is transmitted or propagated through a medium by the vibration of molecules. This vibration of molecules causes them to oscillate about their normal resting position in a line which is in the direction of the propagated wave. Thus, sound waves are **longitudinal waves** (Figure 1.1A). This is in contrast to waves that form when a pebble is dropped into a pond. In this instance, wave motion is perpendicular to the direction of wave motion; these waves are called **transverse waves** (Figure 1.1B).

Pressure variations in the wave cause the molecules to become disturbed which results in oscillation of these molecules. Sound is propagated by "pushing" molecules into another one forming a series of compressions (zones of high pressure) and rarefaction (zones of low pressure) (Figure 1.2).

Properties of Sound Waves

Sound waves are characterised by a number of parameters including (1) amplitude, (2) wavelength, (3) period, (4) frequency, and (5) velocity (Figure 1.3).

1. Amplitude (A): The amplitude of a wave can refer to particle displacement, particle velocity, or acoustic pressure of a sound wave. When referring to particle displacement, the amplitude is a measure of the maximum height of a wave.

2. Wavelength (λ): Wavelength refers to the distance between two successive zones; that is, the distance between two compression zones or between two rarefaction zones. Wavelength is expressed in units of distance (m, cm, mm, or μm).

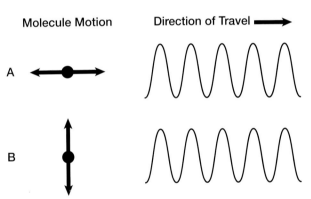

Figure 1.1: Longitudinal Waves and Transverse Waves.
A. Longitudinal waves: particles oscillate in the same direction as the propagated wave.
B. Transverse waves: particles move perpendicularly to the direction of the propagated wave.

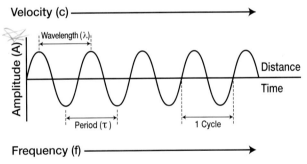

Figure 1.3: Sound Wave Parameters.
Sound waves are characterised by a number of parameters including amplitude, wavelength, period, frequency, and velocity.

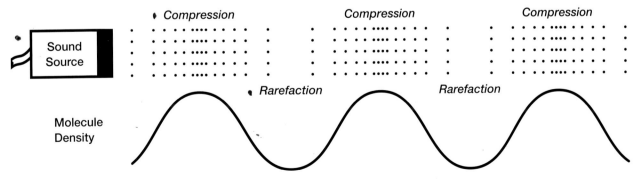

Figure 1.2: Compressions and Rarefaction of a Sound Wave.
Pressure variations in the wave cause the molecules to become disturbed which results in oscillation of these molecules. Sound is propagated by "pushing" molecules into another one forming a series of compressions (zones of high pressure) and rarefaction (zones of low pressure).

3. Period (τ): The period is a measure of the time taken for one complete wave cycle to occur. Period is expressed in units of time (s, ms, μs). Period is inversely related to the frequency (f):

(Equation 1.1)

$$\tau = \frac{1}{f}$$

4. Frequency (f): The frequency of a wave refers to the number of cycles that pass a given point per second; that is, the number of cycles per second. The unit of frequency is the hertz (Hz) where 1 hertz equals one cycle per second. The frequency of human hearing is in the range of 40 Hz to 15 kHz while the frequencies utilised in diagnostic ultrasound are in the order of 2 MHz to 10 MHz. Frequency is inversely related to the period:

(Equation 1.2)

$$f = \frac{1}{\tau}$$

5. Velocity (c): Velocity refers to the speed in which sound waves propagate through a medium. Velocity is measured in units of distance per time (m/s, cm/s). The velocity of sound wave propagation through a medium is determined by the density (β) and compressibility (ρ) of that medium such that as density of a medium increases, the velocity of sound through that medium increases.

(Equation 1.3)

$$c = \frac{1}{\sqrt{\beta\ \rho}}$$

Density and velocity properties of different media are listed in Table 1.1.

Table 1.1: Properties of Different Media

Material	Density (kg/m³)	Velocity (m/s)
Air	1.2	330
Water	1000	1480
• Soft Tissue:		
average	1060	1540
Liver	1060	1550
Muscle	1080	1580
Fat	952	1459
Brain	994	1560
Kidney	1038	1560
Spleen	1045	1570
Blood	1057	1575
Bone	1912	4080

Source: Hedrik, Hykes, and Starchman: *Ultrasound Physics and Instrumentation. 3rd Edition, 1995.* Mosby Year Book Inc. pp: 7.

For diagnostic ultrasound purposes, ultrasound instruments assume that the velocity of sound in soft tissues is 1540 m/s. This is a very important factor as the positioning of echoes on the image display are calculated based on this assumption. Hence, when the velocity of sound through a medium is not 1540 m/s, the position of a structure on the image display will be incorrect.

The Wave Equation:

One of the most important equations in ultrasound is the wave equation which relates frequency (f), wavelength (λ), and velocity (c):

(Equation 1.4)

$$c = \lambda\ f$$

Velocity of sound through soft tissue is assumed to be constant; hence, there is an inverse relationship between wavelength and frequency. Therefore, as frequency increases, wavelength decreases and vice versa. This relationship is very important in diagnostic ultrasound as image resolution is related to wavelength, while the depth of penetration and attenuation of the ultrasound beam is related to frequency.

Interaction of Ultrasound with Tissue

The interaction of ultrasound waves with organs and tissues encountered, along the ultrasound beam, can be described in terms of (1) attenuation, (2) absorption, (3) reflection, (4) scattering, (5) refraction, and (6) diffraction (Figure 1.4).

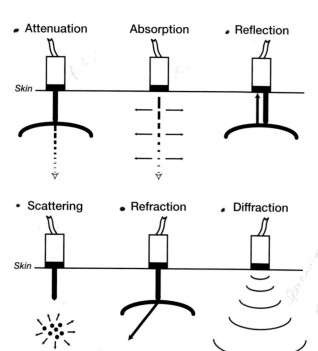

Figure 1.4: Interactions of Ultrasound with Tissue.
The interaction of ultrasound waves with organs and tissues encountered along the ultrasound beam can be described in terms of attenuation, absorption, reflection, scattering, refraction, and diffraction.

1. Attenuation:

Attenuation refers to the reduction in strength of the ultrasound signal as the wave traverses through a medium. As ultrasound travels through a medium, the signal strength is progressively attenuated due to absorption of ultrasound energy as well as by reflection, scattering, and refraction of the ultrasound beam.

The unit for attenuation is decibel (dB). The decibel is simply a unit used to express a relative difference between two acoustic signals and is based on a logarithmic scale. Decibels can be used to describe the relationship between amplitude or intensity of the signal:

(Equation 1.5)

$$dB = 10 \ \log_{10} \left(\frac{I}{I_o} \right)$$

where I = intensity of the beam at any point
I_0 = initial intensity of the beam

Hence, a reduction in the intensity of the original ultrasound signal ($I_0 = 1$) by one-half ($I = 0.5$) equates to - 3 dB:

$$dB = 10 \ \log_{10} \left(\frac{0.5}{1} \right)$$

$$= 10 \times \log_{10} 0.5$$

$$= 10 \times 0.301$$

$$= -3$$

Table 1.2 outlines the relationship between decibels, intensity ratios, and the percentage of intensity remaining in the ultrasound beam and the percentage of intensity lost from the ultrasound beam.

Table 1.2: Relationships between Decibels, Intensity Ratios, the Percentage of Intensity remaining in the ultrasound beam and the Percentage of Intensity lost from the Ultrasound Beam.

dB	I/Io	Percentage of ultrasound remaining (%)	Percentage of ultrasound lost (%)
0	1	100	0
- 3	0.5	50	50
- 6	0.25	25	75
- 10	0.1	10	90
- 20	0.01	1	99
- 30	0.001	0.1	99.9
- 40	0.0001	0.01	99.99

Attenuation is directly related to the frequency of ultrasound and the distance that the pulse travels into the medium. Hence, greater attenuation occurs the further the ultrasound signal has to travel and the higher the frequency. Furthermore, the frequency is also inversely related to the maximum image depth such that higher frequency transducers have shallower imaging depths while lower frequency transducers are able to image deeper into the body. As a rule of thumb, the attenuation of ultrasound in soft tissue is 1 dB/cm/MHz.

2. Absorption:

Absorption is the only process whereby sound energy is actually dissipated within a medium. Other modes of interaction with tissue such as reflection, scattering, refraction and diffraction decrease the intensity of the ultrasound beam by redirecting the energy of the beam. Absorption refers to the transformation of ultrasound energy into heat. Three factors determine the amount of absorption within a medium: (1) the viscosity of the medium, (2) the "relaxation time" of the medium, and (3) the frequency of sound.

Viscosity refers to the amount of particle freedom within a medium or the ability of molecules to move past one another. The higher the viscosity of the medium, the greater the resistance to molecular movement within the medium. Furthermore, high viscosity means that greater frictional forces need to be overcome by the vibrating molecules resulting in greater heat generation. Water is an example of a low viscosity medium and syrup is a high viscosity medium.

The *"relaxation time"* of a medium refers to the time taken for a molecule to return to its resting position after it has been displaced. When a sound wave travels through medium with short relaxation time molecules vibrate and then quickly come to rest before the second wave arrives. However, in media with a long relaxation time, molecules vibrate for a longer period of time. Therefore, when the second wave arrives, the molecules may still be vibrating (usually in the opposite direction to the sound wave). Thus, the second wave must first stop the molecules from vibrating and then reverse the direction of the molecules. This requires additional energy that results in heat generation.

Frequency also affects absorption in relation to both viscosity and the relaxation time. Viscosity of a medium changes with frequency. Increasing the frequency means that molecule motion is increased resulting in more "drag" of the molecules which, in turn, increases friction and generates heat. In addition, increasing the frequency means that the molecules remain in motion longer; hence, more energy is required to stop and redirect the molecules resulting in greater absorption. Thus, the rate of absorption is directly related to the frequency. Doubling the frequency, in effect, doubles the absorption. The degree of absorption limits the depth of penetration of the ultrasound beam. Hence, higher frequency transducers result in greater absorption that reduces the depth of penetration. Lower frequency transducers have a lesser degree of absorption and, therefore, increased depth penetration.

3. Reflection:

The most important interaction of ultrasound imaging is reflection of the transmitted ultrasound beam from internal structures encountered. Ultrasound images are created when there is reflection of the ultrasound beam at the interface between two tissue boundaries or media. The amount of ultrasound reflected depends upon the relative changes in the acoustic impedance between two media or tissues.

Acoustic impedance (Z) is dependent upon tissue density (ρ) and the propagation speed through that tissue or medium (c):

(Equation 1.6)

$$Z = \rho \ c$$

where Z = acoustic impedance (kg/m²/s or the rayl)
       ρ = tissue density (kg/m³)
       c = propagation speed (m/s)

If the acoustic impedance between two media is the same, sound is transmitted from the first medium, through to the second medium without any reflection of the ultrasound beam. When the acoustic impedances between two media differ, some of the ultrasound energy is reflected from the boundary between the two media, and some of the energy is transmitted. The amount of ultrasound energy reflected and transmitted is dependent upon the acoustic mismatch between the two media such that the greater the acoustic mismatch, the greater the degree of reflection and the lesser the degree of transmission (Figure 1.5).

The percentage of transmitted and reflected ultrasound energy can be calculated when the acoustic impedance of two media is known using equations 1.7 and 1.8.

(Equation 1.7)

$$percentage \ reflected(\%) = \left[\frac{\left(Z_2 - Z_1 \right)}{Z_2 + Z_1} \right]^2 \times 100$$

(Equation 1.8)

$$percentage \ transmitted(\%) = \left[\frac{4 \ Z_1 \ Z_2}{\left(Z_1 + Z_2 \right)^2} \right] \times 100$$

where Z_1 = acoustic impedance in medium 1.
where Z_2 = acoustic impedance in medium 2.

Large differences in acoustic impedance are found at bone/soft tissue interfaces as well as at air/soft tissue boundaries. Using acoustic impedance values listed in Table 1.3, it is possible to determine the percentage of reflection and transmission at the bone/soft tissue, and air/soft tissue boundaries (examples 1 and 2).

Table 1.3: Properties of Different Media

Material	Density (kg/m³)	Velocity (m/s)	Acoustic Impedance (kg/m²/s x 10⁻⁶)
Air	1.2	330	0.0004
Soft Tissue (average)	1060	1540	1.63
Bone	1912	4080	7.8

Source: Hedrik, Hykes, and Starchman: Ultrasound Physics and Instrumentation. 3rd Edition, 1995. Mosby Year Book Inc. pp: 7.

Example 1:

Calculation of the Transmission and Reflection of Ultrasound Energy at the Bone/Soft Tissue Interface.

$$percentage \ reflected(\%) = \left[\frac{\left(Z_2 - Z_1 \right)}{Z_2 + Z_1} \right]^2 \times 100$$

$$= \left[\frac{\left(7.8 - 1.63 \right)}{7.8 + 1.63} \right]^2 \times 100$$

$$= \left[\frac{6.17}{9.43} \right]^2 \times 100$$

$$= 0.654^2 \times 100$$

$$= 43\%$$

$$percentage \ transmitted(\%) = \left[\frac{4 \ Z_1 \ Z_2}{\left(Z_1 + Z_2 \right)^2} \right] \times 100$$

$$= \left[\frac{4 \times 7.8 \times 1.63}{\left(7.8 + 1.63 \right)^2} \right] \times 100$$

$$= \left[\frac{50.856}{9.43^2} \right] \times 100$$

$$= \left[\frac{50.856}{88.925} \right] \times 100$$

$$= 57\%$$

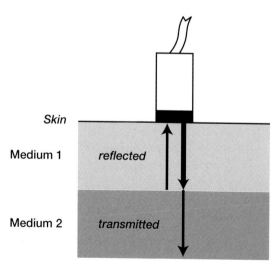

Figure 1.5: Transmission and Reflection of Ultrasound Energy. This illustration demonstrates ultrasound energy passing through medium 1. When the ultrasound beam encounters a medium of different acoustic impedance (medium 2), some ultrasound energy is transmitted and some energy is reflected. The degree of transmission and reflection is related to the amount of acoustic mismatch between these two media.

Example 2:
Calculation of the Transmission and Reflection of Ultrasound Energy at the Air/Soft Tissue Interface.

$$percentage\ reflected(\%) = \left[\frac{(0.0004 - 1.63)}{0.0004 + 1.63}\right]^2 \times 100$$

$$= \left[\frac{-1.63}{1.6304}\right]^2 \times 100$$

$$= 0.999^2 \times 100$$

$$= 99.8\%$$

Percentage transmitted (%):
There is a simpler method of calculating the percentage transmission when the percentage reflection is known. The percentage reflection plus the percentage transmission equals 100%; hence, the percentage transmission is equal to 100% - percentage reflection. Therefore:

percentage transmission (%) **= 100 - 99.8**
= 0.2 %

Due to this poor transmission of ultrasound energy at air/soft tissue boundaries, a coupling medium is required at the transducer/tissue interface.

Types of Reflectors:
Ultrasound reflections or echoes are generated from two types of reflectors: specular reflectors and scatterers.
Specular reflectors are large with respect to the wavelength and present a relatively smooth surface to the ultrasound beam. These reflectors act as a mirror and are highly angle dependent (Figure 1.6). To optimise an ultrasound examination of specular reflectors, the angle of incidence between the ultrasound beam and this reflector should be perpendicular. When these reflectors are parallel to the ultrasound beam, dropout of echoes may occur on the ultrasound image as little or no sound is reflected from them. Examples of specular reflectors include cardiac walls and valves.

4. Scattering:
Scatterers are small with respect to the wavelength (less than 1 wavelength) and have rough or irregular surfaces. When the ultrasound beam strikes the surface of these structures, "scattering" of the ultrasound beam occurs (Figure 1.4). Unlike specular reflectors, scatterers reflect the ultrasound beam in multiple directions and are, therefore, not angle dependent. Reflections occurring from scatterers are very weak compared to those from specular reflectors. However, although the reflections from scatterers are weak, they are ever present and are very important in the visualisation of structures parallel to ultrasound beam. Scatter reflectors are frequency dependent so that increasing the frequency increases backscatter from these reflectors. Examples of scatter reflectors include cardiac myocardium.
Rayleigh scatters are special reflectors that reflect

ultrasound energy concentrically; that is, equally in all directions (like a pebble dropped into a pond). Red blood cells (RBCs) are examples of Rayleigh scatterers. Scattering of ultrasound from these moving RBCs form the basis for Doppler echocardiography (see Chapter 5).

5. Refraction:
The ultrasound beam can be refracted, or deflected from its straight propagation path, when the sound beam encounters tissues of different velocities or propagation speeds. This, in effect, results in the *bending* of the sound wave. The degree of bending of the sound wave as it travels through media of different velocities is dictated by *Snell's law* (Figure 1.7 and equation 1.9):

(Equation 1.9)

$$\frac{\sin \theta_i}{\sin \theta_t} = \frac{c_i}{c_t}$$

where $\sin \theta_i$ = incident angle
$\sin \theta_t$ = transmit angle
c_i = propagation of sound in incident medium
c_t = propagation speed in transmitted medium

Note that refraction of the ultrasound beam is determined by difference in the velocities or propagation speeds through tissues and is not related to differences in acoustic impedance. Awareness of the potential for refraction of the ultrasound beam to occur is an important concept as refraction can produce artefacts whereby returning echoes are located incorrectly.

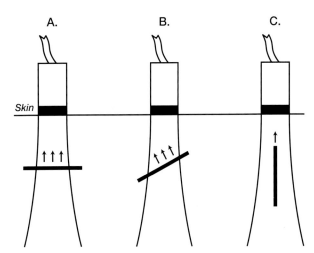

Figure 1.6: Specular Reflectors and their Orientation to the Ultrasound Beam.
Specular reflectors originate from relatively large, smooth, mirror-like structures. These structures are best imaged when they lie in a plane that is directly perpendicular to the ultrasound beam (**A**). When the angle between the specular reflector and the ultrasound beam varies from 90 degrees, some of the returning signals are reflected back to the transducer and some returning signals miss the transducer altogether (**B**). When a specular reflector is parallel to the ultrasound beam, little or no echoes return to the transducer, hence, "drop-out" of these structures occurs (**C**).

A.

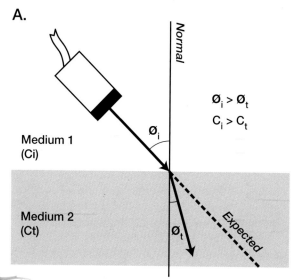

B.

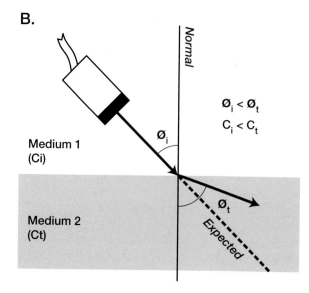

Figure 1.7: Snell's Law.
Refraction of the ultrasound beam occurs when the beam encounters tissues of different velocities. The degree of refraction is determined by Snell's law. The direction of refraction depends on whether the velocity in transmitted medium (C_t) is greater or less than that of the incident medium (C_i). **A.** This example illustrates refraction of the sound beam when C_t is less than C_i, resulting in bending of the beam away from the expected path or toward the normal. **B.** This example illustrates refraction of the sound beam when C_t is greater than C_i, resulting in bending of the beam away from the expected path or away from the normal.

6. Diffraction: ✓

Diffraction refers to the spreading out of the ultrasound beam as it moves farther away from the sound source. When diffraction of the ultrasound beam occurs, the intensity of the beam lessens as the same power is spread over a larger area.

Image Production and Ultrasound Transducers

The Ultrasound Transducer:

Diagnostic ultrasound uses a transducer to emit pulses of sound waves. The principal component of the transducer that produces the ultrasound beam is the piezoelectric crystal. When an alternating electrical current is applied to a piezoelectric crystal, the crystal expands and contracts; thus, generating sound waves. Conversely, when the ultrasound wave returns to the transducer and strikes the piezoelectric crystal, an electric current is generated. Therefore, the transducer acts as both the transmitter and receiver of ultrasound.

The frequency that the transducer emits essentially depends on the propagation speed within the piezoelectric crystal as well as the thickness of the crystal. Crystal frequency is inversely related to thickness and directly related to the propagation speed through the crystal. Hence, the thicker the crystal and the slower the propagation speed through the crystal, the lower the transducer frequency.

Image Production:

Two-dimensional (2-D) image production is obtained by sweeping the ultrasound beam across the imaging plane. The ultrasound image is formed one line at a time. These lines are then added together to form one frame. The frames are then repeated to produce a real-time image. The brightness of the dots displayed on the 2-D image is proportional to the amplitude of the returning echo from the anatomical interfaces. The position of the returning echoes is dependent upon the round-trip time of the pulse and the velocity of the medium. The range equation is used to calculated the distance (D):

(Equation 1.10)

$$D = \frac{c\,t}{2}$$

where   c   = propagation speed through tissue (m/s)
      t   = time taken for the ultrasound signal to return to the transducer (s)
      2   = refers to the fact that the pulse must travel to the structure and then back again

The propagation speed of sound in soft tissue is assumed to be constant at 1540 m/s, hence:

(Equation 1.11)

$$D\,(m) = 770 \times round\ trip\ time$$

where $770 = 1540$ (m/s) $\div 2$

Typically, the time taken for echoes to return to the transducer is in the order of ms and the distance to reflectors is in the range of mm, thus:

(Equation 1.12)

$$D\,(mm) = 0.77 \times round\ trip\ time\ (ms)$$

where $0.77 = 1.54$ (mm/µs) $\div 2$

An increase in the round trip time indicates that the reflector is at a greater distance from the transducer.

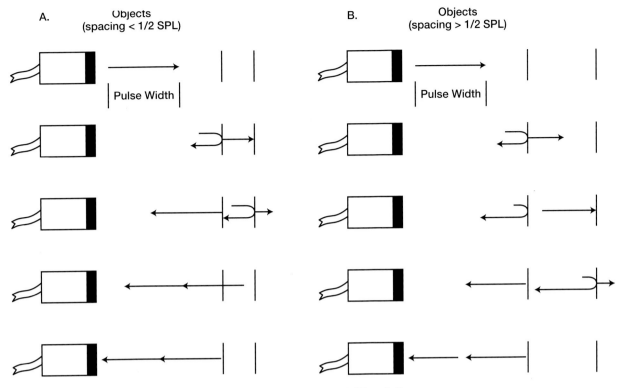

Figure 1.8: The Relationship between the Spatial Pulse Length and Axial Resolution.
A. In this example, two objects are at a distance of less than one-half the spatial pulse length (SPL). Observe that the sound wave that is reflected off the second object, reaches the initial sound wave before it has been totally reflected off the first object. Hence, the two sound waves reach the transducer "end-to-end" and, therefore, are interpreted as a single echo.
B. In this example, the two objects are separated by a distance that is larger than one-half the spatial pulse length (SPL). Hence, the transducer "hears" two distinct echoes and the two objects are resolved and, therefore, displayed as two separate entities.

Spatial Resolution

Spatial resolution refers to the ability of the ultrasound instrument to detect structures that are anatomically separate and to display them as being separate.
Spatial resolution is divided into two separate components: (1) axial resolution: that is the resolution along the axis of the ultrasound beam, and (2) lateral resolution: that is the resolution perpendicular to the ultrasound beam.

1. Axial resolution:

Axial resolution refers to the ability of the ultrasound system to detect echoes from structures at different depths along the axis of the beam and to then display them as separate structures. Axial resolution primarily depends upon the physical length of the pulses being used to form the ultrasound beam. This measurement is the spatial pulse length. In order for two separate structures to be resolved, they must be separated by a distance which is at least half that of the pulse length (Figure 1.8). Therefore:

(Equation 1.13)

$$axial\ resolution = \frac{spatial\ pulse\ length}{2}$$

The spatial pulse length (SPL) is calculated from the wavelength (λ) and the number of cycles within the pulse (n) (Figure 1.9):

(Equation 1.14)

$$SPL = \lambda\ n$$

Hence, the spatial pulse length can be decreased and image resolution improved, by decreasing the wavelength or by decreasing the number of cycles within the pulse. Typically, the number of cycles in the pulse is determined by the manufacturer (between 2 and 4) and, therefore, cannot be altered by the operator. However, the wavelength can be altered by changing the frequency of the transducer.

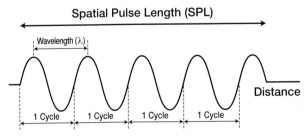

Figure 1.9: The Spatial Pulse Length.
This schematic illustrates a single pulse length or spatial pulse length (SPL). A single pulse is composed of a number of cycles (wavelengths). In this example, there are four cycles. If the distance of each cycle is known, the total length of the pulse can be calculated. As the length of each cycle is the wavelength, the SPL is equal to wavelength multiplied by the number of cycles.

Recall that wavelength is related to frequency and the propagation or velocity of sound within a medium (the wave equation - 1.4):

$$c = \lambda \, f$$

Velocity of sound (c) through tissue is constant, hence, there is an inverse relationship between wavelength (λ) and frequency (f):

(Equation 1.15)

$$\lambda = \frac{c}{f}$$

Thus, as frequency increases, the wavelength becomes shorter; conversely, as the frequency decreases, the wavelength becomes longer. Consider the wavelength, spatial pulse length, and axial resolution for a 5 MHz transducer and a 2 MHz transducer (examples 3 and 4).

Example 3: Determination of the Axial Resolution of a 5 MHz Transducer.
Axial resolution is determined by the spatial pulse length (SPL) which, in turn, is dependent upon the wavelength (λ).

A. Wavelength:

$$\lambda = \frac{1540}{5 \times 10^6} = 0.00031 \; m = 0.31 \; mm$$

B. Spatial pulse length:
Assuming that the pulse consists of 4 cycles:

$$Spatial \; pulse \; length = \; 0.31 \times 4 \; = 1.2 \; mm$$

C. Axial resolution:

$$Axial \; resolution = \; 1.2 \div 2 \; = \; 0.6 \; mm$$

Example 4: Determination of the Axial Resolution of a 2 MHz Transducer.
Axial resolution is determined by the spatial pulse length (SPL) which, in turn, is dependent upon the wavelength (λ).

A. Wavelength:

$$\lambda = \frac{1540}{2 \times 10^6} = 0.00077 \; m = 0.77 \; mm$$

B. Spatial pulse length:
Assuming that the pulse consists of 4 cycles:

$$Spatial \; pulse \; length = \; 0.77 \times 4 \; = 3.1 \; mm$$

C. Axial resolution:

$$Axial \; resolution = \; 3.1 \div 2 \; = \; 1.55 \; mm$$

Technical Consideration:
For a pulse with only two wavelengths, the spatial pulse length and axial resolution can be decreased for a given transducer frequency and the axial resolution can be improved. For the 5 MHz transducer, the spatial pulse length decreases to 0.6 mm and the axial resolution improves to 0.3 mm. Likewise for the 2 MHz transducer, the spatial pulse length decreases to 1.5 mm and the axial resolution improves to 0.75 mm. Hence, although higher frequency transducers have improved axial resolution, it is the spatial pulse length which determines the axial resolution, not the transducer frequency itself.

2. Lateral resolution:
Lateral resolution refers to the ability of the ultrasound system to distinguish two closely spaced reflectors that are positioned perpendicular to the axis of the ultrasound beam; that is, objects which are "side by side". Lateral resolution is generally poorer than the axial resolution. This is because the lateral resolution is related to the beam width.
Ultrasound machines assume that all received echoes have arisen from the central axis of the beam. Therefore, separate objects at the same depth within the width of the ultrasound beam will produce a single echo, and are not resolved. Hence, for separate objects to be displayed as separate, distinct entities, they must be separated by a distance that is greater than the beam width (Figure 1.10). Therefore,

(Equation 1.16)

$$lateral \; resolution = beam \; width$$

Generally, the width of the ultrasound beam increases with lower transducer frequencies; hence, lateral resolution tends to degrade with lower frequency transducers. Lateral resolution of low frequency transducers can be improved by focusing the ultrasound beam (Figure 1.11). Focusing of the ultrasound beam effectively narrows or converges the beam in the focal region; in fact, the ultrasound beam is at its narrowest at the focal zone. Since lateral resolution is equal to the beam width, the focal region will display improved lateral resolution. The magnitude of improvement is dependent upon the degree of focussing.
Therefore, the best spatial or image resolution occurs using high frequency transducers and by optimising the focal zone. However, high frequency transducers increase attenuation and increased attenuation means that there is a reduction in depth penetration. Therefore, the transducer frequency used should be a compromise between attenuation losses and spatial resolution requirements.

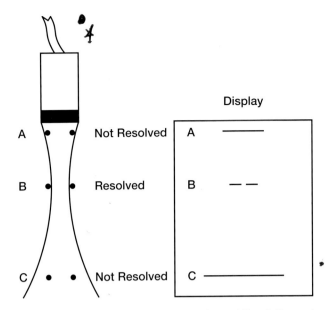

Figure 1.10: The Relationship between Lateral Resolution and the Beam Width.
In this schematic, it can be appreciated that two separate objects at positions **A** and **C** are not resolved on the image display. This is because both objects are encompassed within the ultrasound beam and the instrument assumes that all echoes arise from the central axis of the beam. Observe that "smearing" of these echoes is noted on the image display, this is because each of the imaged objects is effectively summed together. Observe that the two objects at position **B** are resolved as these objects are separated by a distance that is greater than the ultrasound beam width.
From Gent, R.: Applied Physics and Technology of Diagnostic Ultrasound. Milner Publishing pp: 96, 1997. Reproduced with permission from the author.

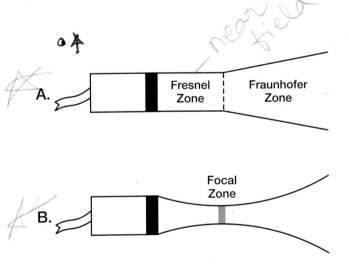

Figure 1.11: Focusing of the Ultrasound Transducer.
A. This is an illustration of a non-focused transducer demonstrating the near-field (Fresnel zone) and the far-field (Fraunhofer zone). In unfocused transducers, the lateral resolution is best within the near-field and poorest in the far-field. Poor lateral resolution in the far-field is explained by the divergence or "widening" of the ultrasound beam in this region.
B. This is an illustration of a focused ultrasound beam. Observe that the ultrasound beam narrows considerably within the focal zone; hence, lateral resolution within this region is greatest.

References and Suggested Reading:

- Bioeffects Committee, American Institute of Ultrasound in Medicine: Bioeffects considerations for the safety of diagnostic ultrasound. *Journal of Ultrasound in Medicine 7 (suppl): S1-S38, 1988.*
- Feigenbaum, H. Echocardiography. Chapter 1. 5th Ed. Lea & Febiger, 1994.
- Gent, Roger.: Applied Physics and Technology of Diagnostic Ultrasound. Milner Publishing (3 Milner Street, Prospect. South Australia 5082), 1997.
- Hedrik,Hykes, and Starchman: Ultrasound Physics and Instrumentation. 3rd Edition, Mosby Year Book Inc., 1995.
- Otto, C.M. and Pearlman, A.S.: Textbook of Clinical Echocardiography. Chapter 1. W.B. Saunders Company. 1995

Chapter 2
The Two-Dimensional Echocardiographic Examination

The real-time, two-dimensional (2-D) examination of the heart allows the assessment of cardiac morphology, pathology, and function. Echocardiography is highly operator dependent. Therefore, it is extremely important that the data obtained is both accurate and reproducible, and that the cardiac sonographer is capable and competent. Accuracy is achieved through thorough education and by a comprehensive knowledge of all aspects of the echocardiographic examination as well as the identification and recognition of the potential pitfalls and limitations of the technique. Reproducibility can be attained through the utilisation of standardised views and techniques. Standardisation, with respect to image orientation and nomenclature, is crucial in the display and understanding of the complex anatomy of the heart. Standardisation of views also aids the acquisition of reproducible data, allows interlaboratory communication, and simplifies the training and understanding of the inexperienced observer [4]. Consequently, a standardisation of techniques improves accuracy and reproducibility.

Optimisation of 2-D Images

The resolution and image quality of 2-D images is dependent upon several technical factors. Each of these factors as well as how they can be adjusted to optimise the 2-D image display is discussed briefly.

Transducer Selection:
The transducer selected for the 2-D examination should be the highest frequency transducer that allows adequate penetration. High frequency transducers increase backscatter and improve resolution but lack depth penetration. Low frequency transducers have broader band pulses that penetrate further but result in reduced image resolution. Hence, the best image resolution occurs with high frequency transducers while the greatest depth penetration occurs with low frequency transducers. Therefore, the transducer selected should be the highest frequency transducer that allows adequate penetration to the structure(s) or region(s) of interest.

Depth:
The depth function adjusts the vertical field of view (FOV) of the image. The depth of imaging affects the frame rate such that the deeper the FOV the greater time required for the signal to return to the transducer and, therefore, the slower the frame rate. Conversely, the shallower the FOV the less time required for the signals to return to the transducer and, therefore, the higher the frame rate. Therefore, in order to maintain the frame rate, the smallest FOV that allows the display of the region of interest should be employed.

Zoom:
The "zoom" function enables magnification of a specified region of interest. The value of this function is in the investigation of valvular morphology and pathology and relatively small masses such as vegetations or thrombus. This function should also be employed to improve measurement accuracy when measuring relatively small structures or masses.

Focus:
The focal zone of the transducer indicates the region of the image at which the ultrasound beam is narrowest; hence, resolution is greatest in this region. Therefore, repositioning of the focal zone is particularly important when performing 2-D measurements and in examination of specific regions of interest.

Gain:
The gain function adjusts the displayed amplitude of all received signals and, therefore, affects the brightness of echoes on the display. Optimal gain settings provide enough signal amplification to produce the desired image without dropout or "blooming" of signals.

Time Gain Compensation (TGC):
Time gain compensation (TGC) or depth gain compensation (DGC) adjusts the amplitude or gain of returning echo signals along the length of the ultrasound beam or at specific image depths. Recall that as the ultrasound beam travels further into the body, the beam is attenuated. Therefore, the primary function of the TGC is to ensure that signals of similar magnitude are displayed at the same amplification. For example, within the heart, the structures imaged in the near field should have the same amplitude as those structures imaged in the far field. The TGC is used in conjunction with the gain control to produce the desired image.

Dynamic range:
The dynamic range represents the ratio of the maximum to minimum signal level and is expressed in decibels (dB). The dynamic range compares one signal level with another on a logarithmic scale. This function allows adjustment of the number of levels of gray displayed in the image. Increasing the dynamic range increases the amount of gray scale displayed so that weaker signals are included and the image is softened; therefore, dynamic range is increased when images are of good quality. Decreasing the dynamic range results in the production of high quality contrast images such that weaker signals are eliminated, noise is reduced, and the strongest echo signals are enhanced; therefore, the dynamic range is decreased when image quality is poor.

4: Henry, et al.: Circulation 62, No. 2, pp 213,1980.

Preprocessing:

Preprocessing refers to the manipulation of data as it is acquired. For example, preprocessing functions may be used to sharpen the edges or borders of structures within the field of view. Hence, manipulation may be used to smooth or sharpen borders.

Persistence:

Persistence refers to the smoothing of the image that is achieved by averaging several consecutive frames. This reduces image noise and, therefore, improves image quality. However, the principal disadvantage of persistence is inferior temporal resolution. This is because sampling occurs over a longer period of time, therefore, averaging of several frames of moving structures results in "blurring" of the real-time image. For this reason, minimal persistence is used in the assessment of the dynamic heart.

Postprocessing:

Postprocessing refers to the manipulation of data after it is stored. Postprocessing curves define the relationship between echo amplitude and the displayed pixel intensity that affects the softness and brightness of gray scale images stored in the memory. Increasing the postprocessing curve smooths the gray scale images by adding more gray shades and, therefore, reduces gray scale contrast. Conversely, decreasing the postprocessing curve increases the contrast of gray scale images by removing gray shades, which in affect increases gray scale contrast.

B-Colour:

Brightness colour (B-colour) assists in improving the contrast resolution by enhancing subtle soft tissue differences. This is achieved by using a colour scale rather than a gray scale display. Theoretically, the human eye can only appreciate a limited number of shades of gray but is able to distinguish a greater number of different hues of other colours. Hence, "changing the colour" of the image allows enhanced appreciation of soft tissue structures.

Technical Consideration:
B-colour does not change the ultrasound information displayed but only improves the perception of that information.

Acoustic Windows

The two-dimensional (2-D) examination attempts to examine the three-dimensional heart using various **acoustic windows** and **imaging planes** to develop a series of **standard two-dimensional images**.

Special acoustic windows are required to image the heart. This is because the heart is mostly covered by bony structures such as the ribs and the sternum as well as by overlying lung tissue. Recall from Chapter 1, transmission of the ultrasound beam is poor at bone/soft tissue interfaces and air/soft tissue interfaces. Dense materials such as bone almost totally absorb sound waves, while air-filled structures such as lungs almost totally reflect sound waves.

Echocardiographic acoustic windows are areas in which the heart does not lie directly beneath bony and lung interfaces. There are four commonly utilised echocardiographic acoustic windows (Figure 2.1). The *parasternal window* is the area bounded superiorly by the clavicle, medially by the sternum and inferiorly by the apical region. The *apical window* is located in the region where the apical impulse is maximal or around the fifth intercostal space in the mid-axillary line. The *subcostal window* is located near the midline of the body under the subxiphoid region. The *suprasternal window* is designated by the suprasternal notch region.

Alternative windows also exist and may be utilised to image the heart and great vessels in certain circumstances. These windows include the right parasternal window and the right apical window. The right parasternal window is utilised in the assessment of certain congenital heart anomalies as well as in the assessment of the ascending aorta. The right apical window is also utilised in the assessment of certain congenital heart anomalies.

In the presence of a large left pleural effusion, the fluid can be used as an acoustic window to the heart. To image the heart utilising the pleural effusion, the patient is placed in a right lateral decubitus position and the transducer is placed on the patients' back. This view is particularly useful in the assessment of the descending thoracic aorta (especially when looking for aortic dissections).

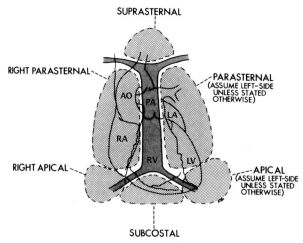

Figure 2.1: Echocardiographic Acoustic Windows.
From Henry, et al.: Report of the American Society of Echocardiography Committee on Nomenclature and Standards in Two-dimensional Echocardiography. Circulation 62, No. 2, pp 213,1980. Reproduced with permission from Lippincott, Williams & Wilkins.
Abbreviations: AO = aorta; **LA** = left atrium; **LV** = left ventricle; **PA** = pulmonary artery; **RA** = right atrium; **RV** = right ventricle

Imaging Planes

Standard nomenclature such as sagittal, transverse or coronal planes, used by anatomists to describe body orientation is not used to describe echocardiographic 2-D imaging planes for two important reasons. Firstly, the heart lies in an oblique position within the chest, and secondly, the orientation and position of the heart is variable between individuals. Therefore, 2-D echocardiographic nomenclature is described with respect to the way in which the imaging plane transects the heart itself.

Three orthogonal planes are routinely employed in 2-D echocardiography (Figure 2.2). The *long axis plane* is the plane perpendicular to the dorsal (posterior) and ventral (anterior) surfaces of the body and parallel to the long axis of the heart. This imaging plane provides anatomic information about the aorta, left atrium, left ventricle, interventricular septum and posterior wall of the left ventricle.

The *short axis plane* is the plane perpendicular to the dorsal (posterior) and ventral (anterior) surfaces of the body and is perpendicular to the long axis plane. Various levels of the short plane can be utilised to examine the heart from its apex, through its base, to the great arteries.

The *four chamber plane* is the plane that runs parallel to the dorsal (posterior) and ventral (anterior) surfaces of the body and transects the heart from its apex to its base encompassing all four cardiac chambers. Thus, from this view, the heart is divided into four chambers by the interventricular and interatrial septa in the longitudinal plane and by the atrioventricular valves (mitral and tricuspid valves) in the transverse plane.

Standard 2-D Images

The three orthogonal planes employed in echocardiography can be obtained from the utilisation of the various echocardiographic acoustic windows and imaging planes described above (Figure 2.3). Long axis views of the heart can be obtained from the parasternal and apical windows. Theoretically, it is also possible to obtain a long axis view of the heart from the suprasternal window; however, in practice, a long axis view of the aorta only is usually attained. Short axis views of the heart can be obtained from the parasternal, subcostal, and suprasternal windows. Four chamber views of the heart can be obtained from the apical and subcostal windows.

Two other views that are routinely used, which are not represented in the above imaging planes or views, include the apical five chamber and apical two chamber views. The apical five chamber view is considered a variation of the apical four chamber view while the apical two chamber view is a variation of the apical long axis view.

The standard 2-D images that are routinely used in an echocardiographic examination are labelled according to transducer location, spatial orientation of the imaging plane, and structure(s) identified. These standard 2-D echocardiographic views are summarised in Table 2.1.

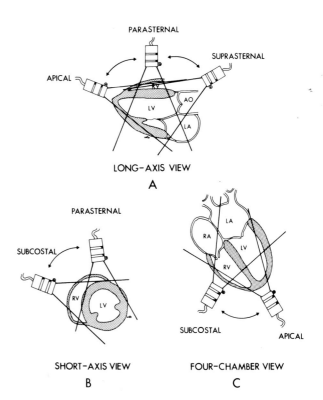

Figure 2.3: Transducer Orientations.
This schematic illustrates the transducer orientations that are utilised in obtaining (**A**) long axis views, (**B**) short axis views and (**C**) four chamber views of the heart.
From Henry, et al.: Report of the American Society of Echocardiography Committee on Nomenclature and Standards in Two-dimensional Echocardiography. Circulation 62, No. 2, pp 215,1980. Reproduced with permission from Lippincott, Williams & Wilkins.
Abbreviations: AO = aorta; **LA** = left atrium; **LV** = left ventricle; **RA** = right atrium; **RV** = right ventricle.

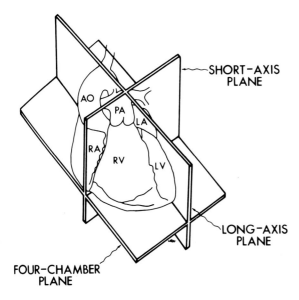

Figure 2.2: Two-dimensional Imaging Planes.
From Henry, et al.: Report of the American Society of Echocardiography Committee on Nomenclature and Standards in Two-dimensional Echocardiography. Circulation 62, No. 2, pp 213,1980. Reproduced with permission from Lippincott, Williams & Wilkins.
Abbreviations: AO = aorta; **LA** = left atrium; **LV** = left ventricle; **PA** = pulmonary artery; **RA** = right atrium; **RV** = right ventricle

The 2-D echocardiographic views that are about to be described are those views that can be commonly acquired in the majority of patients. It should be noted, however, that patient position as well as transducer position, tilting and angulation described to obtain each view necessitate constant modification (sometimes to the extreme) for each individual patient. Inconsistencies in transducer and patient positions are primarily related to the variable position and orientation of the heart within the chest as well as deformities of the chest wall itself.

It should also be recognised that not all echocardiographic views will be attainable in all patients, however, even in the most technically challenging patient, rarely will no diagnostic information be obtained. In the technically challenging patients, as many views as possible should be attempted and emphasis should be placed on answering the clinical question rather than trying to achieve the impossible.

Transducer Terminology:

In the following narration of 2-D echocardiographic views, certain terms will be used to describe the transducer manoeuvres (see Figure 2.4).

Movement: Movement of the transducer implies actual movement of the footprint of the probe on the chest wall along the scan plane without changing the rotation or tilt of the transducer. Movement of the transducer can be inferior (toward the patient's feet), superior (toward the patient's head), lateral (away from the midline of the patient), or medial (toward the midline of the patient).

Tilting: Tilting refers to "rocking" of the transducer up and down from a fixed point on the chest wall. Hence, the footprint of the transducer remains in the same position on the chest wall but the "tail" of the transducer is altered. Tilting of the transducer changes the position of the scan plane. Transducer tilting is typically described as being superior (tilting the tail of the transducer toward the patient's feet), inferior (tilting the tail of the transducer toward the patient's head), anterior (tilting the image plane toward the patient's front), or posterior (tilting the image plane toward the patient's back).

Angulation: Angulation refers to the "side-to-side" movement of the transducer from a fixed point on the chest wall. Hence, the footprint of the transducer remains in the same position on the chest wall. Angulation of the transducer aims to bring structures of interest at the side of the imaging plane into the centre of the image. Transducer angulation is typically described as being either medial (pointing the transducer face toward the midline of the patient), or lateral (pointing the transducer face toward the side of the patient or away from the midline).

Rotation: Rotation simply refers to pivoting or twisting of the transducer from a fixed position on the chest wall. Transducer rotation is described as being either clockwise or counterclockwise. Rotation of the transducer changes the position of the scan plane; for example, from the parasternal long axis view, clockwise rotation of the transducer changes the imaging plane to the parasternal short axis view.

Table 2.1: Standard Two-Dimensional Echocardiographic Imaging Planes.

Transducer Location	Imaging Plane	Structures Identified
Parasternal	Long Axis	• Left Ventricle • Right Ventricular Inflow Tract • Right Ventricular Outflow Tract
	Short Axis	• Pulmonary Artery Bifurcation • Aorta and Left Atrium • Left Ventricular Outflow Tract • Left Ventricle (Mitral Valve) • Left Ventricle (Papillary Muscle) • Left Ventricle (Apex)
Apical	Four Chamber Five Chamber Long Axis Two Chamber	• Four Chambers • Four Chambers + Aorta • Left Ventricle • Left Ventricle & Left Atrium
Subcostal	Four Chamber	• Four Chambers
	Short Axis	• Left Ventricle • Right Ventricular Outflow Tract • Aorta and Left Atrium • Vena Cava and Right Atrium
Suprasternal	Long Axis	• Aortic Arch
	Short Axis	• Aortic Arch

A

C

B

D

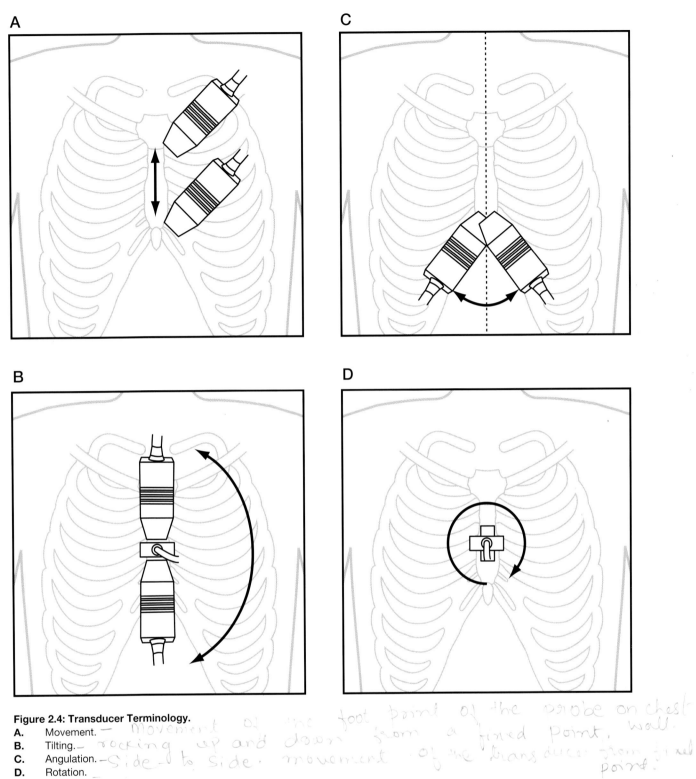

Figure 2.4: Transducer Terminology.

A. Movement. — Movement of the foot point of the probe on chest wall.
B. Tilting. — rocking up and down from a fixed point.
C. Angulation. — Side to side movement of the transducer from fixed point.
D. Rotation.

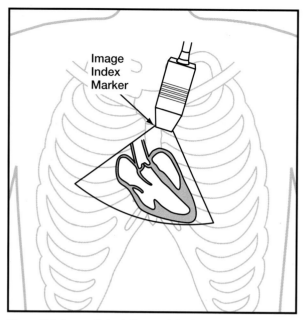
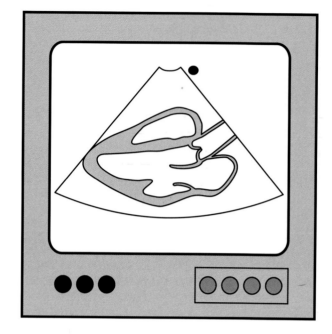

Figure 2.5: Image Orientation and the Image Index Marker.
Left, In this schematic, the image index marker is pointed to the patient's right side.
Right, Based on the standards recommended by the American Society of Echocardiography, the edge of the imaging plane (indicated by the image index marker) is traditionally displayed to the right of the image.

Image Orientation:

All ultrasound transducers have an image index marker that indicates the edge of the imaging plane. The image index marker may be in the form of a groove, external ribbing, or a button.

Based on the standards recommended by the American Society of Echocardiography [5], the image index marker should indicate the part of the scan plane that will appear to the right of the image display (Figure 2.5). Observe that the image (sector) orientation is such that "to the right of the image" refers to the right of the image (sector) as one faces the screen. "To the left of the image" refers to the left of the image or sector as one faces the screen.

The Parasternal Position

Patient Positioning:

The patient is placed in a steep left lateral decubitus position with the patient's left arm extended over their head. The aim of this position is to: (1) drop the left lung away from the mid-line of the chest, (2) allow the heart to fall away from behind the dense bony sternum, and (3) maximise the intercostal spaces, thus, improving transducer accessibility. This view may be further facilitated by held expiration that may further reduce the air-soft tissue interface.

Parasternal Long Axis View of the Left Ventricle

Transducer Position and Angulation: (Figure 2.6)
The transducer is placed in the third, fourth or fifth intercostal space to the left of, and close to, the sternum. The transducer should be perpendicular to the chest wall with the image index marker rotated toward the patient's right clavicle (rotated to approximately 11 o'clock.). The beam is, thus, orientated to the long axis of the left

ventricle with the scan plane running parallel along an imaginary line joining the right shoulder and the left leg.

Sector and Image Orientation:

Anatomic relationships to the sector image are orientated so that anterior structures such as the chest wall and right ventricle are seen at the top of the sector while posterior structures such as the posterior wall of the left ventricle are seen at the bottom of the sector. Superior structures such as the aorta and left atrium are seen to the right of the image and inferior structures such as the ventricles are seen to the left of the image.

Structures Visualised and Normal Echocardiographic Appearances: (Figure 2.6)

The first structure encountered by the ultrasound beam from this view and all subsequent views is the **chest wall**. The **anterior wall of the right ventricle** is seen immediately behind the chest wall and is relatively thin when compared to the thickness of the left ventricular walls and the interventricular septum. The **right ventricular cavity** that is bounded by the anterior right ventricular wall and the interventricular septum appears echo-free; occasionally portions of the tricuspid valve apparatus may be seen within the cavity of this ventricle. During systole, the anterior wall of the right ventricle thickens and the cavity of the right ventricle becomes smaller as the ventricle contracts.

The **proximal ascending aortic root** in its long axis (first 3 to 5 cm) appears as two, relatively thin parallel lines that move anteriorly during systole and posteriorly in diastole. Various levels of the aortic root such as the aortic annulus, trans-sinus and sinotubular diameters can usually be appreciated from this view.

5: Henry, W.L. et al.: Circulation 62(2): 212-217, 1980.

Pace Rhythm.

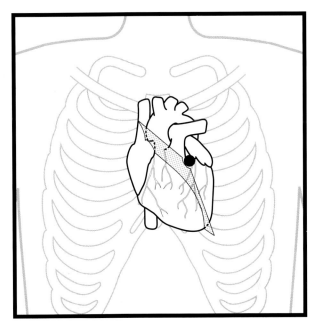

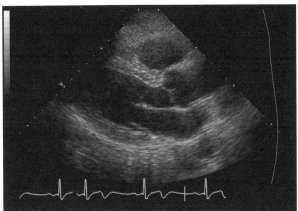

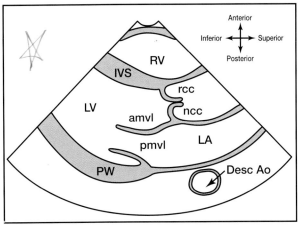

Figure 2.6: The Parasternal Long Axis of the Left Ventricle.
Top, Transducer Position and Imaging Plane.
Middle, Echocardiographic Structures Visualised.
Bottom, Schematic Illustration of Structures Visualised including the Sector Orientation.
Abbreviations: amvl = anterior mitral valve leaflet; **Desc Ao** = descending aorta; **IVS** = interventricular septum; **LA** = left atrium; **LV** = left ventricle; **ncc** = non-coronary cusp; **pmvl** = posterior mitral valve leaflet; **PW** = posterior wall; **rcc** = right coronary cusp; **RV** = right ventricle.

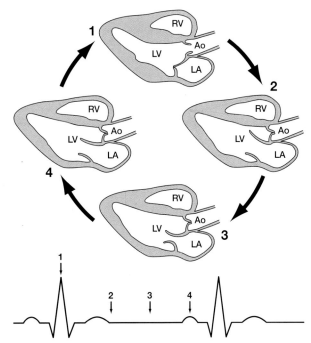

Figure 2.7: Motion of the Mitral Valve Leaflets throughout the Cardiac Cycle.
During the early filling phase of diastole (2), the pressure within the left atrium exceeds that of the left ventricle which causes the mitral leaflets to open. Thus, the anterior mitral leaflet moves anteriorly toward the interventricular septum and the posterior leaflet moves posteriorly. In mid diastole, the period of diastasis occurs (3). During this phase, the pressure gradient between the left atrium and left ventricle approaches zero resulting in minimal flow of blood between these two chambers. Therefore, the mitral valve begins to close. Before the mitral valve can close completely, atrial contraction occurs and the mitral leaflets open again (4). Hence, the mitral valve effectively opens twice during diastole. During systole (1), the mitral leaflets coapt to lie posteriorly within the left ventricular cavity.

The **mitral valve leaflets** along with their **subvalvular apparatus** (chordae tendineae and papillary muscle attachments) are also delineated well from this view. The **anterior mitral leaflet** appears longer and larger than the smaller **posterior mitral leaflet**. Both leaflets should appear thin, produce uniform echoes and be unrestricted in their motion. Movement of the mitral leaflets throughout the cardiac cycle is not as simple as that of the aortic valve leaflets due to the various phases that occur during diastole. In normal sinus rhythm, there are three distinct patterns of mitral valve motion corresponding to three phases that occur during diastole (Figure 2.7).

The subvalvular apparatus of the mitral valve leaflets may also be delineated. The **posterolateral papillary muscle** is identified as a cone-shaped protrusion arising from the endocardial surface of the left ventricular myocardium. **Chordae tendineae** appear as taut, string-like fibres spanning between the papillary muscles and mitral leaflets.

The **left atrium** lies immediately posterior to the aortic root. The cavity of the left atrium should be free of echoes.

The basal and mid portions of the **interventricular septum** and the **posterior (inferolateral) wall** of the left ventricle should be seen to produce uniform echoes. The thickness of the interventricular septum and posterior wall should be symmetric measuring no more than 1.1 cm during diastole. During systole, as the left ventricle contracts, the interventricular septum thickens and moves posteriorly or inward into the left ventricular cavity; during diastole, the septum moves anteriorly or outward.

The posterior wall of the left ventricle moves in the opposite direction to the interventricular septum; that is, during systole, the posterior wall moves anteriorly or upward. During diastole, this wall moves posteriorly or outward.

The **left ventricle**, which is bounded by the interventricular septum and the posterior wall, should appear free of echoes. Note that the cardiac apex of the left ventricle is not normally seen from this view.

The **left ventricular outflow tract (LVOT)** is bounded anteriorly by the basal interventricular septum and posteriorly by the anterior leaflet of the mitral valve. The LVOT should appear widely patent during systole. Continuity between the anterior aortic wall and the interventricular septum as well as between the posterior aortic wall and the anterior mitral leaflet is best appreciated in this view. Delineation of this **aorto-septal** and **mitral-aortic** continuity is extremely important in the assessment of certain congenital heart lesions.

One, two or three circular, echo-free structures can be seen posterior to the left atrium representing the descending thoracic aorta, the coronary sinus and the circumflex coronary artery. The largest of these circular structures, which should always be seen, is the **descending thoracic aorta**. The **coronary sinus** and the **circumflex coronary artery** are not always seen because of their relatively small size. Both the coronary sinus and the circumflex coronary artery lie within the atrioventricular groove and can be easily differentiated from the descending thoracic aorta by their motion throughout the cardiac cycle. The coronary sinus and the circumflex coronary artery are contained within the pericardium while the descending thoracic aorta is extra-pericardial. Therefore, the coronary sinus and circumflex coronary artery move with the atrioventricular groove as the heart contracts while the descending thoracic aorta does not.

Occasionally the **right pulmonary artery**, in its short axis, is seen posterior to the aorta and superior and anterior to the left atrium. When seen, the right pulmonary artery appears as an echo-free, circular structure between the aorta and left atrium.

Abnormalities Detected from the Parasternal Long Axis View of the Left Ventricle:

Abnormalities that may be detected from this view are listed in Table 2.2.

An example of tetrology of Fallot, which is commonly diagnosed from this view, is depicted in Figure 2.8.

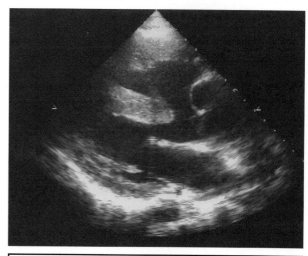

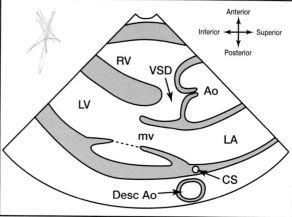

Figure 2.8: Parasternal Long Axis View of the Left Ventricle demonstrating Aorto-septal Discontinuity.

Top, This is an echocardiographic example demonstrating aorto-septal discontinuity in a patient with tetralogy of Fallot.

Bottom, This is a schematic illustrating the echocardographic features seen in A. Observe the presence of a dilated, over-riding aorta, a large ventricular septal defect, and right ventricular hypertrophy. The fourth component that completes the tetralogy of Fallot is infundibular right ventricular outflow tract obstruction which can be identified from the parasternal long or short axis views of the right ventricular outflow tract .

Abbreviations: Ao = aorta; **Desc Ao** = descending aorta; **mv** = mitral valve; **LA** = left atrium; **LV** = left ventricle; **RV** = right ventricle; **VSD** = ventricular septal defect.

Table 2.2: Abnormalities Detected from the Parasternal Long Axis View of the Left Ventricle:

Cardiac Structure	Detectable Abnormalities
Aortic Root	• dilatation • dissection flaps _dissection = tearing_ • ascending aortic aneurysms • sinus of Valsalva aneurysms • supravalvular stenosis
Aortic Valve	• reduced leaflet excursion: valvular stenosis or reduced cardiac output • calcification • prolapse • vegetations • bicuspid valves • systolic doming • premature aortic valve closure: associated with LVOT gradients (for example, with hypertrophic obstructive cardiomyopathy and subaortic membranes)
Left Atrium	• dilatation • thrombus • myxomas • cor triatriatum
Mitral Valve and Supporting Structures	• reduced mobility: valvular stenosis or reduced cardiac output • valvular or annulus calcification • prolapse • flail leaflets • ruptured chordae • failure of leaflet coaptation • vegetations • diastolic mitral valve flutter: associated with aortic regurgitation • systolic anterior motion of the anterior mitral leaflet: associated with hypertrophic obstructive cardiomyopathy
Left Ventricular Outflow Tract	• outflow tract obstruction: muscular, membraneous, or due to systolic anterior motion of the anterior mitral leaflet
Aorto-Septal and Mitral-Aortic Continuity	• discontinuity as seen in certain congenital heart lesions (see Figure 2.8)
Interventricular Septum	• increased thickness or hypertrophy • thinning: associated with myocardial infarction • reduced systolic thickening • hypokinesis or akinesis: associated with ischaemic heart disease • abnormal motion: due to ischaemia or infarction, left bundle branch block, pacemaker rhythm, post open heart surgery, volume or pressure overloaded right ventricle
Inferolateral Wall	• increased thickness or hypertrophy • thinning: associated with myocardial infarction • aneurysm or pseudoaneurysm • reduced systolic thickening • hypokinesis or akinesis: associated with ischaemic heart disease
Left Ventricular Cavity	• dilatation • systolic dysfunction • thrombus • intracavity masses/tumours
Right Ventricular Cavity	• dilatation • impaired systolic function • increased right ventricular wall thickness
Coronary Sinus	• dilatation: most commonly associated with a persistent left superior vena cava
Descending Aorta	• dilatation • aortic dissection flaps • allows differentiation between pleural and pericardial effusions [6]

6: The descending aorta is extra-pericardial; hence, a pericardial effusion will appear as an echo-free space anterior to the descending aorta. Pleural fluid is typically seen inferior and posterior to the descending aorta. Therefore, in the presence of a pleural effusion the aorta maintains its immediate posterior relationship behind the left atrium.

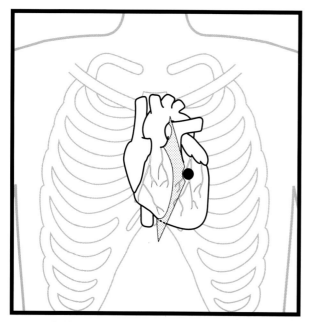

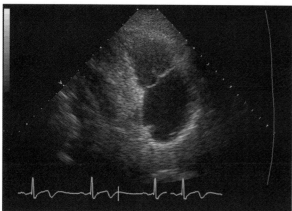

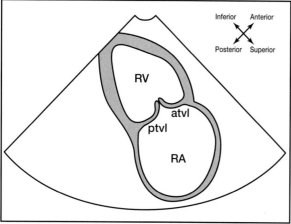

Figure 2.9: The Long Axis of the Right Ventricular Inflow Tract.
Top, Transducer Position and Imaging Plane.
Middle, Echocardiographic Structures Visualised.
Bottom, Schematic Illustration of Structures Visualised including the Sector Orientation.
Abbreviations: atvl = anterior tricuspid valve leaflet; **ptvl** = posterior tricuspid valve leaflet; **RA** =right atrium; **RV** = right ventricle.

Parasternal Long Axis View of the Right Ventricular Inflow Tract

Transducer Position and Angulation: (Figure 2.9)
The transducer position and rotation is similar to that used to obtain the long axis view of the left ventricle. The right ventricular inflow tract view is obtained by tilting the transducer inferiorly while angling medially; that is, by directing the transducer toward the patient's right leg. Minor adjustments which may be required to achieve this view include movement of the transducer laterally or away from the sternum, slight clockwise rotation of the transducer (15 to 20 degrees), and/or movement of the transducer inferiorly or an intercostal space lower.

Sector and Image Orientation:
Anatomic relationships to the sector image are orientated so that inferior structures are seen at the top left of the image while anterior structures are seen at the top right of the image. Superior structures are seen at the bottom right of the image, and posterior structures are seen at the bottom left of the image. Hence, the chest wall appears at the top of the image, the right atrium appears at the bottom right of the image, and the right ventricular apex appears at the top left of the image.

Structures Visualised and Normal Echocardiographic Appearances: (Figure 2.9)
The inferior portion of the right atrium and the right ventricular inflow tract up to and including the right ventricular apex can be visualised. The cavities of the right atrium and ventricle should appear echo free although the chordal and papillary muscle attachments of the tricuspid valve may be seen within the heavily trabeculated cavity of the right ventricle.

The **papillary muscles** of the right ventricle are not as easily distinguished as those of the left ventricle. Typically, there are two principal papillary muscles (anterior and posterior) with a smaller supracristal (or conus) papillary muscle.

Two of the three **tricuspid valve leaflets** are seen toward the centre of the image. The anterior tricuspid leaflet is seen anteriorly while the posterior leaflet appears posteriorly. As with the anterior leaflet of the mitral valve, the anterior leaflet of the tricuspid valve is longer and larger than either the septal or the posterior tricuspid leaflets.

The tricuspid leaflets should appear thin, produce uniform echoes and be unrestricted in their motion. Movement of the tricuspid leaflets throughout the cardiac cycle is identical to that of the mitral leaflets.

The **inferior vena cava (IVC)** is commonly seen draining into the right atrial cavity at the bottom left of the image.

A persistent **eustachian valve** or valve of the IVC may be occasionally seen. This valve is a remnant of the embryonic valve of the IVC that plays an important role in the circulation of blood through the foetal heart [7].

7: In foetal life, oxygenated blood from the placenta travels toward the foetal heart via the inferior vena cava. The eustachian valve acts to direct this oxygen-rich blood through the fossa ovalis, into the left atrium and ultimately to the foetal brain. This ensures that oxygen-rich blood reaches the developing foetal brain.

The eustachian valve can be recognised as a horizontal linear structure spanning from the entrance to the IVC to the inferior border of the right atrium immediately below the tricuspid annulus where it attaches to the interatrial septum. The appearance of this valve may simulate vegetations, thrombus or tumours; however, the relationship of this structure to the inferior vena cava and its attachment to the interatrial septum will allow it to be differentiated from other pathology.

Similar to, but less commonly encountered than the eustachian valve, is the thin, web-like, fenestrated membrane of the **Chiari network**. The Chiari network is simply a redundant eustachian valve. This structure can be differentiated echocardiographically from the eustachian valve by its characteristic chaotic, random motion and by its highly reflective appearance within the right atrium. Like the eustachian valve, this structure is considered a normal variant and should not be confused with tricuspid vegetations, flail leaflets, tumour or thrombi.

Abnormalities Detected from the Parasternal Long Axis View of the Right Ventricular Inflow Tract:

Abnormalities that may be detected from this view are summarised in Table 2.3.

Table 2.3: Abnormalities Detected from the Parasternal Long Axis View of the Right Ventricular Inflow Tract

Cardiac Structure	Detectable Abnormality
Right Atrium	• dilatation • intracardiac masses/tumours
Tricuspid Valve	• reduced mobility: valvular stenosis or reduced cardiac output • systolic doming (stenosis) • prolapse • ruptured chordae • vegetations
Right Ventricle	• dilatation • systolic dysfunction • intracavity masses/thrombus • increased thickening of right ventricular free wall
Inferior Vena Cava	• migratory tumours/thrombus
Eustachian Valve Chiari Network	• these structures are normal variants; however, when large and mobile may be confused with thrombus, tumours, or vegetations

Parasternal Long Axis View of the Right Ventricular Outflow Tract

Transducer Positioning and Angulation:

(Figure 2.10)

The transducer position and rotation is similar to the long axis view of the left ventricle. This view is obtained by tilting the transducer superiorly while angling laterally; that is, the transducer is directed toward the patient's left shoulder. Minor adjustments

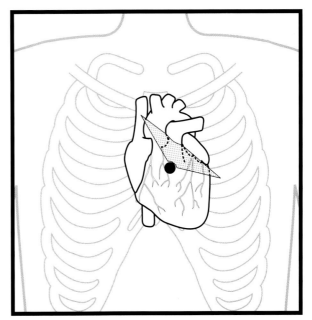

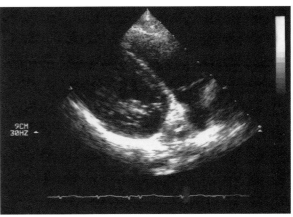

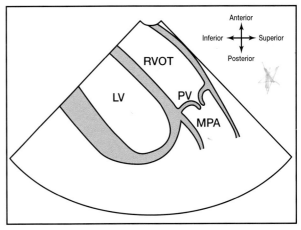

Figure 2.10: The Long Axis View of the Right Ventricular Outflow Tract.

Top, Transducer Position and Imaging Plane.

Middle, Echocardiographic Structures Visualised.

Bottom, Schematic Illustration of Structures Visualised including the Sector Orientation.

Abbreviations: LV = left ventricle; **MPA** = main pulmonary artery; **PV** = pulmonary valve; **RVOT** = right ventricular outflow tract.

which may be required to achieve this view include movement of the transducer laterally or away from the sternum, slight clockwise rotation of the transducer (less than 20 degrees), and/or movement of the transducer superiorly or an intercostal space higher.

Sector and Image Orientation:

Anatomic relationships to the sector image are orientated so that anterior structures such as the chest wall and right ventricular outflow tract (RVOT) are seen at the top of the sector while posterior structures such as the left ventricle are seen at the bottom of the sector. Superior structures such as the pulmonary artery and its branches are seen to the right of the sector, and inferior structures are seen to the left of the sector.

Structures Visualised and Normal Echocardiographic Appearances: (Figure 2.10)

This view allows visualisation of the entire **RVOT** which should remain widely patent throughout the cardiac cycle.

Two of the three **pulmonary valve leaflets** are usually visualised. These leaflets should appear thin, produce uniform echoes, and be unrestricted in their motion. During systole, the pulmonary leaflets snap open and lie nearly parallel to the walls of the main pulmonary artery. Leaflets close abruptly at the onset of diastole.

The **proximal main pulmonary artery** is well seen and should appear widely patent, maintaining a consistent diameter along its length. The lumen of this vessel should be free of echoes. Occasionally, the bifurcation of the main pulmonary artery into right and left branches can also be seen.

Abnormalities Detected from the Parasternal Long Axis View of the Right Ventricular Outflow Tract:

Abnormalities that may be detected from this view are summarised in Table 2.4.

Table 2.4: Abnormalities Detected from the Parasternal Long Axis View of the Right Ventricular Outflow Tract.

Cardiac Structure	Detectable Abnormalities
Right Ventricular Outflow Tract	• dilatation • infundibular narrowing • increased free wall thickness
Pulmonary Valve	• stenosis (± systolic doming) • prolapse • vegetations • dysplasia
Main Pulmonary Artery	• dilatation • supravalvular stenosis • branch or peripheral pulmonary artery narrowing or stenosis

Parasternal Short Axis Views

There are 6 levels of interest in the parasternal short axis position with each level labelled according to the primary cardiac structures identified (Figure 2.11).

Transducer Position and Rotation:

The transducer remains in the parasternal position; that is, within the third, fourth, or fifth intercostal space. The ultrasound beam is directed perpendicular to the long axis view of the left ventricle by rotating the transducer 90 degrees clockwise. Hence, the image index marker is pointed toward the patient's right supraclavicular fossa (rotated to approximately 1 o'clock). The scan plane, therefore, runs almost parallel along an imaginary line joining the left shoulder and the right leg.

Transducer Angulation:

Parasternal short axis views of the heart are obtained through a series of sweeps that transect the heart from the level of the great arteries, through the base of the heart, and to the cardiac apex. When the transducer is perpendicular to the chest wall, a short axis view of the left ventricle at the level of the mitral valve is obtained. When the transducer is tilted superiorly and angled medially, the sector plane passes through the short axis levels of the LVOT, the aorta and left atrium, and the pulmonary artery bifurcation. When the transducer is tilted inferiorly and angled laterally, the sector plane passes though the short axis of the left ventricle at the level of the papillary muscles and apex. Minor adjustments to transducer position may be required to obtain images of the short axis of the left ventricular apex. These adjustments include movement of the transducer an intercostal space lower and angling laterally (away) from the sternum.

Sector Orientation:

Anatomic relationships to the sector image are orientated so that anterior structures are seen at the top of the sector while posterior structures are seen at the bottom of the sector. Right-sided structures are seen to the left of the sector, and left-sided structures are seen to the right of the sector.

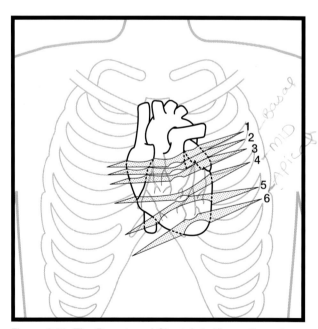

Figure 2.11: The Parasternal Short Axis Views: Transducer Position and Sector Orientation.

Parasternal Short Axis View of the Pulmonary Artery Bifurcation

In order to obtain this view, it may be necessary to move the transducer superiorly or an interspace higher.

Image Orientation:

The RVOT is seen anteriorly. The aorta is visualised in the centre of the image while the main pulmonary artery appears to the right of the image. The right pulmonary artery is seen to the left of the image while the left pulmonary artery appears to the right of the image.

Structures Visualised and Normal Echocardiographic Appearances: (Figure 2.12)

From the parasternal short axis view at the level of the pulmonary artery bifurcation, the following structures can be identified. The **pulmonary valve leaflets** should appear thin, produce uniform echoes and be unrestricted in their motion.

During systole, the pulmonary leaflets snap open and lie parallel to the walls of the main pulmonary artery.

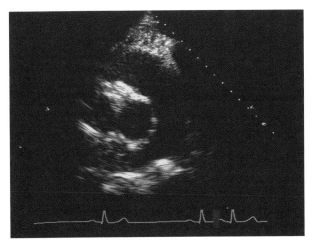

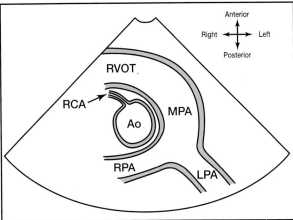

Figure 2.12: Normal Cardiac Structures Visualised from the Parasternal Short Axis View at the Level of the Pulmonary Artery Bifurcation.
Top, Echocardiographic Structures Visualised.
Bottom, Schematic Illustration of Structures Visualised and Sector Orientation.
Abbreviations: Ao = aorta; **LPA** = left pulmonary artery; **MPA** = main pulmonary artery; **RCA** = right coronary artery; **RPA** = right pulmonary artery; **RVOT** = right ventricular outflow tract.

Leaflets close abruptly at the onset of diastole and lie centrally within the main pulmonary artery throughout the diastolic period.

The **main pulmonary artery** is well seen and should appear widely patent, maintaining a consistent diameter along its length. The lumen of this vessel should be free of echoes.

The **proximal right and left pulmonary artery branches** should be of a similar size and their lumens should be echo-free. Only a short portion of the proximal left pulmonary artery can be seen on the right of the image. The proximal right pulmonary artery can be seen coursing posteriorly behind the aorta and to the left of the image.

The **ascending aorta** is seen in its short axis and its lumen should appear free of echoes. At this level, the cusps of the aortic valve are not usually visualised.

The **RVOT** lies anterior to the ascending aorta and should remain widely patent throughout the cardiac cycle.

Parasternal Short Axis View of the Aorta and the Left Atrium

Image Orientation:

The aorta appears as a circle within the centre of the image. The RVOT courses anteriorly above the aorta. The left atrium lies directly behind the aorta. The pulmonary valve is visualised to the right of the image while the right atrium appears to the left of the image.

Structures Visualised and Normal Echocardiographic Appearances: (Figure 2.13)

The **aorta** appears as a circular structure in the centre of the image. All three cusps of the tricuspid **aortic valve** can be visualised in this view. The **right coronary cusp** appears most anterior, the **left coronary cusp** is posterior and to the right of the image while the **non-coronary cusp** is also posterior and to the left of the image. In diastole, when the aortic valve is closed, the cusps produce a "Y" pattern. During systole, the leaflets are seen to snap open up into the aortic root. Identification of the number of aortic valve leaflets is most accurate during systole since a bicuspid valve may appear tricuspid in diastole due to the appearance of a raphe in the position of a normal commissure.

Regions of thickening in the middle of the free edge of each cusp (on the ventricular aspect of the valve) may be observed when the valve is closed. These are the **nodules of Arantius**. These nodules tend to become larger and more prominent with advancing age. Small mobile filaments may also be noted on the ventricular surface of the valve; these are **Lambl's excrescences**. Both the nodes of Arantii and Lambl's excrescences are normal structures that may be seen when image quality is exceptionally good. It is important that these structures are not confused for pathology.

The origins of the **right and left coronary arteries** can often be identified in this view arising from their respective coronary cusps. When visualised, the left coronary cusp can be seen to arise from the level of the aortic valve at approximately 5 o'clock. The right coronary artery usually arises from the aortic root approximately 1 cm above the level of the aortic valve at about 11 o'clock. On occasions, the left main coronary artery can be seen dividing into the left anterior descending and circumflex branches.

The **left atrium** is positioned immediately posterior to the aorta. The cavity of the left atrium should appear free of echoes. Occasionally, the finger-like **left atrial appendage** may be imaged as it extends superiorly and laterally to the right of the image. A thorough examination of this appendage in the setting of atrial fibrillation and mitral stenosis is important. In these conditions, the appendage is predisposed to thrombus formation because of the relative stasis of blood flow.

The **RVOT** crosses anterior to the circular aorta from the left to the right of the image, wrapping around the aorta to produce a "sausage-like" appearance. This "sausage-circle" appearance is an important indicator of the normal anatomic relationship between the great arteries (that is, between the aorta and pulmonary artery).

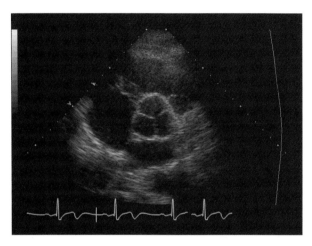

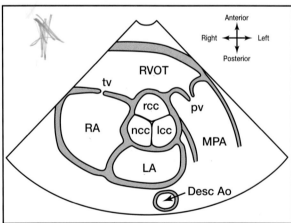

Figure 2.13: Normal Cardiac Structures Visualised from the Parasternal Short Axis View at the Level of the Aorta and Left Atrium.
Top, Echocardiographic Structures Visualised.
Bottom, Schematic Illustration of Structures Visualised including the Sector Orientation.
Abbreviations: Desc Ao = descending aorta; **LA** = left atrium; **lcc** = left coronary cusp; **MPA** = main pulmonary artery; **ncc** = non-coronary cusp; **pv** = pulmonary valve; **RA** = right atrium; **rcc** = right coronary cusp; **RVOT** = right ventricular outflow tract; **tv** = tricuspid valve.

Two of the three **pulmonary valve leaflets** are seen anteriorly and to the right of the aorta. Leaflets snap open in systole to lie parallel to the main pulmonary artery walls. During diastole, leaflets coapt and lie within the centre of the main pulmonary artery.

The **right atrium** appears at the bottom and to the left of the image and its cavity should appear echo-free. The **interatrial septum** (IAS), which separates the right and left atria, runs posteriorly from the non-coronary cusp of the aortic valve. Because the pressure within the left atrium is slightly higher than that of the right atrium, the IAS is seen to bulge from left to right. The IAS may not be seen in its entirety from this view and, hence, may appear defective. This is a result of "drop-out" artefact which occurs as a result of poor backscatter of echoes from this relatively thin structure which lies almost parallel to the ultrasound beam (refer to Chapter 1: "Interaction of Ultrasound with tissue").

Two of the three **tricuspid valve leaflets** are visualised. The anterior tricuspid leaflet appears to the left of the image while the septal leaflet appears medially. Frequently, the **inferior vena cava** and **coronary sinus** can be seen posteriorly to the atria. The **descending thoracic aorta** can also be seen, in its short axis, posterior to the left atrium.

Parasternal Short Axis View of the Left Ventricular Outflow Tract

Image Orientation:

A portion of the RVOT appears anteriorly and to the left of the image. The LVOT is seen in the centre of the image. Segments of the right atrium and tricuspid valve are seen to the left of the image. The left atrial cavity is seen posterior to the LVOT.

Structures Visualised and Normal Echocardiographic Appearances: (Figure 2.14)

The **LVOT**, which is bounded by the basal anterior interventricular septum and anterior mitral valve leaflet, should appear widely patent and unobstructed throughout the cardiac cycle. The echo-free cavity of the **left atrium** appears posterior to the LVOT. Separating the left atrium and the LVOT is the **anterior mitral valve leaflet**, which should appear thin and mobile.

Small sections of the right heart are visualised in this view. A portion of the **RVOT** appears anterior to the LVOT while a portion of the **right atrium** appears to the left of the image. Portions of the **tricuspid leaflets** may also be seen separating the right atrium and right ventricle.

Parasternal Short Axis View of the Left Ventricle - Mitral Valve Level

Image Orientation:

Portions of the right ventricle appear anteriorly. The left ventricle appears posterior. The mitral valve leaflets appear centrally within the cavity of the left ventricle.

Structures Visualised and Normal Echocardiographic Appearances: (Figure 2.15)

The **left ventricle** is transected at the level of the **mitral valve**. When the left ventricle is transected in its short axis, it appears circular in shape. An oval- or egg-shaped cavity indicates that the ventricle is transected obliquely and not in its true short axis. This often results from the transducer being positioned too low on the chest wall. Therefore, by moving the transducer an intercostal space higher, distortion of the ventricle can often be rectified.

At this level, the **basal segments of the interventricular septum, anterior, lateral and inferior walls** can be visualised. The interventricular septum separates the right and left ventricles and is typically concave toward the left ventricle. The septum and other walls of the left ventricle should produce uniform echoes and have a symmetric thickness not exceeding 1.1 cm during diastole. During systole, as the left ventricle contracts, the interventricular septum and other walls thicken and the cavity of the left ventricle diminishes concentrically. During diastole, the walls relax and the cavity of the left ventricle expands. Assessment of these regions for systolic function and regional abnormalities can be determined.

Positioned within the centre of the left ventricular cavity are both **mitral valve leaflets**. As their names suggest, the anterior mitral leaflet appears anteriorly and the posterior

leaflet is posterior. The short axis view of the mitral valve displays a characteristic "fish-mouth" appearance during diastole when the valve is open.

In patients with mitral stenosis, the mitral orifice can be accurately traced to yield the mitral valve area (see Chapter 9). Normally, the leaflets will appear thin and unrestricted, opening to their full excursion during diastole. The points on the mitral annulus where the anterior and posterior leaflets meet are the commissures of the valve. The commissures are classified corresponding to the papillary muscles: the **anterolateral commissure** of the mitral valve appears to the right of the image while the **posteromedial commissure** appears to the left.

A portion of the **right ventricle** is seen anterior to the left ventricle. Sections of the **tricuspid valve** and its supporting apparatus appear to the left of the image and posterior to the right ventricle. Occasionally, the tricuspid valve may be transected in full so that all three leaflets are visualised. In this instance, the tricuspid leaflets produce a round-edge, triangular shape in diastole: the anterior leaflet appears to the left, the septal leaflet appears to the right and the posterior leaflet is seen posteriorly.

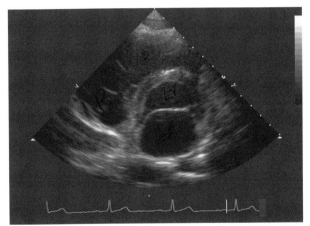

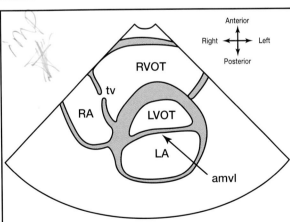

Figure 2.14: Normal Cardiac Structures Visualised from the Parasternal Short Axis View at the Level of the Left Ventricular Outflow Tract.

Top, Echocardiographic Structures Visualised.

Bottom, Schematic Illustration of Structures Visualised including the Sector Orientation.

Abbreviations: amvl = anterior mitral valve leaflet; **LA** = left atrium; **LVOT** = left ventricular outflow tract; **RA** = right atrium; **RVOT** = right ventricular outflow tract; **tv** = tricuspid valve.

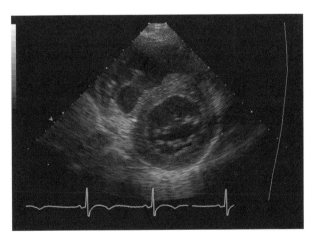

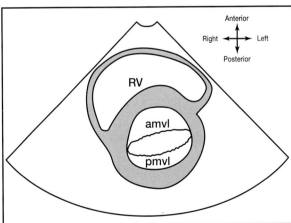

Figure 2.15: Normal Cardiac Structures Visualised from the Parasternal Short Axis View of the Left Ventricle - Mitral Valve Level.

Top, Echocardiographic Structures Visualised.

Bottom, Schematic Illustration of Structures Visualised including the Sector Orientation.

Abbreviations: amvl = anterior mitral valve leaflet; **pmvl** = posterior mitral valve leaflet; **RV** = right ventricle.

Parasternal Short Axis View of the Left Ventricle - Papillary Muscle Level

Image Orientation:

The left ventricle appears in the middle of the image with the papillary muscles projecting into the left ventricular cavity. A portion of the right ventricle appears to the top left of the image.

Structures Visualised and Normal Echocardiographic Appearances: (Figure 2.16)

The **left ventricle** is transected at the level of the **papillary muscles** and appears circular in shape. At this level, the **middle segments of the interventricular septum, anterior, lateral and inferior walls** can be visualised. During systole, as the left ventricle contracts, the interventricular septum and other walls thicken and the cavity of the left ventricle diminishes concentrically. During diastole, the ventricle relaxes and the ventricular cavity expands. Assessment of these regions for systolic function and regional abnormalities can be determined.

The **papillary muscles** are displayed as equal-sized, cone-shaped structures along the lateral and medial aspects of the left ventricular cavity. There are normally two papillary muscles. The position of these muscles is variable, however the anterolateral papillary muscle is typically seen to the right of the image between 3 and 5 o'clock and the posteromedial papillary muscle is displayed to the left of the image between 7 and 9 o'clock.

The apical segment of the **right ventricle** appears anteriorly and to the left of the image. Occasionally, the three papillary muscles of the right ventricle may be depicted. The position and orientation of these papillary muscles is variable.

Parasternal Short Axis View of the Left Ventricle - Apical Level

This view is also known as the apical short axis view. In order to obtain this view, it is often necessary to reposition the transducer laterally (away) from the sternum and one or two intercostal spaces lower. This transducer position is sometimes referred to as the "para-apical" position.

Image Orientation:

The left ventricle appears in the middle of the image. The right ventricular apex, if visualised, appears to the left of the image and is no longer anterior to the left ventricle.

Structures Visualised and Normal Echocardiographic Appearances: (Figure 2.17)

The **left ventricle** appears in the centre of the image as a small, rounded structure with an echo-free cavity. This cavity size should diminish, but not obliterate, in a concentric manner during systole.

At this level, **apical segments of the interventricular septum, anterior, lateral and inferior walls** can be visualised and assessed for systolic function and regional abnormalities.

When imaged from the correct level, no other cardiac structures, with the possible exception of a small segment of the right ventricle, should be seen from this view.

Abnormalities Detected from the Parasternal Short Axis Views:

Abnormalities that may be detected from these views are summarised in Table 2.5. An example of a pressure overloaded right ventricle which is commonly seen from this view is depicted in Figure 2.18.

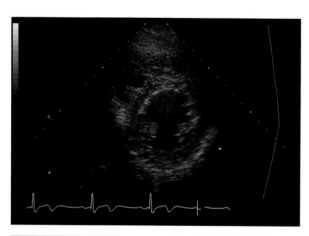

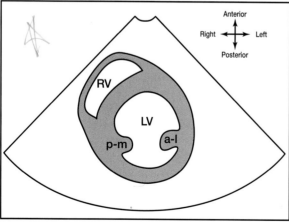

Figure 2.16: Normal Cardiac Structures Visualised from the Parasternal Short Axis View of the Left Ventricle - Papillary Muscle Valve Level.

Top, Echocardiographic Structures Visualised.

Bottom, Schematic Illustration of Structures Visualised including the Sector Orientation.

Abbreviations: a-l = anterolateral papillary muscle; **LV** = left ventricle; **p-m** = posteromedial papillary muscle; **RV** = right ventricle.

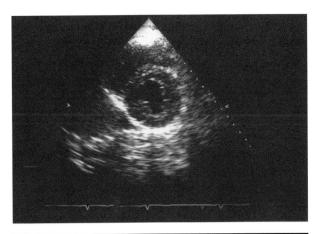

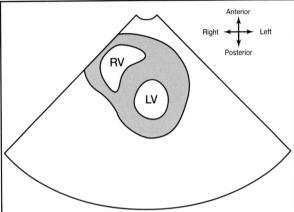

Figure 2.17: Normal Cardiac Structures Visualised from the Parasternal Short Axis View of the Left Ventricle - Apical Level.
Top, Echocardiographic Structures Visualised.
Bottom, Schematic Illustration of Structures Visualised including the Sector Orientation.
Abbreviations: LV = left ventricle; **RV** = right ventricle.

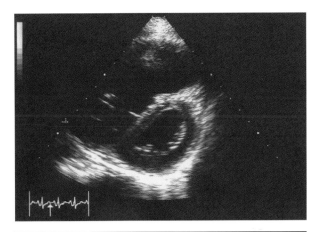

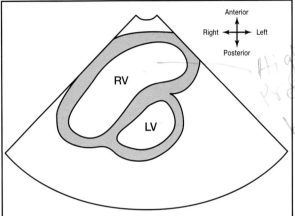

Figure 2.18: Parasternal Short Axis View of the Left Ventricle at the Level of the Papillary Muscles demonstrating Ventricular Distortion due to Pulmonary Hypertension.
Top, Echocardiographic Structures Visualised.
Bottom, Schematic Illustration of Structures Visualised.
This example demonstrates ventricular distortion of the left ventricle that is seen in patients with pulmonary hypertension. Normally, the left ventricle appears circular in shape. In this example, there is flattening or "pancaking" of the interventricular septum during systole which gives the left ventricle a "D-shaped" appearance. This abnormal appearance is the result of increased pressures within the right ventricle during systole. Also observe significant dilatation of the right ventricular cavity.
Abbreviations: LV = left ventricle; **RV** = right ventricle.

Table 2.5: Abnormalities Detected from the Parasternal Short Axis Views:

Short Axis Levels	Detectable Abnormalities
Pulmonary Artery Bifurcation	• dilatation of the main pulmonary artery and its proximal branches • dilatation of the RVOT and ascending aorta • proximal stenosis of right and left pulmonary artery branches • presence of pulmonary artery clots/emboli
Aorta and Left Atrium	*Aortic valve:* • abnormal aortic valve leaflet number: bicuspid, unicuspid, quadracuspid • valvular stenosis • calcification of aortic leaflets • commissural calcification • valvular vegetations *Aortic root:* • sinuses of Valsalva aneurysms/rupture • dilatation of sinuses/root • aortic dissection flaps *Coronary arteries:* • dilatation of the origins of the right and left coronary arteries • aneursyms at origin of the right and left coronary arteries: associated with Kawasaki's disease *Left atrium:* • intracardiac thrombus/tumours • left atrial dilatation *Right ventricular outflow tract:* • increased wall thickness • dilatation • infundibular narrowing *Pulmonary valve:* • stenosis (± systolic doming) • prolapse • vegetations • dysplasia *Interatrial septum:* • abnormal motion: bulges toward left atrium when right atrial pressure increased • atrial septal defects (beware of "drop-out" artefact)
Left Ventricular Outflow Tract	• asymmetric septal hypertrophy • systolic anterior motion of the anterior mitral leaflet • prolapsing aortic valve leaflets • vegetations

Left Ventricle - Mitral Valve	*Mitral valve:*
	• reduced mitral orifice area (mitral stenosis)
	• annular calcification
	• flutter due to aortic regurgitation
	• vegetations
	• redundancy of prolapsing leaflet
	• failure of leaflet coaptation
	
	Left ventricle:
	• systolic dysfunction
	• increased wall thickness: concentric or asymmetric
	• regional wall motion abnormalities
	• distortion of left ventricular shape due to:
	  - ventricular aneurysms
	  - volume or pressure overload of right ventricle
	
	Right atrium and ventricle:
	• dilatation
	• systolic dysfunction of the right ventricle
	• intracavity thrombus

(continued on next page)

Table 2.5: Abnormalities Detected from the Parasternal Short Axis Views:
(continued)

Short Axis Levels	Detectable Abnormalities
Left Ventricle - Mitral Valve	*Tricuspid valve:* • valvular stenosis and thickening • prolapse • vegetations
Left Ventricle - Papillary Muscles	*Left ventricle:* • dilatation • systolic dysfunction • increased wall thickness: concentric or asymmetric • regional wall motion abnormalities • distortion of left ventricular shape due to: - ventricular aneurysms - volume or pressure overload of right ventricle (see Figure 2.18)
	Papillary muscles: • abnormal number (single papillary muscle associated with a parachute mitral valve) • malposition of papillary muscles: associated with hypertrophic obstructive cardiomyopathy • papillary muscle dysfunction • papillary muscle rupture
	Right ventricle: • dilatation • systolic dysfunction of the right ventricle • intracavity thrombus
Left Ventricle - Apex	• regional wall motion abnormalities • apical aneurysms • apical thrombus • apical hypertrophy • systolic obliteration of apex

The Apical Position

Patient Positioning:

The patient remains on their left side at an angle of approximately 60 to 90 degrees. The left arm should also remain extended above the patient's head. A bed that has a cut-out window can be beneficial in examining the heart from this view.

Apical Four Chamber View

Transducer Position and Angulation: (Figure 2.19)
When apical impulse is palpable, the transducer is placed at or in the immediate vicinity of the maximal impulse. This position is often found around the fifth intercostal space in the mid-axilla region (the position of V5 on the 12-lead ECG). The ultrasound beam is directed superiorly towards the patient's head so that the beam is oriented to transect the heart from the apex to the base, including the atria. The image index marker is rotated to approximately 3 o'clock.

Sector and Image Orientation:
Anatomic relationships to the sector image are orientated so that inferior structures such as the cardiac apices of both ventricles appear at the top of the sector and superior structures such as the atria are seen at the bottom of the sector. Left-sided structures such as the left atrium and left ventricle are seen to the right of the sector, and right-sided structures such as the right atrium and right ventricle are seen to the left of the sector.

Structures Visualised and Normal Echocardiographic Appearances: (Figure 2.19)
The apical four chamber view, as the name suggests, allows visualisation of all four cardiac chambers including the cardiac crux. The **cardiac crux or cross** is located in the "centre" of the heart. This anatomical structure is formed by the primum interatrial septum and membraneous interventricular septum, which lie vertically and medially, and by the septal leaflet of the tricuspid valve and the anterior leaflet of the mitral valve which lie horizontally. The identification of the cardiac crux is important in the assessment of congenital heart lesions as the cardiac crux delineates the anatomic relationships between the structures that form this arrangement.

The **long or major axes** of both the left and right ventricles are seen from this view. The **anterolateral wall, inferior septum and apex** of the left ventricle are displayed, as is the **lateral free wall** of the right ventricle. The **left ventricle** appears as a truncated ellipse with a length longer than its width and a tapered apex. Foreshortening of the apical view is recognised when the heart appears "spherical" in shape with minimal tapering at the apex. In such instances, the transducer is usually too high on the chest wall. Movement of the transducer inferiorly or an intercostal space lower often resolves this problem.

The **right ventricle** appears triangular in shape with a cavity about one-half the size of the left ventricle. The apex of the right ventricle is located closer to the base of the heart than that of the left ventricle.

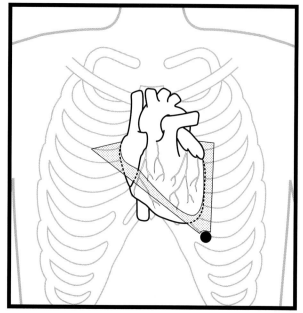

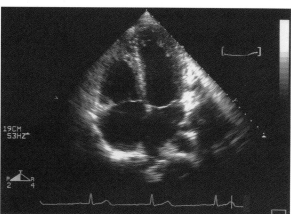

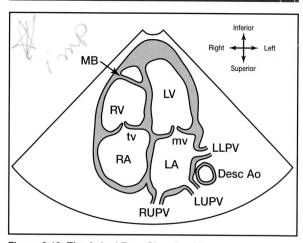

Figure 2.19: The Apical Four Chamber View.
Top, Transducer Position and Imaging Plane.
Middle, Echocardiographic Structures Visualised.
Bottom, Schematic Illustration of Structures Visualised including the Sector Orientation.
Abbreviations: Desc Ao = descending aorta; **LA** = left atrium; **LLPV** = left lower pulmonary vein; **LUPV** = left upper pulmonary vein; **LV** = left ventricle; **MB** = moderator band; **mv** = mitral valve; **RA** = right atrium; **RUPV** = right upper pulmonary vein; **RV** = right ventricle; **tv** = tricuspid valve.

Cavities of both ventricles should appear free of echoes. The right ventricular myocardium may appear more obviously trabeculated than that of the left ventricle, which usually appears relatively smooth. The **moderator band** of the right ventricle can be seen arising from the apical third of the interventricular septum extending across the right ventricular cavity to the right ventricular free wall. This structure as well as the characteristic coarse trabeculation of the right ventricular endocardium and the insertion point of the septal tricuspid leaflet aids in the differentiation of the right ventricle from the left ventricle.

Both atrioventricular (AV) valves, along with their subvalvular apparatus, can be identified and assessed in this view. During diastole, these leaflets open without restriction with their leaflet tips pointing into their respective ventricles. During systole, the AV valves coapt and lie in a plane perpendicular to the atrioventricular ring. The **mitral valve leaflets** can be seen originating from the left atrioventricular ring with the smaller posterior leaflet seen arising from the lateral border. The larger anterior leaflet arises from the medial aspect adjacent to the interventricular septum. Chordal attachments from the mitral leaflets to the anterolateral papillary muscle, located on the lateral wall of the left ventricle, may be appreciated. The **tricuspid valve leaflets** can be identified originating from the right atrioventricular ring with the anterior leaflet arising from the lateral border and the septal leaflet arising from the medial margin. The posterior tricuspid leaflet is not usually seen in this view. Leaflets of both AV valves should appear thin and mobile.

A crucial and distinctive feature of the apical four chamber view is the relationship between the anterior mitral leaflet and the septal tricuspid leaflet. Normally, the left atrioventricular (AV) groove is slightly higher than the right AV groove. Consequently, the anterior mitral leaflet arises from the left AV groove near the superior end of the membraneous interventricular septum while the septal leaflet of the tricuspid valve inserts into the right AV groove close to the mid portion of the membraneous interventricular septum. Thus, the septal tricuspid leaflet is approximately 5 to 10 mm inferior to the insertion point of the anterior mitral leaflet [8]. The position of the insertion points for these two leaflets provide an important anatomic landmark for the identification of the right and left ventricles since the tricuspid valve always leads to the right ventricle and the mitral valve always leads to the left ventricle. Therefore, by correctly identifying the right and left AV valves, the ventricles are easily differentiated.

The portion of septum located between the septal tricuspid leaflet and the anterior mitral leaflets is referred to as the **atrioventricular septum**.

The **interatrial septum** and **interventricular septum** can be clearly delineated in their entirety from this view. As for the parasternal short axis view of the IAS, "drop-out" artefact is commonly seen in the region of fossa ovalis. Due to this potential problem, assessment for defects in the interatrial septum should not be determined from this view alone. The interventricular septum is more muscular and thicker than the interatrial septum (due to the higher pressures within the left ventricle compared to the pressures within the atria). Back-scatter echoes from the interventricular septum are readily detected and "drop-out" artefact is not a problem in the interrogation of this structure.

Pulmonary venous drainage into the left atrium can be appreciated from this view. Visualisation of three of the four pulmonary veins draining into the left atrium is usually possible. The **right upper pulmonary vein** can be seen draining into the supero-medial aspect of the left atrium while the left upper and left lower pulmonary veins are seen draining into the lateral aspect of the left atrium (the left upper vein is located superior to the left lower vein). The right lower pulmonary vein is not usually visualised from this view.

The **descending thoracic aorta** appears as a circular, echo-free structure along the lateral margin of the left atrium. The circular shape of this vessel will differentiate it from the left pulmonary veins, which are usually elongated and of a smaller dimension.

Occasionally, the **left atrial appendage** may be seen as a finger-like projection at the lateral and inferior border of the left atrium. This appendage should be free of echoes.

When the transducer is tilted posteriorly, the **coronary sinus** may be visualised draining into the right atrium. When visualised, the coronary sinus appears as a tunnel-like structure in the atrioventricular groove posterior to the left atrium.

Apical Five Chamber View
Transducer Position and Angulation: (Figure 2.20)
The apical five chamber view is a modification of the apical four chamber view. The transducer position is unchanged. This view is achieved by anterior tilting of the transducer until the LVOT and proximal ascending aorta are visualised. The proximal ascending aorta and the LVOT constitute the "fifth" chamber.

Sector and Image Orientation:
As for the apical four chamber view, the anatomic relationships to the sector image are orientated so that inferior structures such as the cardiac apices of both ventricles appear at the top of the sector and superior structures such as the atria are seen at the bottom of the sector. Left-sided structures such as the left atrium and left ventricle are seen to the right of the sector, and right-sided structures such as the right atrium and right ventricle are seen to the left of the sector. The LVOT is seen in the middle of the image with the proximal ascending aorta appearing superior to the outflow tract.

8: Tajik, A.B. et al.: Mayo Clinic Proceedings 53:285,1978

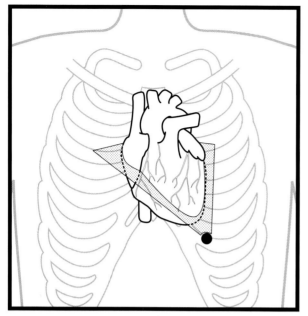

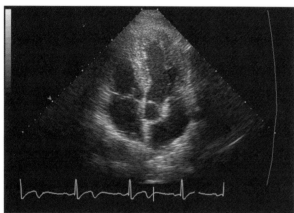

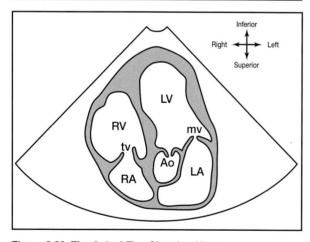

Figure 2.20: The Apical Five Chamber View.
Top, Transducer Position and Imaging Plane.
Middle, Echocardiographic Structures Visualised.
Bottom, Schematic Illustration of Structures Visualised
including the Sector Orientation.
Abbreviations: Ao = ascending aorta; **LA** = left atrium;
LV = left ventricle; **mv** = mitral valve; **RA** = right atrium;
RV = right ventricle; **tv** = tricuspid valve.

*Structures Visualised and Normal Echocardiographic
Appearances:* (Figure 2.20)
In addition to the structures identified in the apical four
chamber view, the **LVOT, proximal ascending aorta**
and **aortic valve leaflets** are also visualised.
The **LVOT** is bounded medially by the interventricular
septum and laterally by the anterior mitral valve leaflet.
The LVOT should appear widely patent throughout the
cardiac cycle.
Two of the three **aortic valve cusps** are seen. The cusps
visualised vary, but typically, it is the left and right
coronary cusps that are seen.
The **left coronary artery** may sometimes be identified
arising from the aorta to the right of the image as it
passes along the left atrioventricular groove.

Apical Long Axis View
Transducer Position and Angulation: (Figure 2.21)
The long axis of the left ventricle is obtained from the
apical position by rotating the transducer 90 degrees
counterclockwise and by tilting the transducer anteriorly
(as required for the apical five chamber view). The
image index marker is, thus, pointed toward the patient's
suprasternal notch (rotated to approximately 12 o'clock).
Minor adjustments may be required, such as slight
lateral or medial angulation, movement of the transducer
medially, and/or movement of the transducer an
intercostal space higher.

Sector and Image Orientation:
Anatomic relationships to the sector image are
orientated so that inferior structures appear at the top
left of the image while anterior structures are seen at the
top right of the image. Superior structures are seen at the
bottom right of the image, and posterior structures are
seen at the bottom left of the image. Hence, the left
ventricle appears at the top left of the image, the left
atrium appears at the bottom right of the image, and the
aorta appears to the right of the image.

*Structures Visualised and Normal Echocardiographic
Appearances:* (Figure 2.21)
Structures visualised in the apical long axis view include
all those described for the parasternal long axis view of
the left ventricle as well as the **true apex of the left
ventricle**. Hence, the structures seen from this view
include:
- anterior wall of the right ventricle
- portion of right ventricular cavity
- proximal ascending aorta
- right and non-coronary cusps of the aortic valve
- left atrium
- anterior and posterior mitral valve leaflets
- subvalvular apparatus of the mitral valve
- left ventricular outflow tract
- interventricular septum
- inferolateral (posterior) wall of the left ventricle
- left ventricular cavity
- descending thoracic aorta
- coronary sinus
- true apex of the left ventricle

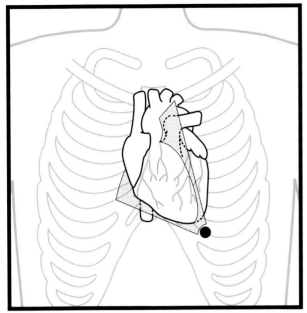

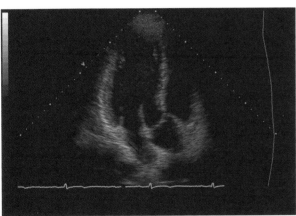

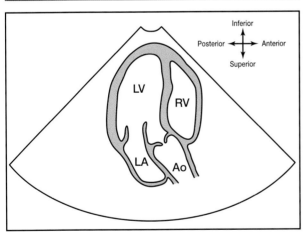

Figure 2.21: The Apical Long Axis View.
Top, Transducer Position and Imaging Plane.
Middle, Echocardiographic Structures Visualised.
Bottom, Schematic Illustration of Structures Visualised including the Sector Orientation.
Abbreviations: Ao = ascending aorta; **LA** = left atrium; **LV** = left ventricle; **mv** = mitral valve; **RV** = right ventricle.

Apical Two Chamber View

Transducer Position and Angulation: (Figure 2.22)
This view is a variation of the apical long axis view and is obtained by rotating the transducer approximately 45 degrees clockwise from the long axis view. Therefore, this imaging plane lies somewhere between the apical four chamber and apical long axis views.

Sector and Image Orientation:
Anatomic relationships to the sector image are orientated so that inferior structures are seen at the top left of the image while anterior structures are seen at the top right of the image. Superior structures are seen at the bottom right of the image; and posterior structures are seen at the bottom left of the image. Hence, the left ventricle appears at the top left of the image and the left atrium appears at the bottom right of the image.

Structures Visualised and Normal Echocardiographic Appearances: (Figure 2.22)
In this view, the cardiac structures that are routinely seen include the **left ventricle, left atrium,** the **mitral valve leaflets,** and the **descending thoracic aorta.**
The importance of this view lies in the assessment of regional wall motion abnormalities as it visualises the **true anterior wall** and the **true inferior wall** of the left ventricle. During systole, as the left ventricle contracts, the ventricular walls thicken and the ventricular cavity decreases in size in a concentric manner. During diastole, the ventricle relaxes and the ventricular cavity expands. Assessment of these regions for systolic function and regional abnormalities can be determined. The cavity of the left ventricle should appear echo-free.
The **mitral valve leaflets** should appear thin and mobile. During diastole, the mitral leaflets should open without restriction with the leaflet tips pointing into the left ventricle. During systole, the mitral leaflets coapt and lie in a plane perpendicular to the atrioventricular ring.
The **descending thoracic aorta** can be opened out onto its long axis by tilting the transducer posteriorly with slight medial angulation and counterclockwise rotation (Figure 2.23). The lumen of this vessel should be widely patent throughout the cardiac cycle and be free of any echoes. This view, although not achievable in some patients, is particularly useful in the assessment of aortic dissections.
Occasionally, the **left atrial appendage** can also be imaged. This appendage appears as a finger-like extension of the left atrium pointing inferiorly and should be echo-free (Figure 2.23).

Abnormalities Detected from the Apical Views:
Abnormalities that may be detected from this view are summarised in Table 2.6. An example of Ebstein's anomaly which is commonly diagnosed from this view is depicted in Figure 2.24.

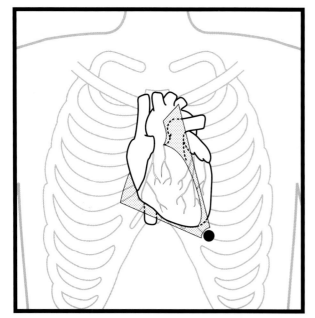

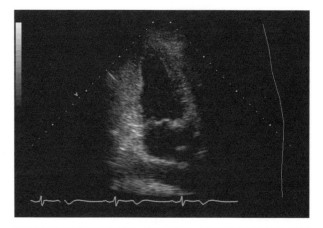

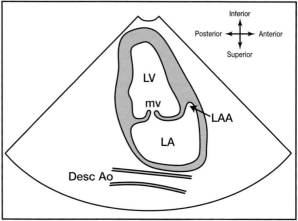

Figure 2.23: The Apical Two Chamber View including the Long Axis of the Descending Thoracic Aorta.
Top, Echocardiographic Structures Visualised.
Bottom, Schematic Illustration of Structures Visualised.
Abbreviations: Desc Ao = descending thoracic aorta; **LAA** = left atrial appendage; **LA** = left atrium; **LV** = left ventricle; **mv** = mitral valve.

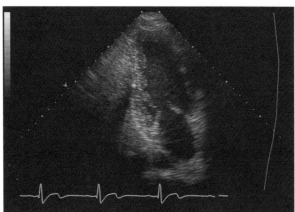

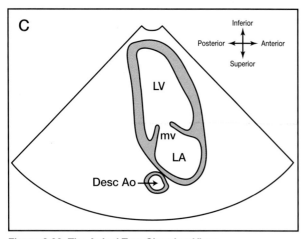

Figure 2.22: The Apical Two Chamber View.
Top, Transducer Position and Imaging Plane.
Middle, Echocardiographic Structures Visualised.
Bottom, Schematic Illustration of Structures Visualised including the Sector Orientation.
Abbreviations: Desc Ao = descending thoracic aorta; **LA** = left atrium; **LV** = left ventricle; **mv** = mitral valve.

Table 2.6: Abnormalities Detected from the Apical Views:

Apical Views	Detectable Abnormalities

Apical 4 Chamber	• dilatation of atria and ventricles
	• abnormal relationships of cardiac crux such as:
	  - mal-alignment of IVS and IAS
	  - Ebstein's anomaly (Figure 2.24)
	  - aortic override of IVS
	• abnormalities of AV valves and subvalvular apparatus:
	  - stenosis, prolapse, flail leaflets
	  - ruptured chordae
	  - annular calcification
	  - vegetations
	• RWMAs
	• ventricular septal defects (eg. congenital, post myocardial infarction)
	• intracardiac masses:
	  - size
	  - point of attachment

Apical 5 Chamber	• LVOT obstruction due to:
	  - asymmetric septal hypertrophy
	  - systolic motion of anterior mitral leaflet
	  - subaortic membrane
	• aortic valve abnormalities:
	  - stenosis
	  - calcification
	  - reduced mobility
	  - prolapse
	  - vegetations

Apical Long Axis	• dilatation of LA and/or LV
	• RWMAs
	• LVOT obstruction due to:
	  - asymmetric septal hypertrophy
	  - systolic motion of anterior mitral valve leaflet
	  - subaortic membrane
	• abnormalities of mitral and aortic valves:
	  - stenosis
	  - calcification
	  - reduced mobility
	  - prolapse
	  - vegetations

Apical 2 Chamber	• dilatation of LA and/or LV
	• RWMAs
	• dilatation of descending aorta
	• identification of dissection flaps
	• abnormalities of mitral and aortic valves:
	  - stenosis
	  - calcification
	  - reduced mobility
	  - prolapse
	  - vegetations

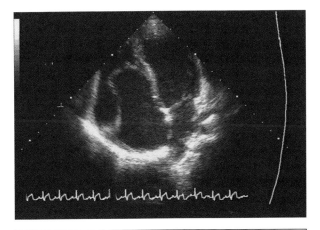

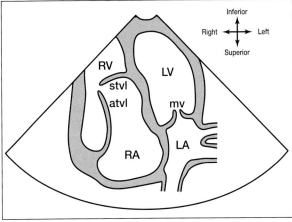

Figure 2.24: Apical Four Chamber View demonstrating Ebstein's Anomaly.

Top, Echocardiographic Structures Visualised.

Bottom, Schematic Illustration of Structures Visualised.

Ebstein's anomaly is a congenital malformation of the tricuspid valve resulting in the characteristic apical displacement of an abnormal, sail-like septal tricuspid leaflet. The diagnostic criterion for this anomaly is a displacement index between the insertion points of the anterior mitral and the septal tricuspid leaflets of ≥ 8 mm/m^2.

When Ebstein's anomaly has been diagnosed, it is very important to assess the interatrial septum, as atrial septal defects are commonly associated with this condition.

Abbreviations: atvl = anterior tricuspid valve leaflet; **LA** = left atrium; **LV** = left ventricle; **mv** = mitral valve; **RA** = right atrium; **RV** = right ventricle; **stvl** = septal tricuspid valve leaflet.

The Subcostal Position

The subcostal views are especially valuable in the assessment of the technically difficult patient where the standard parasternal and apical views are suboptimal. Imaging from the subcostal window is particularly useful in the examination of patients with chronic obstructive airways disease, emphysema, and in the ventilated intensive care patient. In this subset of patients, the subcostal window may sometimes be the only window that provides any diagnostic information.

The subcostal view is also extremely important in the assessment of congenital heart disease. Images recorded from this window often allow better definition of certain cardiac structures such as the interatrial septum.

Patient Positioning:

The patient is supine. Slight bending of the knees is usually required to release tension of the abdominal muscles. The subcostal examination is often facilitated by held inspiration. Inspiration increases the volume of the lungs resulting in inferior displacement of the liver and the heart, thus, bringing the heart into closer proximity with the transducer.

Standard Subcostal Views include the four chamber view and the short axis views at the level of the left ventricle, RVOT, aorta and left atrium, and the vena cava and right atrium.

Miscellaneous Subcostal Views include the subcostal "five" chamber view and the subcostal view of the pulmonary artery. The subcostal five chamber view is a modification of the subcostal four chamber view. This view is achieved by anterior tilting of the transducer to bring the aorta and LVOT into view. In patients who demonstrate exceptionally good subcostal images, further anterior tilting of the transducer from the subcostal five chamber view may display the RVOT and pulmonary valve.

Subcostal Four Chamber View

Transducer Position and Angulation: (Figure 2.25)

The transducer is placed in the subxiphoid position immediately inferior to the sternum along the midline or slightly to the patient's right side. The image index marker is rotated to approximately 3 o'clock. The transducer is tilted slightly anteriorly so that the scan plane is directed towards the region between the suprasternal notch and left clavicle. Minor adjustments, such as slight clockwise or counterclockwise rotations, may be required to obtain all four chambers

Sector and Image Orientation:

Anatomic relationships to the sector image are orientated so that right-sided structures such as the right atrium and right ventricle are seen at the top of the image. Left-sided structures such as the left atrium and left ventricle are seen at the bottom of the image. Inferior structures such as the apices of both ventricles appear to the right

of the image while superior structures such as the atria appear to the left of the image.

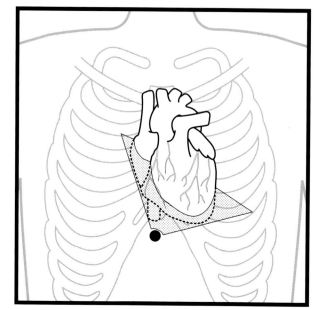

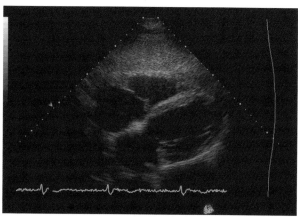

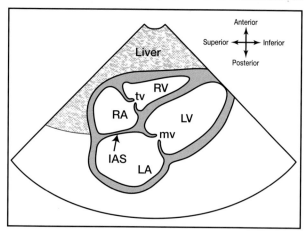

Figure 2.25: The Subcostal Four Chamber View.
Top, Transducer Position and Imaging Plane.
Middle, Echocardiographic Structures Visualised.
Bottom, Schematic Illustration of Structures Visualised including the Sector Orientation.
Abbreviations: IAS = interatrial septum; **LA** = left atrium; **LV** = left ventricle; **mv** = mitral valve; **RA** = right atrium; **RV** = right ventricle; **tv** = tricuspid valve.

9: Shiina, A. et al.: Journal of the American College of Cardiology 3:367,1986.

Structures Visualised and Normal Echocardiographic Appearances: (Figure 2.25)

The **liver** is the first structure transected by the ultrasound beam and appears at the top of the image. The liver is recognised by its characteristic fine mottled appearance. Normally, the liver lies immediately adjacent to the heart so that there is no space between these two organs. Occasionally, a small space containing weak echoes may be seen separating the heart and the liver. This appearance is typical of epicardial fat. From this view, **all four cardiac chambers** can be seen.

The cavity of each chamber should appear free of echoes; although, supporting apparatus of the atrioventricular valves are usually seen within the ventricular cavities.

The **interatrial septum** and **interventricular septum** can be clearly delineated in their entirety from this view. The interatrial septum is best examined from this view. "Drop-out" of the interatrial septum, which may occur from the parasternal and apical views, does not occur from the subcostal view as the septum lies perpendicular to the interrogating ultrasound beam. Normally, thinning of the interatrial septum in the region of the fossa ovalis may be apparent.

Both **mitral valve leaflets** and two of the three **tricuspid valve leaflets** (anterior and posterior leaflets) can also be identified in this view. Leaflets should appear thin and mobile. During diastole, these leaflets open without restriction with their leaflet tips pointing into their respective ventricles. During systole, the atrioventricular valves coapt and lie in a plane perpendicular to the atrioventricular ring.

Subcostal Short Axis Views

As for the parasternal short axis, the heart can also be transected through multiple levels from the subcostal short axis views. In fact, the short views from the subcostal window produce images comparable to those that are obtained from the parasternal window. However, the images from the subcostal window are orientated about 90 degrees clockwise to those acquired from the parasternal views. In addition to the structures seen from the parasternal short axis views, the superior and inferior vena cava, and the abdominal aorta are also visualised.

Transducer Position and Angulation: (Figure 2.26)

The transducer remains in the subxiphoid region. The short axis views are achieved by rotating the transducer approximately 90 degrees counterclockwise from the long axis view so that the scan plane is perpendicular to the four chamber view. The image index marker is directed to about 12 o'clock.

As mentioned, the heart can be transected through several levels. This is achieved by sweeping the scan plane from the patient's left side to their right side.

Sector Orientation:

Orientation of the sector from this view is variable depending on the direction and level of the scan plane. Essentially, anatomic relationships to the sector image are orientated so that anterior structures are seen to the top or right of the sector while posterior structures are seen to the bottom or left of the sector. Inferior and right-sided structures are seen to the top or left of the sector. Superior and left-sided structures are seen to the bottom or right of the sector.

Image Orientation:

Image orientation is similar to that obtained at each parasternal short axis level except the image is rotated 90 degrees clockwise.

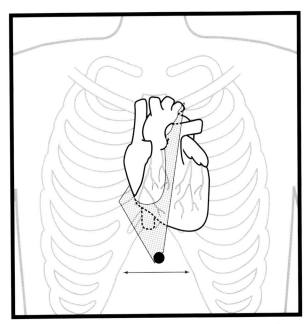

Figure 2.26: The Subcostal Short Axis Views: Transducer Position and Sector Orientation.

Structures Visualised and Normal Echocardiographic Appearances:

Essentially, all levels that can be obtained from the parasternal short axis views can be achieved from the subcostal short axis view. In addition, the long axes of the abdominal aorta, IVC and SVC are also seen.

Left ventricular apex level: (Figure 2.27)

The left ventricular apex can be identified by angling the transducer to the patient's extreme left so that the scan plane is directed toward the patient's left shoulder. The short axis of the left ventricle appears as a small rounded structure with a small echo-free cavity. The cavity of the ventricle should diminish in size, but not obliterate, in a concentric manner during systole.

Abdominal Aorta: (Figure 2.28)

The abdominal aorta in its long axis is visualised by angling the transducer further to the patient's left, past the cavity of the left ventricle. The abdominal aorta can be seen to course from the bottom of the sector (superiorly) to the top of the sector (inferiorly). The lumen of this vessel should be free of echoes and typically demonstrates a characteristic systolic pulse.

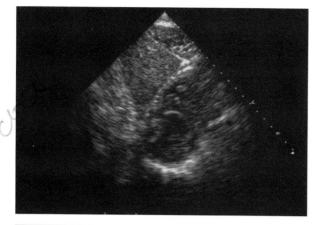

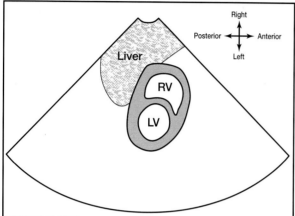

Figure 2.27: Normal Cardiac Structures Visualised from the Subcostal Short Axis View of the Left Ventricular Apex.
Top, Transducer Position and Imaging Plane.
Middle, Echocardiographic Structures Visualised.
Bottom, Schematic Illustration of Structures Visualised and Sector Orientation.
Abbreviations: LV = left ventricle; **RV** = right ventricle.

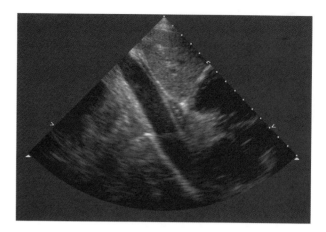

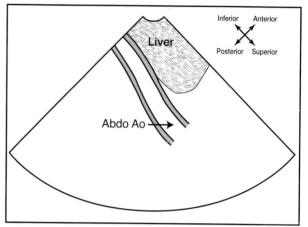

Figure 2.28: Normal Cardiac Structures Visualised from the Subcostal Short Axis View of the Abdominal Aorta.
Top, Echocardiographic Structures Visualised.
Bottom, Schematic Illustration of Structures Visualised and Sector Orientation.
Abbreviations: Abdo Ao = abdominal aorta.

Left ventricle at the level of the papillary muscles:
The left ventricle at the level of the papillary muscles can be visualised when the transducer is swept from the left ventricular apex toward the patient's midline. The **anterolateral papillary muscle** is seen at about 6 o'clock while the **posteromedial papillary muscle** is seen at about 11 o'clock.

Left ventricle at the level of the mitral valve:
The left ventricle at the level of the mitral valve is visualised when the transducer is swept from the papillary muscle level of the left ventricle further towards the patient's midline. The mitral valve leaflets are visualised in the centre of the left ventricular cavity with the anterior mitral leaflet appearing to the right of the image while the posterior mitral leaflet appears to the left of the image.

Right ventricular outflow tract (RVOT) level:
(Figure 2.29)
This view is obtained by sweeping the transducer from the patient's left to the patient's midline so that the scan plane is directed toward the left mid-clavicular line. This view is similar to the parasternal short axis view at the level of the aorta and left atrium; hence, all

structures visualised from this view can also be appreciated from the subcostal short axis view at this level. From this view, the **RVOT, pulmonary valve leaflets** and **main pulmonary artery** appear to the right of the image. The RVOT and main pulmonary artery should remain widely patent throughout the cardiac cycle. The pulmonary valve leaflets should appear thin and mobile, opening during systole and closing with diastole.

Occasionally, the **bifurcation of the pulmonary artery** into right and left branches can be seen. The left branch is seen to the right of the image and while the right branch is seen to the left of the image.

The tricuspid valve is also imaged and appears anterior to the RVOT near the centre of the image. From this view, all three tricuspid leaflets may be visualised. Moving clockwise from 12 o'clock, they are the anterior leaflet, septal leaflet and posterior leaflet.

The short axis of the **aortic root** as well as the **aortic valve cusps** appear in the centre of the image.

Portions of both left and right atria are seen to the left of the image with the **right atrium** appearing above the **left atrium**. The atria are separated by the **interatrial septum**, which appears perpendicular to the ultrasound beam.

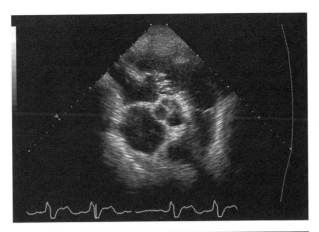

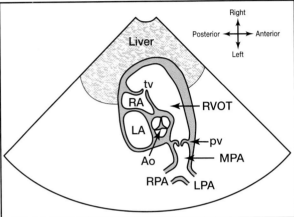

Figure 2.29: Normal Cardiac Structures Visualised from the Subcostal Short Axis View of the Right Ventricular Outflow Tract.
Top, Echocardiographic Structures Visualised.
Bottom, Schematic Illustration of Structures Visualised and Sector Orientation.
Abbreviations: Ao =aorta; **LA** = left atrium; **LPA** = left pulmonary artery; **MPA** = main pulmonary artery; **PV** = pulmonary valve; **RPA** = right pulmonary artery; **RVOT** = right ventricular outflow tract.

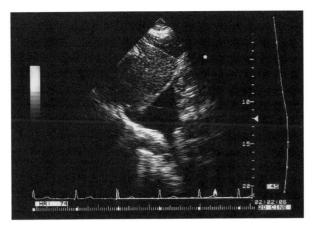

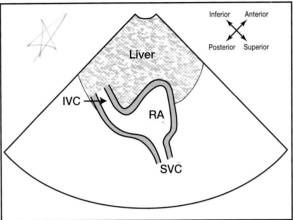

Figure 2.30: Normal Cardiac Structures Visualised from the Subcostal Short Axis View of the Inferior and Superior Vena Cavae.
Top, Echocardiographic Structures Visualised.
Bottom, Schematic Illustration of Structures Visualised and Sector Orientation.
Abbreviations: IVC =inferior vena cava; **RA** = right atrium; **SVC** = superior vena cava.

Inferior and superior vena cava level: (Figure 2.30)
This view is obtained by sweeping the transducer from the patient's midline toward the patient's right side so that the scan plane is directed toward the right midclavicular region. Slight counterclockwise rotation may be required to open out the inferior vena cava so that is can be imaged in its long axis. The **inferior vena cava** can be seen draining into the right atrium. The **eustachian valve**, when present, can be seen in this view guarding the orifice of the inferior vena cava and attaching to the interatrial septum at the level of the fossa ovalis. The **superior vena cava** can be identified draining into the superior aspect of the right atrium. All three **hepatic veins** can often be seen draining into the inferior vena cava from this view (posterior tilting of the transducer may be required).

Abnormalities Detected from the Subcostal Views:
Abnormalities that may be detected from this view are summarised in Table 2.7. An example of a secundum atrial septal defect which is commonly diagnosed from this view is depicted in Figure 2.31.

Table 2.7: Abnormalities Detected from the Subcostal Views.

Subcostal Views	Detectable Abnormalities

Subcostal Four Chamber View	• dilatation of cardiac chambers
	• increased wall thickness of both right and left ventricles
	• defects of the interatrial septum (localisation, size) - see Figure 2.31
	• defects of the interventricular septum (localisation, size)
	• lipomatous hypertrophy (fat infiltration) of interatrial septum:
	  - produces a characteristic dumb-bell appearance with sparing of the fossa ovalis
	• mitral and tricuspid valve abnormalities:
	  - stenosis
	  - calcification
	  - reduced mobility
	  - prolapse
	  - vegetations
	• presence and size of pericardial effusions
	• presence of intracardiac masses (especially atrial myxomas):
	  - determining their point of attachment
	  - size

Subcostal Short Axis	• pulmonary and aortic valve abnormalities:
	  - stenosis
	  - calcification
	  - reduced mobility
	  - prolapse
	  - vegetations
	• RVOT obstruction
	• left ventricular systolic dysfunction
	• abdominal aorta abnormalities:
	  - dilatation
	  - presence of intimal flaps (dissection)
	  - aneurysms
	• dilatation or obstruction of the inferior and/or superior vena cava
	• dilatation of hepatic veins

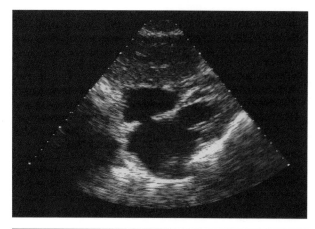

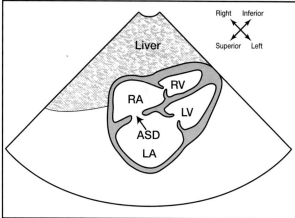

Figure 2.31: Subcostal Four Chamber View demonstrating a Secundum Atrial Septal Defect.

Top, Echocardiographic Structures Visualised.
Bottom, Schematic Illustration of Structures Visualised.

This example demonstrates an atrial septal defect in the secundum septum (arrow). The interatrial septum is best interrogated from the subcostal views as the septum lies in a plane perpendicular to the ultrasound beam. Hence, backscatter from this structure is maximised and "drop-out" artefacts, which may occur from the parasternal and apical views where the septum is parallel to the ultrasound beam, do not occur.

Abbreviations: ASD = atrial septal defect; **LA** = left atrium; **LV** = left ventricle; **RA** = right atrium; **RV** = right ventricle.

The Suprasternal Position

Patient Positioning:

The patient is supine. This view is often facilitated with neck extension over a pillow, which is placed behind the patient's shoulders. This manoeuvre allows greater access to the suprasternal notch region.

Suprasternal Long Axis View

Transducer Position and Angulation: (Figure 2.32)
The transducer is placed in the suprasternal notch with the image index marker pointing toward the patient's left supraclavicular fossa (rotated to approximately 1 o'clock). The transducer is tilted steeply inferiorly and angled anteriorly so that the transducer is almost parallel to the trachea. Slight rotations may be required to view the long axis of the aortic arch.

Sector and Image Orientation:
Anatomic relationships to the sector image are orientated so that superior structures such as the head and neck vessels appear at the top of the image while inferior structures are seen at the bottom of the image. Anterior structures such as the ascending aorta are seen to the left of the image, and posterior structures such as the descending aorta are seen to the right of the image.

Structures Visualised and Normal Echocardiographic Appearances: (Figure 2.32)
The **ascending aorta, aortic arch** and **descending thoracic aorta** are best evaluated from this view and produce a "candy-cane" or "question mark" appearance. The ascending aorta should appear widely patent, maintaining a consistent diameter along its length. Likewise, the aortic arch and descending aorta should also appear widely patent. The descending aorta should be seen to taper slightly as it extends inferiorly. The lumen of this vessel should be free of echoes. A characteristic systolic pulsation of this vessel is also normally apparent.

The origins of the three head and neck vessels can be seen arising from the aortic arch. From anterior to posterior, these vessels are the **innominate (brachiocephalic) artery, left common carotid artery,** and **left subclavian artery.** It is important to note that not all three vessels may be seen to arise from the same imaging plane.

The **left innominate vein** can often be seen superior to the aortic arch as it courses posteriorly and anteriorly. Recognition of this vessel is important as it can sometimes be confused with an aortic dissection flap.

The **right pulmonary artery**, in its short axis, is seen to the posterior (to the right) of the ascending aorta, and inferior to the aortic arch.

Occasionally, the **left atrium** can be identified inferior to the right pulmonary artery. The **aortic valve** and **LVOT** may also be occasionally seen directly inferior to the ascending aorta

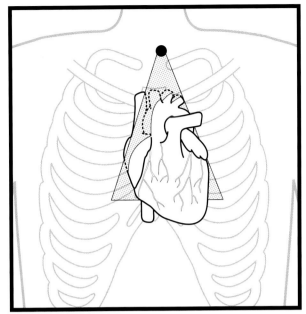

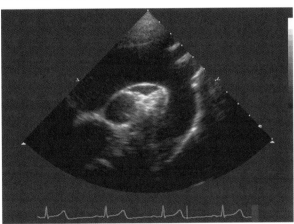

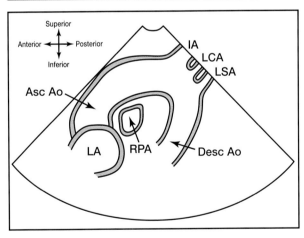

Figure 2.32: The Suprasternal Long Axis View of Aortic Arch.
Top, Transducer Position and Imaging Plane.
Middle, Echocardiographic Structures Visualised.
Bottom, Schematic Illustration of Structures Visualised including the Sector Orientation.
Abbreviations: Asc Ao = ascending aorta; **Desc Ao** = descending aorta; **IA** = innominate artery; **LA** = left atrium; **LCC** = left common carotid artery; **LSA** = left subclavian artery; **RPA** = right pulmonary artery.

Suprasternal Short Axis View

Transducer Position and Angulation: (Figure 2.33)
The transducer position remains in the suprasternal notch position. The transducer is then rotated 90 degrees clockwise from the suprasternal long axis view so that the image index marker is at approximately 4 o'clock.

Sector and Image Orientation:
Anatomic relationships to the sector image are orientated so that superior structures appear at the top of the image while inferior structures are seen at the bottom of the image. Right-sided structures are seen to the left of the image, and left-sided structures are seen to the right of the image. Hence, the superior vena cava appears to the left of the image, the aortic arch appears in the centre of the image, and the right pulmonary artery appears at the bottom of the image.

Structures Visualised and Normal Echocardiographic Appearances: (Figure 2.33)
This view is not routinely employed in the standard 2-D examination of the adult patient but is very useful in the assessment of infants and children with congenital heart lesions.

From this view, the **aortic arch** is transected in its short axis and appears circular and echo-free. The **right pulmonary artery**, in its long axis, is seen inferior to the short axis of the aortic arch running from right to left across the image display. Occasionally, the **bifurcation of the right pulmonary artery** can be visualised to the left of the image.

The **left innominate vein** may also be seen superior to the short axis of the aortic arch.

The **superior vena cava** can be imaged in its long axis and is seen to the left of the short axis of the aortic arch. Slight counterclockwise rotation and lateral or rightward angulation of the transducer is often required to obtain the long axis of this vessel. Movement of the transducer into the right supraclavicular fossa may also be required. When seen, the **left atrium** appears inferior to the right pulmonary artery. On occasions (particularly in children and rarely in the adult), **all four pulmonary veins** can be seen draining into the left atrium in the so-called "crab" view (Figure 2.34). From this view, the right pulmonary veins appear to the left of the image with the right upper vein superior to the right lower vein. The left pulmonary veins appear to the right of the image with the left upper vein superior to the left lower vein.

Abnormalities Detected from the Suprasternal Views:
Abnormalities that may be detected from this view are summarised in Table 2.8. An example of a coarctation of the aorta, which is commonly diagnosed from this view, is depicted in Figure 2.35.

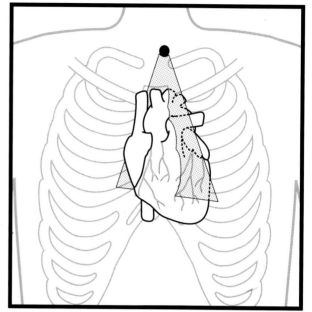

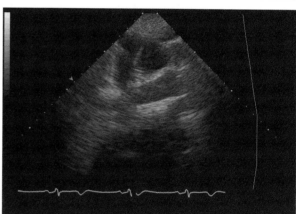

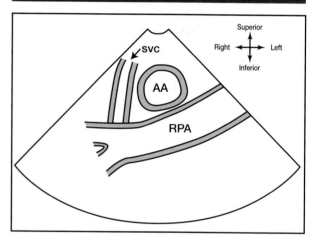

Figure 2.33: The Suprasternal Short Axis View of Aortic Arch.
Top, Transducer Position and Imaging Plane.
Middle, Echocardiographic Structures Visualised.
Bottom, Schematic Illustration of Structures Visualised including the Sector Orientation.
Abbreviations: AA = aortic arch; **RPA** = right pulmonary artery; **SVC** = superior vena cava.

43

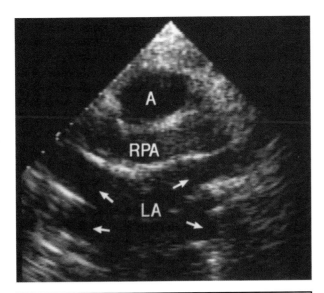

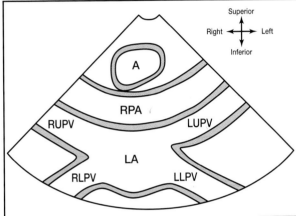

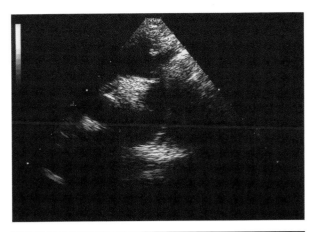

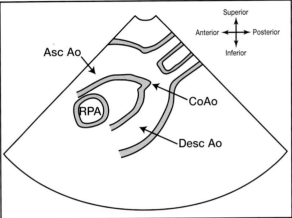

Figure 2.34: The Suprasternal Short Axis of the Pulmonary Venous Drainage into the Left Atrium.
Top, Echocardiographic Structures Visualised.
Bottom, Schematic Illustration of Structures Visualised including the Sector Orientation.
Abbreviations: A = aortic arch; **RPA** = right pulmonary artery; **LA** = left atrium; **LLPV** = left lower pulmonary vein; **LUPV** = left upper pulmonary vein; **RLPV** = right lower pulmonary vein; **RUPV** = right upper pulmonary vein.
From Oh, J.K., Seward, J.B., Tajik, A.J.: The Echo Manual. Little, Brown and Company. pp: 13, 1994. Reproduced with permission from the Mayo Foundation.

Figure 2.35: Suprasternal Long Axis View of the Aorta demonstrating Coarctation of the Aorta.
Top, Echocardiographic Structures Visualised.
Bottom, Schematic Illustration of Structures Visualised including the Sector Orientation.
This example demonstrates the characteristic coarctation shelf, which appears as a "pinching in" of the descending thoracic aorta (arrows).
Abbreviations: Asc Ao = ascending aorta; **CoAo** = coarctation of the aorta; **Desc Ao** = descending aorta; **RPA** = right pulmonary artery.

Table 2.35: Abnormalities Detected from the Suprasternal Views:

Suprasternal Views	Detectable Abnormalities
Suprasternal Long Axis	• dilatation of aorta (various levels) • identification of aortic dissection flaps • abnormalities of the aorta and aortic arch: - coarctation of the aorta (Figure 2.35) - dysplasia - increased pulsatility of the aorta (seen with severe aortic regurgitation) • dilatation of the right pulmonary artery
Suprasternal Short Axis	• superior vena caval abnormalities such as a persistent left superior vena cava (seen from the left supraclavicular fossa) • anomalous pulmonary venous drainage • certain aorto-pulmonary surgical shunts

References and Suggested Reading:

- American Society of Echocardiography: Recommendations for continuous quality improvements in echocardiography. *Journal of the American Society of Echocardiography 8: S1-S28, 1995.*

- Edler, I and Hertz, C.H.: The use of ultrasonic reflectoscope for the continuous recording of the movements of heart walls. *Kungliga Fysuigrafiska Sallskapets I Lund Forhanlinger Bd 24: 1-19,1954.*

- Feigenbaum, H.: Echocardiography. 5th Ed. Lea & Febiger, 1994.

- Henry, W.L. et al.: Report of the American Society of Echocardiography Committee on Nomenclature and Standards in Two-Dimensional Echocardiography. *Circulation 62: 212-217, 1980.*

- Otto, C.M. and Pearlman, A.S.: Textbook of Clinical Echocardiography. W.B. Saunders Company. 1995.

- Reynolds, T. et al.: "Rib-hooks", "pressure points", and "hugs": Technical hints for improving two-dimensional echocardiographic imaging. *Journal of the American Society of Echocardiography. 6: 312-318, 1993.*

- Salcedo, E.: Atlas of Echocardiography. Chapter 2. 2nd Ed. W.B. Saunders Company, 1985.

- Shiina, A. et al.: Two-dimensional echocardiographic spectrum of Ebstein's anomaly: detailed anatomic assessment. *Journal of the American College of Cardiology. 3: 356-370, 1986.*

- Tajik, A.J., Seward, J.B., Hagler, D.J., Mair, D.D., Lie, J.T.: Two-dimensional real-time ultrasonic imaging of the heart and great vessels: Technique, image orientation, structure identification and validation. *Mayo Clinic Proceedings 53:271-303, 1978.*

Chapter 3
Basic Principles of M-Mode Echocardiography

Isolated motion-mode (M-mode) echocardiography was initially used in the early 1960's in the examination of cardiac structures and cardiac pathology. With the advent of real-time, two-dimensional (2-D) imaging and Doppler-derived haemodynamic data, the role of M-mode as the primary diagnostic tool in the echocardiographic examination has diminished considerably. Despite this, M-mode remains a fundamental part of the routine echocardiographic examination.

Basic Principles of M-Mode

M-mode echocardiography produces one-dimensional information on a time-motion graph. Information is displayed along a line representing the ultrasound beam direction. By sweeping this single line of information across the display, a graph of the motion of intracardiac structures transected by the beam, with respect to time, can be achieved (Figure 3.1). Therefore, the M-mode trace records the position and motion of echoes arising from intracardiac structures relative to time.

Three types of information can be obtained from the M-mode examination: (1) motion or time which is displayed on the horizontal axis, (2) distance or depth which is displayed on the vertical axis, and (3) echo strength which is represented as the brightness of structures appearing on the image display. This echo brightness is directly proportional to the strength of the reflected echoes so that blood-filled cavities produce no echoes and solid structures such as cardiac valves and walls produce strong echoes.

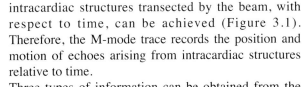

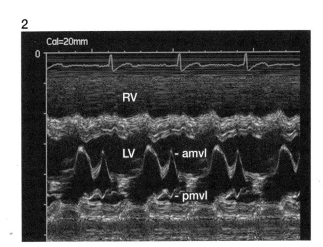

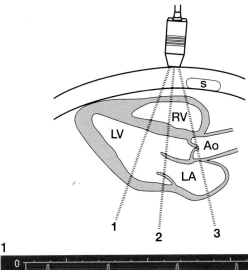

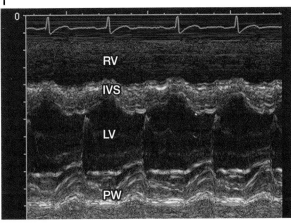

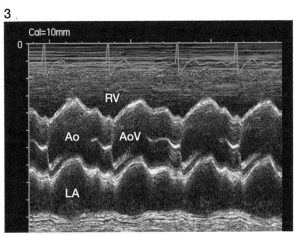

Figure 3.1: The Basic Principles of M-Mode.
This schematic illustrates a cross-section of the heart. The M-mode cursor is depicted transecting the heart through the left ventricular cavity **(1)**, through the mitral valve **(2)**, and through the aorta and left atrium **(3)**. Motion of the structures transected by the ultrasound beam can be displayed throughout the cardiac cycle by sweeping this single line of information across the image display.
Abbreviations: Ao = aorta; **AoV** = aortic valve; **amvl**= anterior mitral valve leaflet; **IVS** = interventricular septum; **LA** = left atrium; **LV** = left ventricle; **pmvl** = posterior mitral valve leaflet; **PW** = posterior wall; **RV** = right ventricle; **S** = sternum.

The principal application of M-mode in the echocardiographic examination is in the assessment and measurement of cardiac chamber dimensions, valvular motion and cardiac function. M-mode echocardiography is also useful for the specific evaluation of the timing of events occurring throughout the cardiac cycle

The optimum window selected for M-mode interrogation is the view in which the ultrasound beam passes perpendicular to the structure(s) of interest.

Advantages of M-Mode Echocardiography

The principal advantage of M-mode echocardiography over other echocardiographic modalities such as 2-D imaging and Doppler, is its superior temporal resolution and rapid sampling frequency. The repetition rate for M-mode is approximately 1000 to 2000 cycles per second, which is far greater than 2-D echo frame rate of between 30 to 100 frames per second. Therefore, M-mode provides valuable information regarding fast moving structures such as cardiac valves. Furthermore, subtle changes in valvular or wall motion are also more readily appreciated with M-mode. Examples of the subtleties detected by M-mode include the high frequency vibrations produced by vegetations, early systolic closure of the aortic valve due to sub-aortic obstruction, and diastolic flutter of the mitral valve and/or interventricular septum due to aortic regurgitation (Figure 3.2). Detection of subtle changes may also aid the semiquantitation of the severity of the lesion; for example, early closure of the mitral valve and premature opening of the aortic valve as seen in acute severe aortic regurgitation may only be appreciated by M-mode.

M-mode also provides good interface definition enhancing the accuracy of measurements of cardiac chambers and great vessels. This accuracy has been further enhanced by utilising 2-D guidance. 2-D imaging allows the display of spatial information, which assists precise alignment of the M-mode cursor as well as allowing the identification of anatomical structures transected by the cursor.

Colour M-mode which incorporates both colour flow Doppler imaging (CFI) and M-mode has also become valuable in the timing of cardiac events which may not be readily appreciated by 2-D and CFI alone. The graphical display of colour M-mode allows the rapid and careful evaluation of time-related events. An example where colour M-mode is particularly helpful is the recognition of diastolic mitral regurgitation which is seen in certain conduction abnormalities such as complete heart block as well as with acute, severe aortic regurgitation (Figure 3.3).

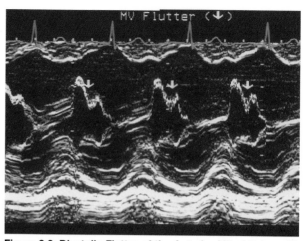

Figure 3.2: Diastolic Flutter of the Anterior Mitral Valve with Aortic Regurgitation.
This is an M-mode example of diastolic flutter of the anterior mitral leaflet because of the aortic regurgitant jet slamming into this leaflet (arrows). Observe the fine, high frequency vibrations displayed on this leaflet during diastole.

Disadvantages of M-Mode Echocardiography

The predominant limitation of M-mode is its lack of spatial information and its one dimensional nature such that only the structure(s) transected by the M-mode cursor are displayed. This lack of spatial orientation has since been overcome with the advent of 2-D guidance of the M-mode cursor.

Acquisition of data from a single dimension also poses significant limitations in the derivation of information about a three-dimensional structure. When the left ventricle is uniformly shaped with a long (major) axis to short (minor) axis ratio of 2:1, the M-mode-derived ejection fraction is relatively reliable. However, in most pathological states such as coronary artery disease, the long axis to short axis ratio is altered. In this instance, the M-mode-derived ejection fraction is often misleading. Furthermore, accuracy of M-mode measurements is also dependent on the recognition of clearly defined borders, which are often ambiguous.

Another disadvantage of M-mode is that many of the M-mode measurements used to indirectly assess left ventricular performance are affected by many variables and are, therefore, unreliable. In addition, many of the M-mode "signs" of cardiac diseases such as those described for pulmonary hypertension, vegetations and aortic valvular disease, are not specific or sensitive. Furthermore, these signs have since been superseded by more reliable and accurate Doppler techniques.

Due to these major limitations, the sole utilisation of M-mode in the assessment and diagnosis of these pathological states is no longer employed; thus, avoiding the potential of false negative and false positive results.

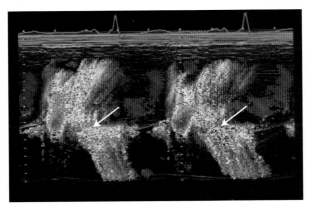

Figure 3.3: Diastolic Mitral Regurgitation.
This is a colour M-mode example of diastolic mitral regurgitation (arrows) in a patient with first degree heart block. This trace was obtained from the apical four chamber view with the M-mode cursor transecting through the mitral valve leaflets which are depicted by the white, linear echo in the centre of the M-mode trace. Observe the timing of the colour flow Doppler signal with the ECG. Mitral regurgitation (the mosaic jet under the mitral leaflets) begins in mid-diastole, well before the Q wave of the ECG.

References and Suggested Reading:

- Feigenbaum, H.: <u>Echocardiography</u>. Chapter 1. 5th Ed. Lea & Febiger, 1994.
- Weyman, A.: <u>Principles and Practice of Echocardiography</u>. Chapter 14. 2nd Ed. Lea & Febiger, 1994.

Chapter 4
The M-Mode Examination of the Heart

2-D guided M-mode can be used in the examination of all four cardiac valves as well as in the evaluation of the left ventricle. As previously mentioned, the role of M-mode in the routine echocardiographic examination of the heart has diminished since the introduction of 2-D real-time imaging and Doppler techniques. However, M-mode still has an important, but limited, place in the routine echocardiographic assessment of the heart. M-mode examination of the left heart structures such as the aortic root, aortic and mitral valves, left atrium and left ventricle should be routinely performed. M-mode measurements of chamber dimensions as well as M-mode calculations such as the fractional shortening and ejection fraction, remain an integral part of the routine and comprehensive echocardiographic examination. While the M-mode examination of the pulmonary valve is not routinely performed, it does offer some helpful information in the assessment of patients with pulmonary hypertension (see Chapter 10). The M-mode examination of the tricuspid valve is rarely useful.

M-Mode Examination of the Aorta, Aortic Valve and Left Atrium

Imaging Plane and Position of M-mode cursor:
The aorta, aortic valve, and left atrium can be examined from either the parasternal long or short axis views. From the parasternal long axis view of the left ventricle, the cursor is directed perpendicular to the long axis of the aorta and through the aortic root at the level of the aortic valve leaflets (Figure 4.1).
From the parasternal short axis view at the level of the aorta and left atrium, the cursor is directed perpendicular through the short axis of the aorta and the left atrium.

Structures transected by the M-mode cursor:
From anterior to posterior, the ultrasound beam passes through the anterior chest wall, the anterior right ventricular wall, the right ventricular cavity, the anterior aortic wall, the right coronary and non-coronary cusps of the aortic valve, the posterior wall of aorta, the left atrial cavity, and the posterior wall of left atrium. Occasionally, the descending thoracic aorta, which lies posterior to left atrium, may also be transected by the M-mode cursor. Hence, the potential exists for confusing the descending aorta for part of the left atrial cavity. This confusion can be avoided by observing the relationship of these two structures on the 2-D image.

Motion of these structures during cardiac cycle:
(Figure 4.1)
Aortic root:
The anterior and posterior walls of the aortic root move in parallel throughout the cardiac cycle. During systole, aortic root moves anteriorly as left atrial volume

increases with the pulmonary venous return. During diastole, the aortic root moves posteriorly as the left atrial volume decreases as blood flows from the left atrium into the left ventricle. Hence, the motion of the aortic root throughout the cardiac cycle reflects left atrial dimensions.

Aortic valve leaflets:
With the onset of ventricular ejection, the aortic valve leaflets snap open. The right coronary cusp moves anteriorly and the non-coronary cusp moves posteriorly. Both leaflets remain separated throughout the left ventricular ejection period and lie parallel to the anterior and posterior aortic walls. Fine systolic fluttering of the aortic leaflets may be seen in the normal individual. With the onset of diastole, the leaflets close abruptly and coapt in the centre of the aortic root producing a single linear echo. Throughout the remainder of diastole the leaflets remain together and follow the posterior motion of the aortic root. This diastolic and systolic motion of the aortic leaflets form a characteristic "box" within the aortic root.

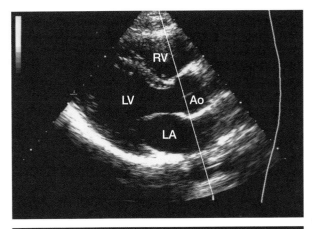

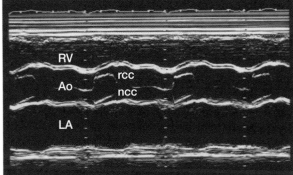

Figure 4.1: M-Mode Examination of the Aorta, Aortic Valve and Left Atrium.
Top, Imaging plane, cursor position and structures transected.
Bottom, Motion of these structures throughout the cardiac cycle.
Abbreviations: Ao = aorta; **LA** = left atrium; **LV** = left ventricle; **mv** = mitral valve; **ncc** = non-coronary cusp; **rcc** = right coronary cusp; **RV** = right ventricle.

Left atrium:

The left atrium lies directly behind the aorta. Although the anterior left atrial wall and the posterior wall of the aortic root are anatomically separate structures, their close proximity results in the production a single echo. Therefore, the anterior left atrial wall follows the same phasic motion as that of the posterior aortic wall throughout the cardiac cycle. The posterior left atrial wall displays minimal motion and so remains relatively immobile during the cardiac cycle.

M-Mode Examination of the Mitral Valve Leaflets

Imaging Plane and Position of M-mode cursor:

The mitral valve leaflets can be examined from either the parasternal long or short axis views. From the **parasternal long axis view** of the left ventricle, the cursor is directed perpendicular to the long axis of the left ventricle and through the tips of the mitral valve leaflets (Figure 4.2).

From the **parasternal short axis view** of the left ventricle at the level of the mitral valve, the cursor is positioned perpendicular to the short axis of the left ventricle and is directed through the tips of the mitral valve leaflets

Structures transected by the M-mode cursor:

From anterior to posterior, the ultrasound beam passes through the anterior chest wall, the anterior wall of the right ventricle, the right ventricular cavity, the basal interventricular septum, the anterior and posterior leaflets of the mitral valve, the basal posterior wall of the left ventricle, and the pericardium.

Motion of the mitral valve during the cardiac cycle:

(Figure 4.2)

As previously mentioned, motion of the mitral valve throughout the cardiac cycle is not as simple as that of the aortic valve (refer to Figure 2.7 in Chapter 2). During diastole, the mitral leaflets separate widely with the anterior leaflet approaching the interventricular septum and the posterior leaflet moving toward the posterior wall of the left ventricle. When the patient is in normal sinus rhythm, the anterior mitral leaflet produces an "M-shaped" configuration while the posterior leaflet, which moves in the reverse direction to the anterior leaflet, forms a "W-shaped" pattern. During systole, the two mitral leaflets close posteriorly within the left ventricular cavity producing multiple linear echoes that move slightly anteriorly throughout the systolic period. The larger anterior mitral leaflet has a greater diastolic excursion than that of the smaller posterior leaflet; hence, the anterior leaflet features more prominently on the M-mode trace.

Each characteristic point which forms the pattern of the anterior mitral leaflet throughout the cardiac cycle has been designated a letter:

D point marks position of the mitral valve leaflets at the onset of diastole;

E point reflects the maximal opening point of the leaflet due to the rapid filling phase of the left ventricle;

F point is the most posterior position of the leaflet immediately following the E point. The posterior motion of the leaflet at this stage of the cardiac cycle occurs in response to the decline in initial diastolic filling; that is, when the pressure gradient between the left atrium and left ventricle lessens;

E-F slope, therefore, represents the initial diastolic closing motion of the anterior leaflet. This slope is an indicator of the rate of left atrial emptying and/or left ventricular filling. Normally, left atrial emptying is rapid resulting in a steep E-F slope;

A point reflects the point of leaflet re-opening that occurs in response to atrial contraction;

B point denotes the position of the anterior leaflet at the onset of ventricular systole and is normally absent;

C point denotes the final position of leaflet coaptation immediately following ventricular systole.

The posterior mitral leaflet can be labelled in the same manner as the anterior leaflet with the addition of an apostrophe (for example, the E' point reflects the maximum posterior deflection of the posterior leaflet occuring in early diastole).

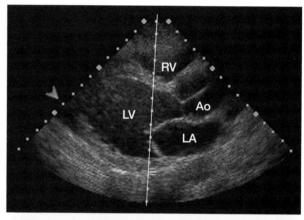

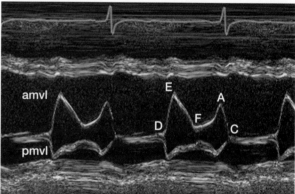

Figure 4.2: M-Mode Examination of the Mitral Valve Leaflets.
Top, Imaging plane, cursor position and structures transected.
Botttom, Motion of these structures throughout the cardiac cycle.
Abbreviations: Ao = aorta; **LA** = left atrium; **LV** = left ventricle; **amvl** = anterior mitral valve leaflet; **pmvl** = posterior mitral valve leaflet; **RV** = right ventricle.

M-Mode Examination of the Left Ventricle

Imaging Plane and Position of M-mode cursor:
Correct cursor position is crucial in the M-mode examination of the left ventricle as many important quantitative values are measured from this trace which may be required for serial evaluation.

M-mode interrogation of the left ventricle can be assessed from the parasternal long view (Figure 4.3), the parasternal short axis view at the level of the papillary muscles, and from the subcostal four chamber and short axis views. The cursor is positioned perpendicular to the long or short axis of the left ventricle just distal to the tips of the mitral valve leaflets.

Structures transected by the M-mode cursor:
From anterior to posterior, the ultrasound beam transects the anterior chest wall, the anterior wall of the right ventricle, the right ventricular cavity, the basal interventricular septum (parasternal long axis view) or anterior wall (parasternal short axis view), the left ventricular cavity, the basal segment of the posterior (inferolateral) left ventricular wall, and the posterior pericardium. The epicardial-visceral pericardial interface is identified by its much brighter echo appearance. Recognition of the true posterior (epicardial) border of the left ventricle is particularly important when assessing the posterior wall thickness of the left ventricle.

Motion of these structures during cardiac cycle:
(Figure 4.3)

As the right ventricle contracts during systole, the anterior right ventricular wall moves posteriorly. As the right ventricle fills during diastole, the anterior right ventricular wall moves anteriorly.

The motion of left ventricular walls reflect changes in ventricular geometry (expansion and contraction) which occurs during the cardiac cycle. Following the onset of systole, the basal interventricular septum moves rapidly posteriorly. During the early filling phase of diastole, there is a sharp anterior movement of the interventricular septum; this anterior motion continues through diastasis (passive filling phase). Following atrial contraction, a further abrupt anterior motion of the interventricular septum may be observed.

The posterior wall of the left ventricle moves anteriorly during systole, to peak slightly after the lowest point of interventricular septum. This later peaking of the posterior wall of the left ventricle can be explained by the fact that the interventricular septum is the first region of the ventricle to be depolarised with ventricular systole. The diastolic motion of the posterior wall mirrors that of the interventricular septum. During the initial filling phase, the posterior wall moves rapidly posteriorly and gradually continues this posterior motion throughout diastasis with a slight, abrupt dipping of the wall with atrial contraction.

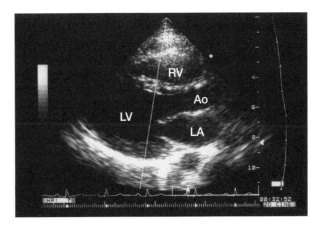

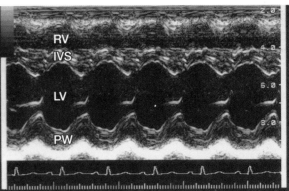

Figure 4.3: M-Mode Examination of the Left Ventricle.
Top, Imaging plane, cursor position and structures transected. *Bottom,* Motion of these structures throughout the cardiac cycle.
Abbreviations: Ao = aorta; **IVS** = interventricular septum; **LA** = left atrium; **LV** = left ventricle; **mv** = mitral valve; **PW** = posterior wall of the left ventricle; **RV** = right ventricle.

M-Mode Examination of the Tricuspid Valve

Imaging Plane and Position of M-mode cursor:
(Figure 4.4)

From the parasternal long axis of the right ventricular inflow tract, the cursor is positioned to transect the bodies of the anterior and posterior tricuspid leaflets. Note that in the majority of cases, however, only one of the tricuspid leaflets can be transected (usually the anterior leaflet).

Structures transected by the M-mode cursor:
The only structure of interest transected by the ultrasound beam is the tricuspid valve leaflet itself.

Motion of the tricuspid valve leaflets during the cardiac cycle: (Figure 4.4)
The motion of the tricuspid valve leaflets throughout the cardiac cycle is similar to the motion of the mitral valve leaflets. Therefore, the pattern of motion of the tricuspid leaflets can be labelled in the same manner and with the same letter as the mitral leaflets.

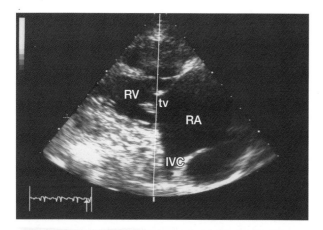

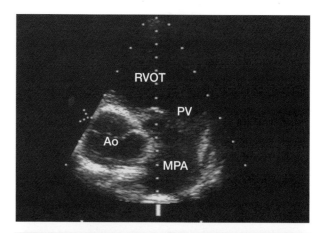

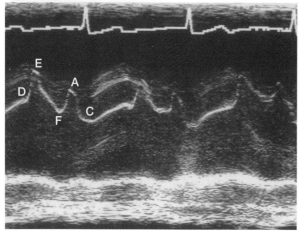

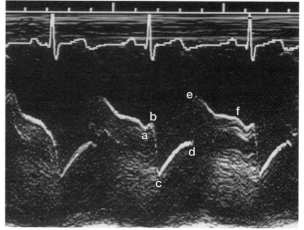

Figure 4.4: M-Mode Examination of the Tricuspid Valve Leaflets.

Top, Imaging plane, cursor position and structures transected.
Bottom, Motion of theanterior tricuspid leaflet throughout the cardiac cycle.

Abbreviations: IVC = inferior vena cava; **RA** = right atrium; **RV** = right ventricle; **tv** = tricuspid valve.

Figure 4.5: M-Mode Examination of the Pulmonary Valve Leaflets.

Top, Imaging plane, cursor position and structures transected.
Bottom, Motion of these structures throughout the cardiac cycle. Observe that the M-mode pattern of the pulmonary valve leaflet produces one-half of the "box" seen on the aortic valve M-mode trace.

Abbreviations: Ao = aorta; **MPA** = main pulmonary artery; **PV** = pulmonary valve; **RVOT** = right ventricular outflow tract.

M-Mode Examination of the Pulmonary Valve

Imaging Plane and Position of M-mode cursor:
(Figure 4.5)
Two of the three pulmonary valve leaflets can be visualised from the parasternal long and/or short axis views of the RVOT but only one leaflet can be transected by the M-mode cursor at any one time. The cursor is usually directed through the posterior leaflet rather than through the anterior leaflet, as the posterior leaflet is less likely to be overshadowed by lung tissue.

Structures transected by the M-mode cursor:
The only structure of interest that is transected by the ultrasound beam is the pulmonary valve leaflet itself.

Motion of the pulmonary valve leaflets during the cardiac cycle: (Figure 4.5)
During systole, the pulmonary valve opens and is seen to move posteriorly while in diastole the leaflets move anteriorly to their closed position in the middle of the

pulmonary artery. The principal points which form the pattern of pulmonary valve motion throughout the cardiac cycle have been designated letters:
a wave reflects the small posterior deflection immediately following atrial contraction;
b point denotes the small anterior deflection occurring at onset of ventricular systole;
c point is the large posterior deflection immediately following ventricular ejection;
d point reflects the gradual anterior motion of the leaflet during the ventricular ejection period;
e point refers to the closed position of the leaflet upon completion of ventricular ejection;
f point represents the slight posterior movement of the leaflet during diastole and is the point immediately prior to atrial contraction and the next **a point.**

Abnormalities detected from the M-mode examination:
Abnormalities that may be detected from the M-mode examination are summarised in Table 4.1 and illustrated in Figure 4.6.

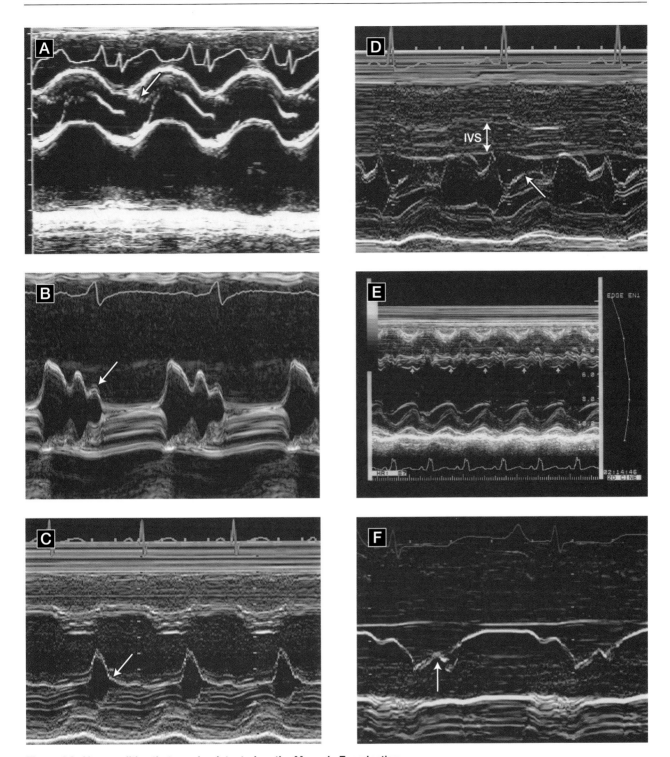

Figure 4.6: Abnormalities that may be detected on the M-mode Examination.

All abnormalities are depicted by the arrows.

A. Mid-systolic closure of the aortic valve associated with LVOT obstruction.

B. B-notch on the anterior mitral valve leaflet is indicative of an increased left ventricular end-diastolic pressure

C. Early diastolic closure of the mitral valve associated with severe aortic regurgitation.

D. Systolic anterior motion of the anterior mitral leaflet associated with hypertrophic obstructive cardiomyopathy.

E. Abnormal motion of the interventricular septum associated with left bundle branch block.

F. Mid-systolic notching on the pulmonary valve associated with pulmonary hypertension.

Table 4.1: Abnormalities detected from the M-mode examination.

Structures Transected	Detectable Abnormalities
Aortic Root, Left Atrium, Aortic Valve Leaflets	• dilatation of the aortic root and/or left atrium • reduced aortic root motion: associated with low cardiac output states • increased aortic root motion: associated with increased left atrial filling (for example, mitral regurgitation) • reduced cusp separation of the aortic leaflets: associated with aortic stenosis, low cardiac output states • mid-systolic closure of the aortic valve: associated with LVOT obstruction
Mitral Valve Leaflets	• diastolic flutter: associated with aortic regurgitation • "B-notch" : associated with increased left ventricular end-diastolic pressures • reduced EF slope: associated with mitral stenosis, reduced left ventricular compliance • early closure: associated with acute severe aortic regurgitation, and first degree heart block • systolic anterior motion of the anterior mitral leaflet: associated with hypertrophic obstructive cardiomyopathy
Left Ventricle, Right Ventricle	• dilatation • reduced systolic function • increased wall thickness: associated with hypertrophy • decreased wall thickness: myocardial scarring following myocardial infarction • abnormal septal motion: due to ischaemia or infarction, left bundle branch block on the ECG, pacemaker rhythm, post open heart surgery, volume or pressure overload of the right ventricle • diastolic flutter of interventricular septum: associated with aortic regurgitation • pericardial effusion
Pulmonary Valve	• increased a wave: associated with pulmonary stenosis • decreased a wave: associated with pulmonary hypertension • mid systolic notching between the c-d slope: associated with pulmonary hypertension

References and Suggested Reading:

• Ambrose, J.A., et al.: Premature closure of the mitral valve: Echocardiographic clue for the diagnosis of aortic dissection. *Chest 73:121-123,1978.*

• Botvinick, E.H., et al.: Echocardiographic demonstration of early mitral valve closure in severe aortic insufficiency: its clinical applications. *Circulation 51:836-847,1975.*

• Cope, G.D., et al.: Diastolic vibration of the interventricular septum in aortic insufficiency. *Circulation 51:589-593,1975.*

• Davis, R.H., et al.: Echocardiographic manifestations of discrete subaortic stenosis. *American Journal of Cardiology 33:277-280,1974.*

• Feigenbaum, H.: Echocardiography. Chapter 2. 5th Ed. Lea & Febiger, 1994.

• Johnson, A.D. and Gosink, B.B.: Oscillation of left ventricular structures in aortic regurgitation. *Journal of Clinical Ultrasound 5:21-24,1977.*

• Krueger, S.K. et al.: Echocardiography in discrete subaortic stenosis. *Circulation 59:506-513,1979.*

• Minz, G.S., et al.: Comparison of two-dimensional and M-mode echocardiography in the evaluation of patients with infective endocarditis. *American Journal of Cardiology 43:738-742, 1979.*

• Otto, C.M. and Pearlman, A.S.: Textbook of Clinical Echocardiography. Chapter 2. W.B. Saunders Company. 1995

• Pietro, D.A., et al.: Premature opening of the aortic valve: An index of highly advanced aortic regurgitation. *Journal of Clinical Ultrasound 6:170-172,1978.*

• Pridie, R.B., et al.: Echocardiography of the mitral valve in aortic valve disease. *British Heart Journal 33:296-304,1971.*

• Salcedo, E.: Atlas of Echocardiography. Chapter 2. 2nd Ed. W.B. Saunders Company, 1985.

• St. John Sutton, M and Oldershaw, P. Textbook of Adult and Pediatric Echocardiography and Doppler. Blackwell Scientific Publications. 1989. pp 47.

• Strunk, B.L., et al.: The posterior aortic wall echogram - Its relationship to left atrial volume change. *Circulation 54:744-750,1976.*

• Weaver, W.F., et al.: Mid-diastolic aortic valve opening in severe acute aortic regurgitation. *Circulation 55:145-148,1977.*

• Weyman, A.: Principles and Practice of Echocardiography. Chapter 14. 2nd Ed. Lea & Febiger, 1994.

• Winsberg, F. et al.: Fluttering of the mitral valve in aortic insufficiency. *Circulation 41:225-229,1971.*

Chapter 5
Basic Principles of Spectral Doppler

Doppler techniques have become a fundamental element in the routine echocardiographic examination offering haemodynamic data to the anatomical information provided by the 2-D examination. Understanding of basic Doppler principles is an important prerequisite for performing the Doppler examination of the heart.

There are two principal types of Doppler utilised in the echocardiographic examination:

1) spectral Doppler (including pulsed-wave and continuous-wave Doppler) and,
2) colour flow Doppler imaging or mapping.

Normal and Abnormal Blood Flow

Before addressing the principles of Doppler, it is important to understand the basic concepts of the physics of blood flow.

Haemodynamics:
Haemodynamics refers to the investigation of the physical principles of blood flow and circulation. Blood flow is a very complex phenomenon. Blood is not a uniform liquid, it contains solid matter such as blood cells and proteins. Furthermore, blood flow is pulsatile (not steady flow) and blood vessel walls are not solid, they are elastic tubes that expand and contract.

Flow characteristics of blood also depend upon a range of factors including: (1) the type of blood vessel (artery or vein), (2) the size of the vessel, (3) resistance to flow offered by the vessel, (4) the phase of the cardiac cycle in which blood flow occurs, and (5) the disease processes which result in narrowing of the vessel.

Properties of Blood:
There are two important characteristics of blood flow that require particular attention: **density** and **viscosity**.

Density of blood refers to the mass of blood per unit volume (expressed in units of g/ml). Density provides a measure of an objects resistance to **acceleration** such that the greater the mass, the greater the resistance to flow.

Viscosity refers to the resistance of flow offered by fluid in motion (expressed in units of the poise). Viscosity describes the ability of molecules to move past one another by overcoming frictional forces. Water has a low viscosity while syrup has a high viscosity. Blood has a viscosity of **0.035 poise at 37ºC** while the viscosity of water is **0.0069 poise at 37ºC**.

Pressure/Flow relationship:
Pressure is the driving force behind all fluid flow. Therefore, a pressure difference is required for flow to occur. If pressure is greater at one end of the vessel than it is at the opposite end, flow will occur from the higher pressure end to the **lower** pressure end. The same principle also applies to flow through the heart. Blood flow from one location to another occurs when the pressure in one chamber or vessel is greater than that in the another chamber or vessel. For example, blood flows from the left atrium into the left ventricle when the pressure in the left atrium exceeds that of the left ventricle.

The flow rate is determined, not only by the pressure difference between two regions, but also by the resistance to flow. Resistance to flow is determined by the viscosity of blood (v), the radius of the vessel lumen (r), and the length of the vessel (L) and is expressed by the following equation:

(Equation 5.1)

$$R = \frac{8\,L\,v}{\pi\,r^4}$$

The relationship between flow rate (Q), pressure difference (DP) and resistance (R) is described by *Poiseuille's law*:

(Equation 5.2)

$$Q = \frac{\Delta P}{R}$$

Thus, by substituting equation (5.1) for the resistance to equation 5.2, flow rate can be derived by the following equation:

(Equation 5.3)

$$Q = \frac{\Delta P\,\pi\,r^4}{8\,L\,v}$$

where Q = flow rate (cc/s)
      ΔP = pressure difference (dyne/cm²)
      R = resistance (g/cm⁴/s)
      v = viscosity (poise)
      r = radius (cm)
      L = length (cm)

Typically, the viscosity of blood and the length of vessels within the cardiovascular system do not change; hence, the flow rate is primarily determined by pressure difference or vessel radius:

(Equation 5.4)

$$Q = \Delta P\,\pi\,r^4$$

From this relationship, it can be appreciated that an increase in the pressure difference and/or the radius will increase flow; conversely, a reduction in the pressure difference and/or radius will reduce flow.

Types of flow:
There are two primary categories of blood flow profiles:
(1) laminar, and (2) turbulent.

1. Laminar flow:
Laminar flow is normal flow. The flow profile of laminar flow forms the shape of a parabola (Figure 5.1). This profile occurs because the velocity of blood flow is not uniform across the vessel lumen. As blood flows through a long straight blood vessel, concentric layers of flow are formed with each layer remaining parallel to the vessel wall and to each other (that is, the layers do not mix). The velocity of each layer is not the same due to friction between the layers and the vessel wall. The maximal flow velocity occurs at the centre of the vessel and minimal or zero flow occurs at the vessel walls. This results in a decreasing profile of flow velocities from the centre to the vessel wall producing the parabolic flow profile. In arteries, this laminar flow profile is affected by flow acceleration, the curvature of the vessel, and converging and diverging flow (Figure 5.2).

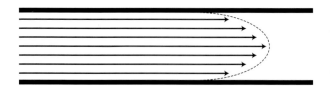

Figure 5.1: Laminar Flow Profile.
Laminar flow profile forms the shape of a parabola. Observe that maximal flow velocity occurs at the centre of the vessel, with flow decreasing in velocity closer to the vessel walls.

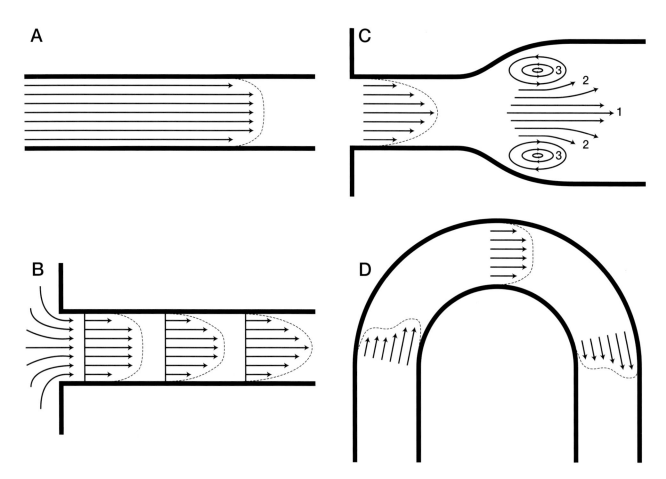

Figure 5.2: Alterations to the Laminar Flow Profile.
A. Acceleration of flow: When blood flow is accelerated, the laminar flow profile is converted into a more uniform distribution or flat flow profile. This is known as plug flow.
B. Converging flow: When a large artery branches into a smaller one, laminar flow is converted into a flat profile. This uniform profile gradually reverts to a laminar, parabolic profile as blood flow moves along the vessel.
C. Diverging flow: Diverging flow occurs as the blood vessel diameter increases. In this instance, the flow profile consists of multiple flow patterns: region 1 - uniform high velocity flow; region 2 - stagnant flow; region 3 - eddy flow.
D. Vessel curvature: As blood flow travels around a bend, the flow profile becomes asymmetric with increased velocities occurring in the inner part of the curve (on the ascending limb of the curve) and on the outer part of the curve (on the descending limb of the curve).

2. Turbulent (Abnormal) flow:

Turbulent flow typically occurs when blood flow passes through an obstruction or narrowed area. Thus, turbulent flow occurs in the presence of valvular stenosis, valvular regurgitation and/or septal defects. Obstruction to flow creates increased velocities and associated flow vortices (whirlpool or circular flow patterns). These flow vortices shed off jets in multiple directions which travel at variable velocities; thus, blood flow becomes random and chaotic (Figure 5.3).

Turbulent flow is predicted by **Reynold's number** which is determined by the density of blood (ρ), vessel diameter (d), velocity of flow (c), and the viscosity (v) and is expressed by the equation:

(Equation 5.5)

$$Re = \frac{\rho\,c\,d}{v}$$

Turbulent flow typically occurs when the Reynold's number exceeds 2000.

The Continuity Principle:

When turbulent flow exists, the velocity of blood flow across the narrowed orifice increases. The basis for this increase in velocity is explained by the continuity principle, which is based on the conservation of mass. This principle states that "whatever mass flows in, must flow out". Therefore, in order for the flow volume to be maintained, the velocities at the stenosis must be greater than the velocities proximal and distal to the stenosis.

Volumetric flow rate is related to the average flow velocity (V) and the cross-sectional area (CSA) and can be expressed by the following equation:

(Equation 5.6)

$$Q = V \times CSA$$

where Q = volumetric flow rate (L/s)
  V = mean velocity (cm/s)
  CSA = cross-sectional area (cm²)

Based on the continuity principle, the flow rate proximal to a stenosis (Q1) must equal the flow rate through the stenosis (Q2). Therefore, if the stenosis is an area one-half that of the proximal area of the tube, the average flow speed at the stenotic site must be double in order to maintain flow (Figure 5.4).

The Doppler Principle

The Doppler principle is applied in echocardiography to enable the determination of the absence or presence of blood flow, flow direction, flow velocities, and flow characteristics.

The **Doppler effect** describes the assumed change in frequency (f) or wavelength (λ) that occurs due to relative motion between the wave source, the receiver, and the reflector of the wave. In diagnostic ultrasound, the reflectors of the wave are the red blood cells (RBCs). When the ultrasound beam is directed toward moving RBCs, there are two separate frequencies detected by the ultrasound transducer: (1) the transmit frequency of the transducer (ft or fo), and (2) the received frequency (fr). Depending on the relative motion of RBCs to the ultrasound beam (that is, motion of the RBCs **toward** or **away** from the transducer), there **may** or **may not** be a discernible change between the transmitted frequency and the received frequency. Typically, the following three situations may occur (Figure 5.5):

1. When the RBCs are **stationary** compared to the transducer, the received frequency (f_r) is equal to the transmitted frequency (f_t), and, therefore, there is a **zero Doppler shift**;

2. When the RBCs are moving **toward** the transducer, the received frequency (f_r) is greater than transmitted frequency (f_t), and there is a **positive Doppler shift**;

3. When the RBCs are moving **away** from the transducer, the received frequency (f_r) is less than the transmitted frequency (f_t), and there is a **negative Doppler shift**.

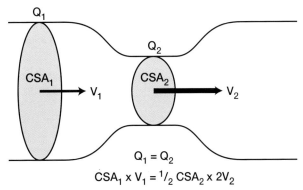

Figure 5.4: The Continuity Principle.
Based on the continuity principle, the flow rate through region Q1 must equal the flow rate through region Q2. Therefore, when the cross-sectional area at Q2 (CSA2) is decreased by half, the velocity at Q2 (V2) must double to maintain equal flow rate through both regions.

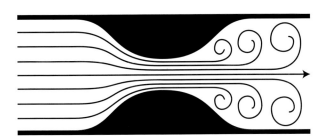

Figure 5.3: Turbulent Flow Profile.
Turbulent flow profiles occur when normal flow is interrupted. This results in the creation of flow vortices in which multiple jets of varying velocities are shed off in multiple directions.

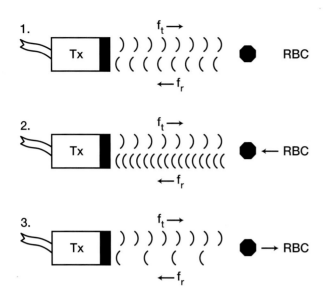

Figure 5.5: The Doppler Effect.
1.   When the RBCs are stationary compared to the
      transducer (Tx):
      ● received frequency (fr) is identical to the transmitted
        frequency (ft)
      ● zero Doppler shift

2.   When RBCs are moving toward the transducer (Tx):
      ● received frequency (fr) is greater than the transmitted
        frequency (ft)
      ● positive Doppler shift

3.   When RBCs are moving away from the transducer (Tx):
      ● received frequency (fr) is less than the transmitted
        frequency (ft)
      ● negative Doppler shift

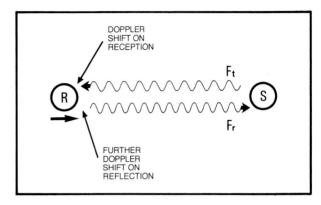

Figure 5.6: The Double Doppler Shift.
This schematic illustrates the "double Doppler shift" between
the transducer, which is the source (S), and the red blood cells
(RBCs) which are the receivers (R). The first Doppler shift
occurs with transmission of the pulse from the transducer. In
this first instance, a Doppler shift results between the
transducer (acting as the stationary source) and moving RBCs
(acting as the moving receiver). The second Doppler shift
occurs upon reception of the returning signal to the transducer.
In this instance, a Doppler shift results between the moving
RBCs (acting as the moving source) and the transducer (acting
as the stationary receiver).
From Gent, R.: <u>Applied Physics and Technology of Diagnostic
Ultrasound</u>. Milner Publishing pp: 225, 1997. Reproduced with
permission from the author.

The Doppler Shift:

The ***Doppler shift*** or frequency shift represents the
difference between the received and transmitted
frequencies, which occurs due to motion of RBCs relative
to the ultrasound beam. The resultant frequency shift is
directly proportional to the relative velocity of the moving
column of RBCs. Therefore, the **greater** the velocity or
speed that the RBCs move within a column of blood, the
greater the frequency shift detected. This Doppler shift
may be **positive** or **negative** depending upon the direction
of blood flow in relation to the ultrasound beam. A
positive Doppler shift occurs when blood flow is **toward**
the transducer while a **negative** Doppler shift occurs
when blood flow is **away** from the transducer.

By observing the reflected frequency from moving RBCs,
it is possible to determine the motion of the column of
blood. As mentioned, a Doppler or frequency shift occurs
when the ultrasound beam strikes a moving blood cell.
The **velocity** and **direction** of blood flow can be
calculated by determining the **frequency shift** created.

The Doppler Equation

The degree of increase or decrease in the Doppler shift is
dependent on three important factors: (1) the frequency of
sound transmitted from the transducer, (2) the velocity of
motion of the column of blood, and (3) angle between the
direction of blood flow and ultrasound beam. The

relationship of these factors to the Doppler shift can be
expressed by the Doppler equation:

(Equation 5.7)

$$\pm \Delta f = \frac{2 \, f_0 \, V \, \cos\theta}{C}$$

where $\pm$ Δf = Doppler frequency shift (Hz)
       f_0 = known transmitted frequency (Hz)
       V   = velocity of blood flow (m/s)
       c   = speed of sound in tissue (m/s)
       $\cos\theta$ = angle between the ultrasound beam
               and blood flow
       2   = accounts for the "double Doppler
               shift" (see Figure 5.6)

In clinical practice, the Doppler shift (Δf), transducer
frequency (f_0), and the speed of sound in tissue (c) is
known; hence, this equation can be rearranged to
calculate the velocity (V) of blood flow:

(Equation 5.8)

$$V = \frac{C \, (\pm \Delta f)}{2 \, f_0 \, \cos\theta}$$

Factors affecting the Doppler equation:

Angle of Incidence: The most important limitation of the Doppler equation in the estimation of blood flow velocity is the ***incident angle*** between the ultrasound beam and the direction of blood flow (Figure 5.7). When a moving column of RBCs is aligned directly **parallel** to the ultrasound beam, the maximum Doppler shift and, therefore, **maximum** velocity is obtained. However, when a moving column of blood is aligned perpendicular to the ultrasound beam, **no** Doppler shift is detected and no blood flow velocities are recorded. Therefore, the maximum detectable velocity of blood flow is highly dependent upon the Doppler angle.

As stated in the Doppler equation, the angle of incidence between the ultrasound beam and blood flow is a function of cosine. Table 5.1 lists the cosine values for various angles and the percentage error that occurs when the ultrasound beam is not aligned parallel to the direction of blood flow. Figure 5.8 also illustrates the importance of a parallel angle of incidence between the ultrasound beam and the direction of blood flow. Therefore, Table 5.1 and Figure 5.8 explain by example that as long as the angle between the ultrasound beam and blood flow is less than or equal to 20 degrees, cosine is close to 1 and the percentage error is less than or equal to 7%, and, therefore, the angle can be ignored. However, once the angle exceeds 20 degrees, cosine becomes significantly less than 1 and the percentage error increases significantly.

The incident angle is particularly important when evaluating cardiac haemodynamics where the maximal velocity is crucial to the diagnosis or the identification of velocity jets as well as in ascertaining haemodynamic information.

Observe that the importance of a parallel angle of incidence in the Doppler interrogation is in contrast to 2-D echocardiography where the best images are obtained when the ultrasound beam is perpendicular (90 degrees) to the structure investigated.

Table 5.1: Cosines for Various Angles and Percentage Error.

Angle θ (degrees)	Cos θ	Percentage Error (%)
0	1.00	0
10	0.98	2
20	0.94	7
30	0.87	13
40	0.77	23
50	0.64	36
60	0.50	50
70	0.34	66
80	0.17	83
90	0.00	100

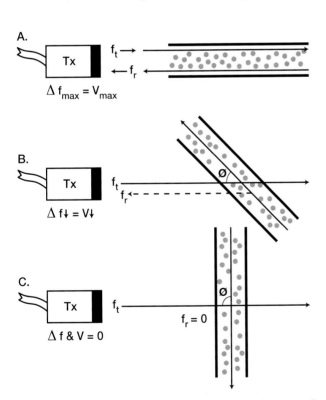

Figure 5.7: The Incident Angle between the Ultrasound Beam and the Direction of Blood Flow.
A. When blood flow is directly parallel to the ultrasound beam, the maximum Doppler shift (Δfmax) and, therefore, maximal velocity (Vmax) is obtained.
B. As the angle between the direction of blood flow and the ultrasound beam increases, the Doppler shift (Δf) decreases and the true velocity (V) is underestimated.
C. When the angle between the ultrasound beam and blood flow direction is perpendicular, there is no Doppler shift detected and, therefore, velocity equals zero.

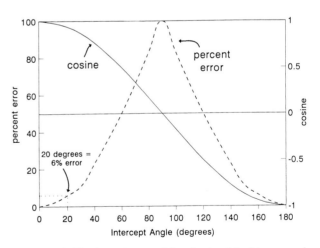

Figure 5.8: The Importance of the Angle of Incidence and the Direction of Blood Flow.
Observe that cosine (solid line) equals 1 when the intercept angle (X-axis) is either 0° or 180°; that is, when the ultrasound beam is aligned parallel to blood flow direction. In this instance, the percentage error (dashed line) is 0%; therefore, the true maximal velocity is determined.
Observe that cosine equals 0 when the intercept angle is 90°; that is, when the ultrasound beam is aligned perpendicular to blood flow direction. In this instance, the percentage error is 100% so that no velocities are recorded.
When the intercept angle between the direction of blood flow and the ultrasound beam is 20° or less, cosine approaches 1 and the percentage error is ≤ 6%.
From Otto and Pearlman: <u>Textbook of Clinical Echocardiography.</u> pp: 22, W B Saunders Company, 1995. Reproduced with permission from W.B. Saunders.

Technical Consideration:
In clinical practice, it is possible to "correct" for the angle. However, this is not recommended as in most cases it is possible to align the direction of blood flow parallel to the ultrasound beam by using multiple echocardiographic views. Furthermore, the use of angle correction makes the serial assessment of patients difficult unless the same angle correction is applied. Hence, it is simpler to avoid this potential problem by always assuming that flow is parallel to the ultrasound beam.

Therefore, in echocardiography because angle correction is not utilised, the ultrasound system always assumes that the angle between the ultrasound beam and the direction of blood flow is parallel. Hence, the determination of the velocity of blood flow using the Doppler equation can be simplified to:

(Equation 5.9)

$$V = \frac{C\,(\pm \Delta f)}{2\,f_0}$$

Effect of Frequency: The Doppler equation also indicates that the maximum detectable velocity is a function of the transmitted frequency (transducer frequency). Lower frequency transducers have the ability of yielding higher velocities. Consider the maximum detectable velocity for a 5 MHz transducer and a 2 MHz transducer with a frequency shift of 5 kHz (examples 1 and 2).

Example 1: Determination of the Maximum Detectable Velocity for a 5 MHz Transducer.

$$V = \frac{C\,(\pm \Delta f)}{2\,f_0}$$

$$= \frac{(1540)\,(5\times10^3)}{(2)\,(5\times10^6)}$$

$$= \frac{7.7\times10^6}{10\times10^6}$$

$$= 0.77\,m/s$$

Example 2: Determination of the Maximum Detectable Velocity for a 2 MHz Transducer.

$$V = \frac{(1540)\,(5\times10^3)}{(2)\,(2\times10^6)}$$

$$= \frac{7.7\times10^6}{4\times10^6}$$

$$= 1.9\,m/s$$

Observe that the use of lower frequency transducers in the Doppler interrogation is in contrast to 2-D imaging which utilises higher frequency transducers in order to improve image resolution.

Pressure Determination

Probably the most important application of Doppler ultrasound is in the estimation of intracardiac pressure gradients. As mentioned, movement of blood within the cardiovascular system is primarily determined by pressure differences between two locations. These pressure differences can be derived by application of the conservation of energy principle. This principle states that in the absence of applied forces, the total energy of a system is constant; that is, energy flowing into the system is equal to the total energy flowing out of the system. The conservation of energy principle is expressed by the *Bernoulli equation*:

(Equation 5.10)

$$\Delta P = \tfrac{1}{2}\rho\,(V_2^2 - V_1^2) + \int_1^2 \frac{d\vec{v}}{dt}\times d\vec{s} + R(\vec{v})$$

$$\begin{array}{ccccccc}
\text{Pressure} & = & \text{convective} & + & \text{flow} & + & \text{viscous}\\
\text{decrease} & & \text{acceleration} & & \text{acceleration} & & \text{friction}
\end{array}$$

where ΔP = the pressure difference between 2 points (mm Hg)
V_1 = velocity at proximal location (m/s)
V_2 = velocity at distal location (m/s)
ρ = density of fluid (g/cm³)
dv = change in velocity over the time period (dt)
ds = distance over which pressure decreases (cm)
R = viscous resistance in the vessel (g/cm⁴/s)
V = velocity of blood flow (m/s)

From the above equation, it can be seen that there are three important components involved in the determination of the pressure gradient:
1. convective acceleration which occurs whenever there is a change in the CSA of flow
2. flow acceleration which refers to the pressure drop required to overcome inertial forces
3. viscous friction which refers to the loss of velocity due to friction between blood cells and vessel walls

In most clinical situations, the following assumptions can be made:
a. flow acceleration can be ignored as at peak velocities, acceleration is zero,
b. viscous friction is negligible as the flow profile within the centre of the lumen is generally flat and losses are minimal toward the centre of the vessel,
c. mass density ($\tfrac{1}{2}\rho$) for normal blood equals 4,
d. there is conservation of energy; that is, there is no energy transfer.

The Simplified or Modified Bernoulli Equation:
Accounting for the factors above, the Bernoulli equation can be modified or simplified to:

(Equation 5.11)

$$\Delta P = 4\left(V_2^2 - V_1^2\right)$$

Furthermore, flow velocity proximal to fixed orifice (V_1) is usually much lower than the peak velocity through the orifice (V_2), therefore, V_1 can be ignored, further simplifying the Bernoulli equation to:

(Equation 5.12)

$$\Delta P = 4V^2$$

The application of the Bernoulli equation in Doppler haemodynamic calculations is discussed in greater detail in Chapter 11 (see "Determination of Pressure Gradients").

The Spectral Doppler Display

Spectral analysis of the Doppler shifts provides a graphic display of blood flow velocities plotted over time. Information displayed on the Doppler spectrum includes: (1) flow velocity, (2) direction of flow, (3) timing of the signal, and (4) the intensity of the signal (Figure 5.9).

1. Velocity: Flow velocity is displayed on the Y-axis. The velocity of RBCs within the sampled column of blood is calculated using the Doppler equation. The absence of flow velocity is represented by the zero baseline.

2. Direction of flow: Flow direction is also displayed on the Y-axis and is determined by the Doppler equation. A positive Doppler shift indicates that flow is toward the transducer. Positive Doppler shifts are traditionally displayed **above** zero baseline. Negative Doppler shifts indicate that flow is directed away from the transducer. Negative Doppler shifts are traditionally displayed **below** zero baseline. It is important to recognise that these velocities above and below the baseline actually represent flow toward and away from the transducer and do not represent forward or backward flow in the circulation.

3. Intensity or amplitude of signal: Blood cells do not move at equal velocities and, therefore, they create many different frequency shifts. The amplitude or intensity of the Doppler signal reflects the number of blood cells moving within a range of the velocities at a particular point in time. Hence, intensity of the signal is proportional to the number of blood cells moving at that velocity, at that particular time. Intensity of the Doppler signal is represented by the brightness of the signal as displayed on the gray scale image. Therefore, **bright regions** indicate a strong Doppler shift frequency at a particular instant in time indicating that numerous blood cells are moving at velocities corresponding to that Doppler shift. Conversely, **darker regions** indicate that the Doppler shift frequency at that point in time is weak, thus, indicating that very few blood cells are travelling at velocities corresponding to that Doppler shift.

4. Timing of signal: Timing of the Doppler signal is displayed on the X-axis along with the ECG. Therefore,

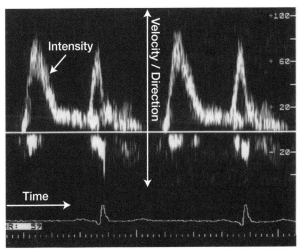

Figure 5.9: The Spectral Doppler Display.
This is a pulsed-wave (PW) Doppler example of mitral inflow. Timing of flow is depicted on the X-axis while direction and velocity are both depicted on the Y-axis. The intensity of the signal is represented by the gray scale. See text for details.

the change in blood flow velocity, flow direction, and flow intensity throughout the cardiac cycle can be easily determined.

Other information which can be determined from the spectral Doppler display includes the differentiation between laminar and turbulent flow on the pulsed-wave (PW) Doppler spectrum, and the differentiation between PW and continuous-wave (CW) Doppler. The spectral display of these signals will be discussed in the following sections.

Doppler Audio Signals

Doppler shift frequencies are in the audible range and, therefore, can be represented as an audible signal. The audio signal during the Doppler examination is very important as it provides valuable information about the quality and type of the Doppler signal. The audio signal should be used as a guide for localising blood flow and for aligning the ultrasound beam parallel to flow direction. Optimal audio signals will be reflected in the spectral display by strong, well-defined signals. The audible characteristics of the Doppler signal also indicate the type of flow encountered. Laminar flow has a smooth tone whereas turbulent flow has a harsh, raspy sound.

Doppler Modalities and Principles

The primary Doppler modalities utilised in echocardiography include: (1) spectral Doppler (PW Doppler and CW Doppler), and (2) colour flow Doppler imaging (CFI). The principles of CFI are covered separately in Chapter 7.

Most ultrasound systems combine 2-D imaging and CW and PW Doppler and are referred to as Duplex systems. A "stand alone" non-imaging CW Doppler transducer is also available and has certain advantages over the Duplex systems. Table 5.2 lists the comparisons between PW and CW Doppler.

Continuous-Wave Doppler Principles.
Continuous-wave (CW) Doppler refers to the **continuous** transmission of the Doppler signal toward the moving RBCs and the continuous reception of the returning signals reflected from the moving RBCs. Using this modality, blood flow along the entire beam is observed. Therefore, there is **no range resolution**; that is, there is no indication of the depth from which the signals have been generated. This lack of range resolution is the primary disadvantage of this modality. Due to the loss of range resolution, interpretation of flow signals may be confusing. However, Doppler signals from within the heart and great vessels demonstrate characteristic flow profiles that can be recognised by observation of several factors including: (1) the timing and duration of flow signals from the onset to the cessation of flow, (2) flow direction relative to the ultrasound beam, (3) the velocity of the blood flow signal, and (4) the typical flow profiles of the semilunar and atrioventricular valves.
The principal advantage of CW Doppler is in its ability to display high velocities (up to 15 m/s).

Pulsed-Wave (PW) Doppler Principles:
With PW Doppler, ultrasound signals are sent out in short bursts or pulses. Through range gating, PW Doppler has the ability to select Doppler information from a particular location within the heart or great vessels utilising a **sample volume**.
The sample volume has a three-dimensional tear-drop shape. The **length** of the sample volume determines the length of time that the transducer is activated to receive information from the sample volume location. The **width** of the sample volume depends upon the profile of the transducer beam. Sample volume length and location (depth into tissue) are operator controlled. Unlike CW Doppler in which there is continuous reception of Doppler signals, with PW Doppler, the transducer will only function as a receiver for a limited period of time. This time period corresponds to the interval required for the sound to return to the transducer from a specified area designated by the sample volume (all other information outside of the sample volume is ignored). Another burst of sound waves **will not** be transmitted until the transducer has received echoes corresponding to the sample volume location. The **pulse repetition frequency (PRF)**, which refers to the frequency at which the PW transducer transmits pulses, determines when the next burst of sound waves are emitted. In other words, the PRF determines the sampling rate. This phenomenon creates a major disadvantage to PW Doppler as the PRF effectively limits the maximum velocity detectable.

The Nyquist Limit:
The Nyquist limit is the maximum velocity that can be measured by PW Doppler. This limit is determined by the PRF. The Nyquist limit is equal to one-half of the pulse repetition frequency (PRF):

(Equation 5.13)

$$Nyquist\ Limit = \frac{PRF}{2}$$

Therefore, the maximum velocity which can be detected by PW Doppler as determined by the Nyquist limit and the Doppler equation (equation 5.8) is explained by the following equation::

(Equation 5.14)

$$\frac{PRF}{2} = \pm\,\Delta f = \frac{2\,f_0\,V\cos\theta}{C}$$

$$V = \frac{C\,PRF}{4\,f_o\,\cos\theta}$$

Aliasing:
Aliasing is the phenomenon that occurs when the Nyquist limit is exceeded. As mentioned above, there is a limit to the maximum velocity that can be detected by PW Doppler instruments. The maximal velocity is determined by the Nyquist Limit which is equal to one-half the PRF. Therefore, signals need to sampled at least twice per cycle of their highest Doppler frequency shift in order to be unambiguously resolved. Aliasing of Doppler signals refers to the erroneous or ambiguous display of velocities that have exceeded the Nyquist limit. This results in the display of improper Doppler shift or velocity information (Figure 5.10). Another simple analogy is displayed in Figure 5.11.

In clinical practice, when the blood flow velocity is high, the PRF may not be great enough to sample the returning frequencies twice per cycle. Therefore, the instrument "misses" some of the shifted waves and misinterprets the Doppler shift frequency as well as the velocity. If the "perceived" returning frequency is lower than the transmitted frequency, it will be plotted below the zero baseline as a negative Doppler shift even though it may actually be a higher positive Doppler shift. This results in the "wrap around" of the displayed Doppler signal as each of the Doppler frequencies above the Nyquist limit are ambiguously displayed and plotted. It is important to note that the Doppler information itself is retained but is incorrectly displayed.
A commonly encountered example of this phenomenon is seen in the PW Doppler examination of the LVOT in the presence of aortic regurgitation (Figure 5.12).

Avoiding Aliasing:
In order to avoid aliasing, certain factors can be adjusted to increase the Nyquist limit and, therefore, the maximum velocity detected. Techniques that can be employed include: (1) altering variables in the Doppler equation, (2) introducing an offset, (3) utilising "high" PRF mode, and (4) changing from PW to CW Doppler.

Original Signal

Displayed Signal
(sampled $>^1/_2$ PRF)

A.

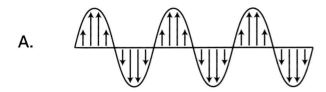

Original Signal

Displayed Signal
(sampled $<^1/_2$ PRF)

B.

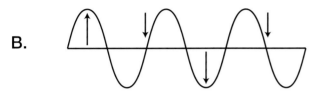

Figure 5.10: Aliasing of Doppler Information.
A. When a signal is sampled at a sufficiently high frequency ($>^1/_2$ PRF) as indicated by the arrows, the **displayed** signal closely resembles that of the **original** signal.
B. When a signal is sampled at a frequency that is too low ($<^1/_2$ PRF) as indicated by the arrows, the **displayed** signal appears at a lower frequency than the original signal. Therefore, the resultant signal is reconstructed **erroneously**.

1. Altering Variables in the Doppler Equation:

Recall that the maximum velocity detected by PW Doppler is derived by equation (5.14):

$$\frac{PRF}{2} = \pm \Delta f = \frac{2 f_0 V \cos\theta}{C}$$

$$V = \frac{C \, PRF}{4 \, f_o \, \cos\theta}$$

From this equation, it can be appreciated that the maximum velocity can be increased by altering the following variables:
i)   increasing the PRF
ii) decreasing the transmitted frequency
iii) increasing the speed of sound in tissue

iv) decreasing cos θ (that is, by increasing the angle of incidence between the transducer and blood flow direction)

The speed of sound in tissue is constant at 1540 m/s and cannot be altered and, as previously mentioned, angle correction in echocardiography should be avoided. Therefore, of the variables listed above, only i) and ii) can be manipulated in echocardiography.

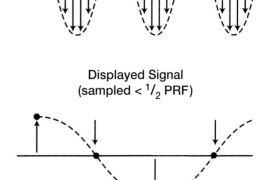

Figure 5.12: Aliasing of the Pulsed-wave (PW) Doppler Signal in the Left Ventricular Outflow Tract in the Presence of Aortic Regurgitation.
This is an example of a PW Doppler signal recorded from the apical five chamber view in a patient with aortic regurgitation. Observe that during diastole an ambiguous Doppler signal is displayed both above and below the zero baseline (*arrows*). From this view, aortic regurgitation is actually directed toward the transducer and, therefore, should be displayed above the zero baseline. However, as the velocity of this signal is higher than the Nyquist limit, this velocity has "wrapped around" the baseline and is displayed ambiguously (displayed both above and below the baseline).

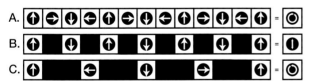

Figure 5.11: The Aliasing Phenomenon.
The aliasing phenomenon can be visually illustrated on the diagrams above using a rotating arrow.
A. Observe that the arrow, which is rotating clockwise, is accurately seen to rotate clockwise on the film when sampled each frame.
B. When the frame rate of the film is halved (blacked out frames), the arrow rotation is ambiguous and the direction of the arrow cannot be determined.
C. When the frame rate is reduced further (blacked out frames), the direction of arrow rotation is falsely displayed; in this instance, the arrow appears to rotate counterclockwise.

i) Increasing the Pulse Repetition Frequency (PRF):

The PRF is determined by the range equation. Recall that in 2-D imaging, the range equation is used to determine the depth to an object (Chapter 1) and is calculated by the following equation:

(Equation 1.10)

$$D = \frac{c\,t}{2}$$

where D = distance to the structure or region of interest (m)

    c = propagation speed through tissue (m/s)

    t = time taken for the ultrasound signal to return to the transducer (s)

    2 = refers to the fact that the pulse must travel to the structure and then back again

By rearranging equation (1.10), the time or period taken for a pulse to travel to a specified depth into the body and to return to the transducer is given by the following equation:

(Equation 5.15)

$$T = \frac{2\,D}{C}$$

Recall from Chapter 1, that frequency and, therefore, the PRF, is inversely related to the period (equation 1.2), therefore:

(Equation 5.16)

$$PRF = \frac{1}{T} = \frac{C}{2\,D}$$

Since the speed of sound in soft tissue (C) is assumed to be constant, the only way to increase the PRF is by *decreasing* the depth (D). Therefore, since the maximum detectable velocity with PW Doppler is equal to one-half the PRF, the maximum detectable velocity in terms of the PRF, the Nyquist limit, and the Doppler equation can be written as:

(Equation 5.17)

$$V = \frac{C}{2\,f_o} \times \frac{PRF}{2}$$

$$= \frac{C}{2\,f_o} \times \frac{C}{2 \times 2\,D}$$

$$= \frac{C^2}{8\,f_o\,D}$$

Therefore, the maximal detectable velocity can be increased by reducing the depth to the region of interest. This can be accomplished by changing transducer positions so that the desired region of interest is closer to the transducer.

ii) Decreasing the Transmitted Frequency:

The selection of a lower frequency transducer will increase the maximum velocity measured at any depth. From equation 5.17, it can be seen that by decreasing the transmitted frequency, the maximum velocity detected will be increased. Consider the maximum velocity which can be detected using a 5 MHz transducer and a 2 MHz transducer at a depth of 10 cm and a PRF of 7700 pulses per second (examples 3 and 4).

Example 3: Determination of the Maximum Detectable Velocity for a 5 MHz Transducer at a depth of 10 cm and a PRF of 7700 pulses per second.

$$V = \frac{C^2}{8\,f_o\,D}$$

$$= \frac{(1540)^2}{(8)\,(5 \times 10^6)\,(0.1)}$$

$$= \frac{2.4 \times 10^6}{4 \times 10^6}$$

$$= 0.6\ cm/s$$

Example 4: Determination of the Maximum Detectable Velocity for a 2 MHz Transducer at a depth of 10 cm and a PRF of 7700 pulses per second.

$$V = \frac{(1540)^2}{(8)\,(2 \times 10^6)\,(0.1)}$$

$$= \frac{2.4 \times 10^6}{1.6 \times 10^6}$$

$$= 1.5\ cm/s$$

2. Introducing an Offset:

Introducing an offset simply refers to an electronic "cut and paste" technique that moves the "wrapped around" or aliased Doppler signal upward or downward (depending on the direction of the signal). Therefore, by repositioning the zero baseline, the peak of the Doppler signal may be "unwrapped". Repositioning of the zero baseline effectively increases the maximum velocity in one direction (toward or away flow) at the expense of the other direction. Figure 5.13 illustrates how offsetting the zero baseline can increase the maximum detectable velocity.

3. Utilising High PRF Mode:

High PRF can be used to overcome the maximum velocity limitations by using a higher than normal PRF; for example, twice the normal PRF. In this instance, the transmission of any given pulse occurs before the reception of all the echoes from the previous pulse. To do this, high PRF utilises multiple sample gates at various locations (Figure 5.14). Therefore, signals are received from multiple gates at different depths simultaneously.

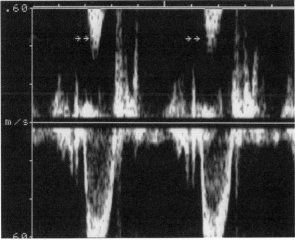
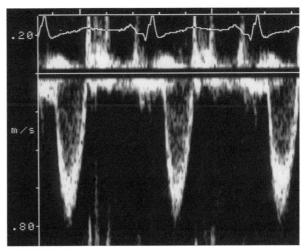

Figure 5.13: Repositioning of the Zero Baseline to Increase the Maximum Velocity.
Left, This is a PW Doppler signal obtained in the LVOT from the apical five chamber view. From this view, blood flow through the LVOT is directed away from the transducer and, therefore, appears below the zero baseline. The maximum velocity that can be detected is 0.6 m/s. As the Doppler signal is greater than this velocity, the signal has aliased with flow appearing to wrap around onto the top of the spectral display (*double arrows*).
Right, By simply repositioning the zero baseline upward, the maximum velocity that can be detected has been increased to 0.8 m/s and the signal is now displayed unambiguously.

By increasing the number of sample gates, the maximum velocity is also increased. For example, by adding or inserting a **second** sample gate, the pulse repetition frequency is increased by two; this essentially increases the Nyquist limit or the maximum velocity detected by a factor of two. The primary disadvantage of high PRF mode is that the exact location of the Doppler shift is not known.

4. Changing from Pulsed-Wave (PW) Doppler to Continuous-Wave (CW) Doppler:
CW Doppler does not have the sampling limitations of PW Doppler; therefore, aliasing will not be a problem. However, as mentioned, the limitation of CW Doppler is that there is no range resolution, hence, it is not possible to determine the exact depth from which the Doppler signal has originated.

Spectral Doppler Display of PW and CW Doppler
Laminar Flow Versus Turbulent Flow (Figure 5.15):
PW Doppler signals are described by their *spectral broadening* patterns and by the presence or absence of a *spectral window*.

Spectral broadening is defined as the widening or vertical thickness of the Doppler shift spectrum. In the presence of laminar flow, RBCs are moving at the same velocity. Therefore, a small range of Doppler shift frequencies are represented resulting in a narrow band of spectral signals being displayed. As flow becomes turbulent, there is a greater variation in blood flow velocities which produces a greater range of Doppler shift frequencies. This results in increased spectral broadening on the spectral display. Spectral broadening may also be increased by using excessive Doppler gains and by widening of the sample gate such that a wider range of velocities are displayed.

Spectral window refers to the echo-free area under the spectral Doppler trace. In the presence of laminar flow, there is a large spectral window under the spectral Doppler trace. As flow becomes turbulent, spectral broadening occurs and the spectral window size is diminished or eliminated.

Pulsed-wave (PW) Doppler Versus Continuous-wave (CW) Doppler (Figure 5. 16):
Pulsed-wave (PW) Doppler Trace:
As mentioned above, in a typical PW Doppler trace of laminar blood flow, there is minimal spectral broadening

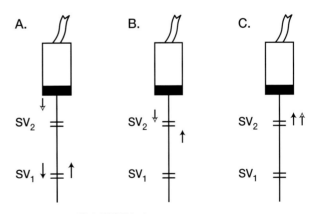

Figure 5.14: High PRF Mode.
High PRF increases the maximum detectable velocity by using more than one sample volume.
A. In this example, two sample volumes are used (SV_1 and SV_2) so that two pulses are sent out one after the other.
B. Observe that the returning signal from SV_1 and the second transmitted signal both reach SV_2 position at the same time.
C. Returning signals from both SV_1 and SV_2 return to the transducer at the same time. This results in range ambiguity, which means that it is not always possible to determine from which depth or sample volume the Doppler signal has originated.

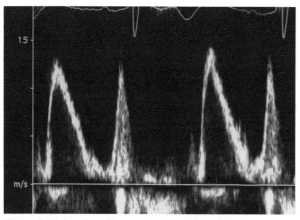 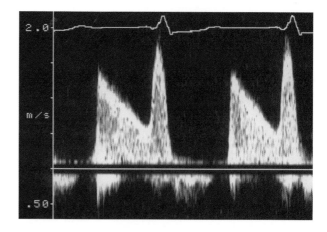

Figure 5.15: Laminar Flow versus Turbulent Flow.
Left, This is an example of laminar flow through a normal mitral valve. Note that there is minimal spectral broadening with an obvious spectral window (dark area under the spectral Doppler curve)..
Right, This is an example of spectral broadening through a stenotic mitral valve. Note the increase in spectral broadening and the absence of the spectral window caused by turbulent flow through the stenotic valve.

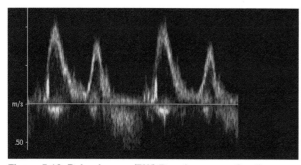 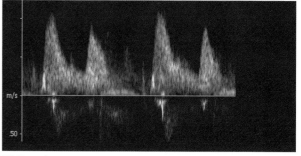

Figure 5.16: Pulsed-wave (PW) Doppler versus Continuous-wave (CW) Doppler.
Left, This is an example of a PW Doppler trace through a normal mitral valve. Note that there is minimal spectral broadening with an obvious spectral window (dark area under the spectral Doppler curve).
Right, This is an example of a CW Doppler trace through a normal mitral valve. Note the increase in spectral broadening and the absence of the spectral window.

with a large spectral window. This appearance is due to the narrow band of blood flow velocities obtained from a single sample volume.

Continuous-wave (CW) Doppler Trace:
On the typical CW Doppler trace, spectral broadening occurs as a large range of blood flow velocities and directions are encountered by the sound beam along the entire beam path. The spectral window is absent with CW Doppler.

Table 5.2: Comparison between Pulsed-Wave (PW) and Continuous-Wave (CW) Doppler.

	CW	PW
● Depth Resolution	**No**	Yes
● Sample Volume	Large	*Small*
● Detection of High Velocities	*Yes*	**No**
● Aliasing	*No*	**Yes**
● Spectral Content	**Wide**	*Narrow*
● Use in Duplex Instruments	Yes	Yes
● Sensitivity	*More*	**Less**
● Transducer Power	*Lower*	**Higher**
● Control of Sample Volume Placement	**Poor**	*Good*

Note: *Advantage*   **Disadvantage**

References and Suggested Reading:

● Feigenbaum, H.: <u>Echocardiography.</u> Chapter 1. 5th Ed. Lea & Febiger, 1994.
● Gent, Roger.: <u>Applied Physics and Technology of Diagnostic Ultrasound.</u> Milner Publishing (3 Milner Street, Prospect. South Australia 5082), 1997.
● Hatle, L. and Angelson, B.: <u>Doppler Ultrasound in Cardiology: Physical Principles and Clinical Application.</u> 2nd Ed. Lea & Febiger, 1985.
● Otto, C.M. and Pearlman, A.S.: <u>Textbook of Clinical Echocardiography.</u> Chapter 1. W.B. Saunders Company. 1995
● Weyman, A.: <u>Principles and Practice of Echocardiography.</u> Chapters 7 - 10. 2nd Ed. Lea & Febiger, 1994.

Chapter 6
The Spectral Doppler Examination

In the routine echocardiographic examination, spectral Doppler interrogation of antegrade flow through the inflow tracts, outflow tracts and cardiac valves can be performed. Blood flow through each of these regions has a characteristic pattern which is identified by its direction, velocity, duration, and timing of flow throughout the cardiac cycle. The normal blood flow velocities through each region are listed in Table 6.1 at the end of this chapter.

Spectral Doppler interrogation of blood flow of these regions is ordinarily performed using PW Doppler so that blood flow velocities within a specific location can be examined. An exception to the use of PW Doppler is in the interrogation of blood flow across the aortic valve where CW Doppler is used. CW Doppler rather than PW Doppler is utilised in this instance for two important reasons. Firstly, the correct placement of the sample volume distal to the aortic valve is often difficult and secondly, blood flow velocities across the aortic valve may exceed the Nyquist limit (especially from the apical window). CW Doppler is also used in any other circumstances in which the velocities exceed the Nyquist limit resulting in signal aliasing. For example, CW Doppler is used in the assessment of stenotic or regurgitation valve lesions, and in some intracardiac shunt lesions.

Optimisation of Doppler Signals
Accurate measurement of flow velocities is dependent upon several technical factors. Each of these factors, as well as how they can be adjusted to optimise the Doppler display, is discussed briefly.

Angle dependency:
The most important technical factor which affects the optimal display of Doppler signals is the parallel alignment between blood flow and the ultrasound beam. Hence, the Doppler interrogation is performed from echocardiographic views in which blood flow is aligned as parallel to the ultrasound beam as possible.

Sample volume position:
As mentioned above, Doppler interrogation is optimised when blood flow is aligned parallel to the ultrasound beam. Hence, during the PW Doppler examination, the sample volume should be positioned where blood flow is most parallel to the ultrasound beam. The position of the sample volume also affects the maximal velocity displayed. Increasing the depth of the sample volume reduces the pulse repetition frequency and, therefore, lowers the maximum detectable velocity that can be displayed (refer to equation 5.17).

Velocity scale and baseline:
The *velocity scale* adjusts the maximum velocity that can be displayed. When using PW Doppler, this scale is limited by the Nyquist limit or pulse repetition frequency. The *baseline* is the horizontal line on the spectral display representing zero Doppler shift. Both the velocity scale and baseline are adjustable. Traditionally, Doppler signals are displayed so that velocities toward the transducer are displayed above the zero baseline while velocities away from the transducer are displayed below the zero baseline. Both the zero baseline and velocity scale should be adjusted so that the velocity spectrum is optimally displayed.

Wall filters:
Wall filters allow the elimination of low frequency Doppler shifts that typically occur due to motion of the cardiac valves or heart walls. Wall filters should be set as low as possible to allow the delineation of the commencement and cessation of flow, thus, improving the accuracy of time interval measurements.

Gain:
The *gain* function adjusts the degree of amplification of received Doppler signals. The gains should be adjusted to optimally display the entire Doppler spectrum without excessive background noise.

Sample volume length:
The *sample volume* is the volume from which Doppler signals are received and processed. The length or gate of this sample volume can be adjusted. Sample volume length should be between 2 to 5 mm to minimise spectral broadening of the signal. Narrow sample volume lengths allow more specific positioning and generally produce "cleaner" spectral signals. Widening of the sample volume length increases the range of velocities detected but also results in increased spectral broadening.

Electrical Events versus Mechanical Events:
Another important concept that should be understood when performing the Doppler examination is that mechanical and electrical events do not occur simultaneously. In fact, there is a short phasic delay following an electrical event before the mechanical event follows. For example, atrial contraction as depicted on the mitral valve inflow signal will occur slightly after the P wave on the ECG.

Doppler Examination of Mitral Valve Inflow
Imaging Plane and Position of Sample Volume:
Doppler interrogation of mitral inflow is best evaluated from the apical four chamber view because flow is usually parallel to the ultrasound beam from this view. The PW Doppler sample volume (1 to 2 mm length) is placed at the tips of the open mitral valve leaflets on left ventricular side of the valve. At this point, it is important to be aware

of the fact that blood flow through the mitral valve is actually directed posterolaterally and not toward the cardiac apex. This is particularly important when assessing mitral inflow in the dilated left ventricle (Figure 6.1).

Normal Spectral Doppler Display:
Normally, blood flow through the mitral valve occurs during diastole with no blood flow occurring during systole. From the apical four chamber view, diastolic flow from the left atrium, through the mitral valve, into the left ventricle is directed towards the transducer and is, therefore, displayed above the zero baseline.

The transmitral velocity profile appears similar to the M-shaped configuration exhibited on the M-mode recording through the anterior mitral valve leaflet; as for the M-mode recording, the mitral inflow signal reflects ventricular filling during diastole.

The derivation of the mitral inflow Doppler signal is an important concept to the understanding of the haemodynamic events that occur during the cardiac cycle, in particular, during diastole. Comprehension of these stages will allow easier interpretation of this signal.

Diastole can be divided into four phases, all of which can be depicted on the mitral inflow Doppler signal (Figure 6.2). These four phases include: (1) the isovolumic relaxation period, (2) the early or rapid filling phase, (3) diastasis, and (4) atrial contraction.

1. Isovolumic relaxation period:

The **isovolumic relaxation phase** occurs following the

closure of the aortic valve and prior to opening of the mitral valve. During this phase, the left ventricular pressure falls rapidly and the ventricle begins to relax. The **isovolumic relaxation time (IVRT)**, the time interval between aortic valve closure and mitral valve opening, can be measured by displaying both the mitral inflow signal and the LVOT signal on the same spectral trace. This is accomplished, using either PW or CW Doppler, by aligning the beam so that is intercepts flow between these two regions. The IVRT is optimally displayed when the closing click of the aortic valve is depicted both above and below the zero baseline. Delineation of this closing click is important as it coincides with the cessation of systolic blood flow.

2. Early and rapid filling phase:

When the pressure within the left ventricle falls below that of the left atrium, continued relaxation and "suction", cause the mitral valve leaflets to open and a "driving" pressure is created. This driving pressure propels blood forward into the left ventricle resulting in early and rapid filling of the ventricle. The **early and rapid filling** phase creates the **peak E wave** of the mitral inflow Doppler trace.

Following the early and rapid filling phase, the diastolic pressure gradient between the left atrium and left ventricle decreases. This results in a rapid and steady fall in the Doppler velocities. The rate of decline in pressures and, thus, Doppler velocities, is reflected by the **deceleration rate or slope**.

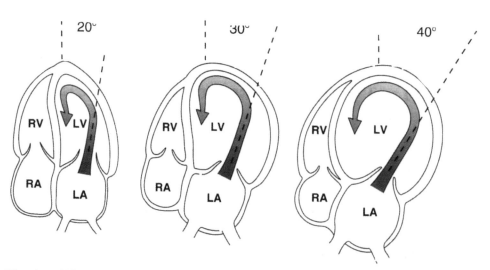

Figure 6.1: The Direction of Mitral Inflow in the Normal-Sized and Enlarged Heart.
This schematic illustrates the direction of mitral inflow within the normal-sized heart and the enlarged heart from the apical four chamber view. Understanding of flow direction is crucial to the alignment of the PW Doppler sample volume so that an accurate velocity profile can be obtained.
Left, In normal individuals, mitral inflow is directed approximately 20 degrees laterally to the cardiac apex. Flow then continues down the lateral wall, around the apex and up to the left ventricular otflow tract (*curved arrow*).
Middle and Right, As the left ventricle enlarges, mitral inflow is directed progressively more laterally such that optimal transducer position for alignment with mitral inflow may be 40 degrees or more from the standard apical imaging position.
Abbreviations: LA = left atrium; **LV** = left ventricle; **RA** = right atrium; **RV** = right ventricle.
Adapted from Appleton, C.P. et al.: Doppler evaluation of left and right ventricular diastolic function: A technical guide for obtaining optimal flow velocity recordings. *Journal of the American Society of Echocardiography 10: 271-291, 1997.* Reproduced with permission from Mosby Inc., St. Louis, MO, USA.

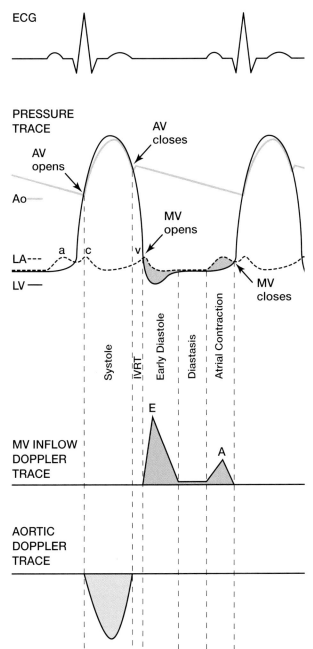

Figure 6.2: Diastole and the Mitral Inflow Doppler Signal.
This schematic illustrates the relationship between the mitral inflow Doppler signal and diastole (see text for details).
Abbreviations: Ao = aorta; **AV** = aortic valve; **IVRT** = isovolumic relaxation time; **LA** = left atrial pressure trace; **LV** = left ventricular pressure trace; **MV** = mitral valve.

3. Diastasis:

During diastasis, the pressures within the left atrium and left ventricle begin to equalise. Despite this equilibrium of pressures, a small amount of blood continues to flow across the mitral valve due to inertia. On the Doppler spectral trace, this decreased flow is reflected as low, uniform velocities close to the zero baseline.

4. Atrial filling phase:

Following atrial contraction, there is a small increase in the left atrial-left ventricle pressure gradient resulting in a further bolus of blood being propelled into the left ventricle. Forward blood flow from the left atrium to the

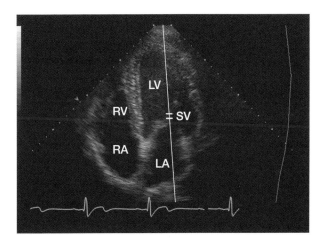

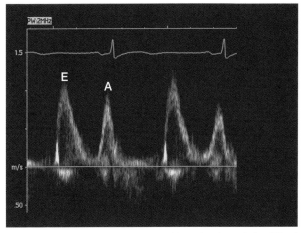

Figure 6.3: The Spectral Doppler Examination of the Mitral Inflow from the Apical Four Chamber View.
Top, Imaging plane and sample volume position.
Bottom, Spectral Doppler display.
Abbreviations: LA = left atrium; **LV** = left ventricle; **RA** = right atrium; **RV** = right ventricle; **SV** = sample volume.

left ventricle is reflected on the Doppler spectral trace as a second peak on the mitral inflow trace referred to as the **peak A wave**.

Technical Consideration:
The normal spectral Doppler display of mitral inflow including sample volume position is demonstrated in Figure 6.3. It is also important to note that correct placement of the sample volume is crucial for the accurate display of the Doppler signal as this signal will vary depending upon the sample volume position (Figure 6.4). When assessing left ventricular diastolic function and filling parameters, the sample volume is placed at the tips of the mitral valve leaflets. When calculating the stroke volume through the mitral valve, the sample volume is placed at the level of the mitral annulus.

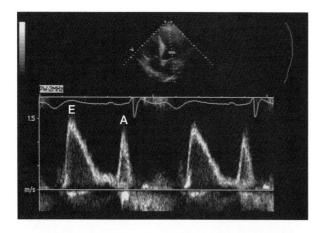

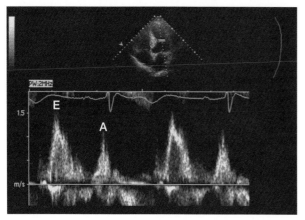

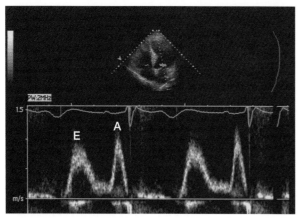

Figure 6.4: The Effect of Sample Volume Position on the Transmitral Doppler Signal.

The Doppler velocity spectrum of mitral inflow changes with the alteration of sample volume position.

Top, This example depicts the typical Doppler spectrum seen when the sample volume is positioned at the tips of the mitral valve leaflets.

Middle, This example illustrates the typical Doppler spectrum seen when the sample volume is positioned too far into the left ventricle. Observe the "feathering" of the Doppler trace which reflects the greater diameter and less laminar flow in the mid ventricle compared with flow between the mitral leaflets.

Bottom, This example illustrates the typical Doppler spectrum seen when the sample volume is at the level of the mitral annulus. Observe that the peak velocities are lower and the relationship between the E wave and the A wave has changed such that the E wave velocity decreases proportionally more than the A wave velocity.

Note: When assessing left ventricular diastolic function and filling parameters, the sample volume is placed at the tips of the mitral valve leaflets. When calculating the stroke volume through the mitral valve, the sample volume is placed at the level of the mitral annulus.

Doppler Examination of the Left Ventricular Outflow Tract and the Aorta

Imaging Plane and Position of Sample Volume:

Left Ventricular Outflow Tract (LVOT):

(Figure 6.5.)

Doppler interrogation of blood flow within the LVOT is best evaluated from the apical five chamber or apical long axis views. The PW Doppler sample volume (3 to 5 mm gate) is placed just proximal to the aortic valve (on the left ventricular side of the valve).

Ascending Aorta:

Doppler interrogation of blood flow within the ascending aorta is best evaluated from the apical five view, apical long axis view, the suprasternal notch window, or from the right sternal border. From any of these positions, it is possible to align the ultrasound beam parallel to the direction of blood flow.

CW Doppler is the method of choice for interrogation of aortic flow. Either the 2-D, guided CW Doppler modality, or the non-imaging, dedicated CW Doppler probe can be utilised. The latter is preferred for evaluation of blood flow from the suprasternal and right parasternal positions due to the difficulty of obtaining satisfactory 2-D images from these views. Furthermore, the smaller footprint of the non-imaging probe improves access to the smaller suprasternal window and, hence, allows easier angulation and manipulation of the probe.

Descending Aorta: (Figure 6.6)

Doppler interrogation of blood flow within the descending aorta is best evaluated from the suprasternal long axis view of the aorta. The PW Doppler sample volume (3-5 mm gate) placed approximately 1 cm distal to origin of left subclavian artery.

Normal Spectral Doppler Trace:

Apical Views: (Figure 6.5)

Blood flow within the LVOT, the aorta, and across the aortic valve occurs during systole, with no flow detectable during diastole. From the apical window, blood flow in the LVOT and ascending aorta, and across the aortic valve is directed away from the transducer and is, therefore, displayed below the zero baseline.

Blood flow detected within the LVOT is displayed in a V-shaped configuration representing steep acceleration and deceleration slopes (the deceleration slope is usually not as steep as the acceleration slope). An aortic valve closing click should be seen immediately following end-ejection. Flow within the LVOT may not be entirely related to systolic flow. Other currents may also be detected within this region. A commonly encountered example relates to the transmission of flow from atrial contraction to the LVOT producing a "J" wave.

Suprasternal and Right Sternal Windows:

(Figure 6.6)

Blood flow within the ascending and descending aorta occurs during systole, with little or no flow detectable during diastole. From these views, blood flow within the ascending aorta is directed toward the transducer and is, therefore, displayed above the zero baseline. Blood flow within the descending aorta from the suprasternal view is directed away from the transducer and, therefore, appears below the zero baseline. As for the LVOT, systolic signals within the ascending and descending aorta are displayed in a V-shaped configuration.

In the Doppler examination of the descending aorta from the suprasternal window, a short period of low velocity flow reversal is normally detected in early diastole. This flow represents the retrograde movement of the blood flow back toward the aortic valve. This flow is directed toward the transducer and, hence, is displayed above the zero baseline (Figure 6.6). The duration of this flow should not exceed the first third of diastole. Recognition of this normal pattern of diastolic flow reversal is important as this may be confused for abnormal pan-diastolic flow reversal which is a characteristic finding of moderate to severe aortic regurgitation (see Chapter 13).

Doppler Examination of Pulmonary Venous Flow

Imaging Plane and Position of Sample Volume:
(Figure 6.7)
Doppler interrogation of pulmonary venous flow is best achieved from the apical four chamber view utilising the

right upper pulmonary vein which lies almost parallel to the ultrasound beam. A slightly larger PW Doppler sample volume of between 3 to 5 mm is placed 1-2 cm into the pulmonary vein, proximal to its entrance into the left atrium.

As for the assessment of the mitral inflow signal, correct positioning of the sample volume is crucial. Correct sample volume placement is often facilitated by the use of CFI. With CFI, red laminar flow from the right upper pulmonary vein as it drains into the left atrium can be readily appreciated in most cases.

Normal Spectral Doppler Display: (Figure 6.7)
As with all venous flow, pulmonary venous flow is continuous throughout the cardiac cycle; that is, throughout diastole and systole. Normal pulmonary venous flow is characterised by three distinct waveforms: (1) systolic forward flow, (2) diastolic forward flow, and (3) atrial flow reversal.

Systolic forward flow occurs as a result of left atrial relaxation and the descent of the mitral annulus toward the cardiac apex with ventricular systole. Systolic forward flow is biphasic in approximately 37% of normal individuals [10].

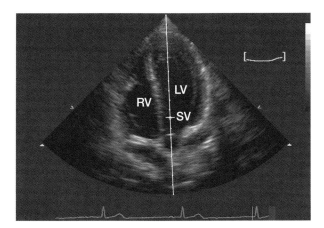

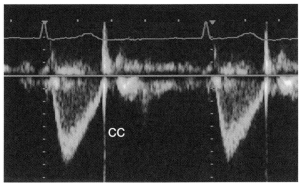

Figure 6.5: The Spectral Doppler Examination of the Left Ventricular Outflow Tract from the Apical Five Chamber View.
Top, Imaging plane and sample volume position.
Bottom, Spectral Doppler display.
Abbreviations: CC = closing click; **LV** = left ventricle; **RV** = right ventricle; **SV** = sample volume.

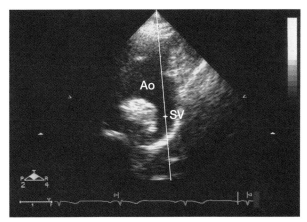

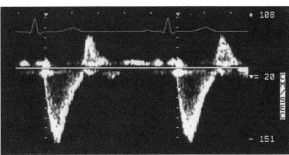

Figure 6.6: The Spectral Doppler Examination of the Descending Thoracic Aorta from the Suprasternal Long Axis View.
Top, Imaging plane and sample volume position.
Bottom, Spectral Doppler display. Observe the short duration diastolic flow reversal.
Abbreviations: Ao = aorta; **SV** = sample volume.

10: Klein, A.L. et al.: Mayo Clinic Proceedings 69:212-224,1994.

Flow is toward the transducer and, therefore, is displayed above the zero baseline. **Diastolic forward flow** occurs in diastole when there is an open conduit between the pulmonary veins, the left atrium, the open mitral valve, and the left ventricle. Diastolic forward flow is usually of a lesser velocity than systolic forward flow. Flow is toward the transducer and, therefore, is displayed above the zero baseline. **Atrial flow reversal** refers to retrograde flow back into the pulmonary vein secondary to atrial contraction. Flow is directed away from the transducer and, therefore, appears below the zero baseline. Normally, atrial reversal velocities are very small (less than 35 cm/s) [11].

Doppler Examination of Tricuspid Valve Inflow

Imaging Plane and Sample Volume Positioning:
(Figure 6.8)
Doppler interrogation of tricuspid inflow is best achieved from the parasternal long axis view of the right ventricular inflow tract or from the apical four chamber view.
The PW Doppler sample volume (3 to 5 mm gate) is positioned centrally between the open tricuspid valve

leaflets tips on the right ventricular side of the valve.

Normal Spectral Doppler Display: (Figure 6.8)
Normally, blood flow through the tricuspid valve occurs during diastole with no blood flow detectable during systole. From either the parasternal long axis view of the right ventricular inflow tract or from the apical four chamber view, diastolic flow from the right atrium, through the tricuspid valve, into the right ventricle is directed towards the transducer and is, therefore, displayed above the zero baseline.
The Doppler velocity profile is identical to that described for the mitral valve except that the velocities are usually lower and vary slightly with respiration.

Respiratory variation of tricuspid inflow venous signals:
It is important to recognise that the flow velocities of the tricuspid inflow vary throughout respiration. During inspiration, there is a slight increase in the E and A waves while during expiration, these velocities are seen to decline.

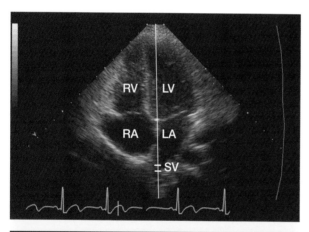
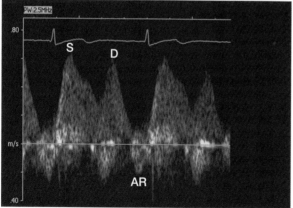

Figure 6.7: The Spectral Doppler Examination of the Right Upper Pulmonary Vein from the Apical Four Chamber View.
Top, Imaging plane and sample volume position.
Bottom, Spectral Doppler display.
Abbreviations: AR = atrial reversal; **D** = diastolic forward flow; **LA** = left atrium; **LV** = left ventricle; **RA** = right atrium; **RV** = right ventricle; **S** = systolic forward flow; **SV** = sample volume.

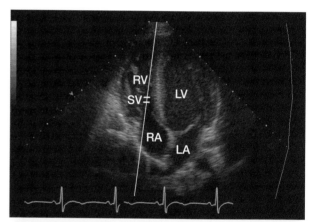
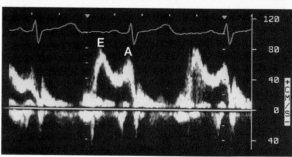

Figure 6.8: The Spectral Doppler Examination of Tricuspid Inflow from the Apical Four Chamber View.
Top, Imaging plane and sample volume position.
Bottom, Spectral Doppler display.
Abbreviations: LA = left atrium; **LV** = left ventricle; **RA** = right atrium; **RV** = right ventricle; **SV** = sample volume.

Doppler Examination of the Right Ventricular Outflow Tract and the Pulmonary Artery

Imaging Plane and Sample Volume Positioning:
Doppler interrogation of the right ventricular outflow tract (RVOT) and pulmonary artery is best achieved from the parasternal long axis or short axis views of the RVOT.

Right Ventricular Outflow Tract (RVOT):
(Figure 6.9)
For interrogation of blood flow within the RVOT, the PW Doppler sample volume (3 to 5 mm gate) is positioned within the outflow tract approximately 1 cm proximal to the pulmonary valve leaflets.

Pulmonary Artery:
For interrogation of blood flow within the pulmonary artery, the PW Doppler sample volume (3 to 5 mm gate) is positioned within the centre of the pulmonary artery 1 cm below the pulmonary valve.

Normal Spectral Display: (Figure 6.9)
Blood flow within the RVOT and pulmonary artery occurs during systole. Direction of blood flow is away from the transducer and, therefore, the signal is displayed below the zero baseline. The Doppler velocity spectrum appears similar to the LVOT signal except that the peak velocity is lower and the duration of the signal is longer. During diastole, there is usually little or no detectable flow. Occasionally, however, a small amount of low velocity retrograde flow of short duration may be detected in early diastole representing the retrograde blood flow back toward the pulmonary valve. This flow is directed toward the transducer and, hence, is displayed above the zero baseline. The duration of this flow is typically less than 50% of the diastolic period and should not be mistaken for pulmonary regurgitation, which is usually holosystolic [12].

Doppler Examination of the Hepatic Veins

Imaging Plane and Position of Sample Volume:
(Figure 6.10)
Doppler interrogation of hepatic venous flow is best achieved from the subcostal long axis view of the inferior vena cava (IVC). From this view, the right or middle hepatic vein can be imaged parallel to the ultrasound beam as it drains into the IVC. The PW Doppler sample volume (2 mm gate) is placed 1 to 2 cm into the hepatic vein proximal to its junction with the IVC. The hepatic vein can be seen to move within the plane of the ultrasound beam during respiration, thus, maintaining the sample volume position within this vein may sometimes prove difficult.

Normal Spectral Doppler Display: (Figure 6.10)
Blood flow within the hepatic vein is continuous throughout the cardiac cycle; that is, throughout systole and diastole. Normal hepatic venous flow is characterised by three distinct waveforms: (1) systolic forward flow, (2) diastolic forward flow, and (3) atrial reversal of flow. Occasionally, a fourth waveform is seen representing reversal of flow due to ventricular systole.
Systolic forward flow occurs as a result of right atrial relaxation with ventricular systole. Flow is directed away from the transducer and, therefore, is displayed below the zero baseline. **Diastolic forward flow** occurs during the rapid filling phase of diastole when the tricuspid valve is open. Diastolic forward flow is usually of a lesser velocity compared with systolic forward flow. Flow is directed away from the transducer and, therefore, is displayed below the zero baseline. **Atrial flow reversal** refers to the retrograde flow of blood back into the hepatic veins secondary to atrial contraction. Normally, these velocities are very small. Flow is directed toward the transducer, therefore, appears above the baseline.
Ventricular flow reversal refers to the retrograde flow of blood back into the hepatic vein occurring in late systole which corresponds to the atrial V wave on the right atrial pressure curve. This flow is of a lesser velocity than the atrial flow reversal velocity. When present, this flow is directed toward the transducer and, therefore, is displayed above the zero baseline.

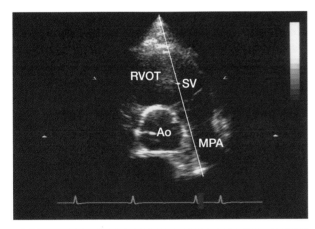

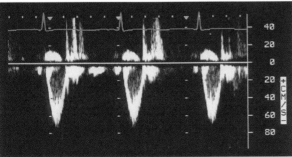

Figure 6.9: The Spectral Doppler Examination of the Right Ventricular Outflow Tract from the Parasternal Short Axis View.
Top, Imaging plane and sample volume position.
Bottom, Spectral Doppler display.
Abbreviations: Ao = aortal; **MPA** = main pulmonary artery; **RVOT** = right ventricular outflow tract; **SV** = sample volume.

12: Nishimura, R.A. et al.: Mayo Clinic Proceedings 60:337,1985.

> **Respiratory variation of hepatic venous signals:**
> It is important to recognise that the flow velocities of the hepatic veins vary throughout respiration. During inspiration, there is an increase in the systolic and diastolic forward velocities as well as in the atrial reversal velocity. Upon expiration, a decrease in the ventricular reversal velocity is seen.

Doppler Examination of the Superior Vena Cava

Imaging Plane and Position of Sample Volume:
(Figure 6.11)
Doppler interrogation of the superior vena cava (SVC) is best achieved from the suprasternal notch or from the right supraclavicular fossa. The PW Doppler sample volume (3-5 mm gate) is positioned at a depth of 5 to 7 cm into the SVC. Correct placement of the sample volume may be facilitated by the use of CFI. With CFI, blue laminar flow down the SVC toward the right atrium can be readily appreciated in most cases.

Normal Spectral Doppler Display: (Figure 6.11)
Blood flow within the SVC is continuous throughout the cardiac cycle; that is, throughout systole and diastole. Normal SVC flow is characterised by three distinct waveforms: (1) systolic forward flow, (2) diastolic forward flow, and (3) atrial reversal of flow. Rarely, a fourth waveform, representing ventricular reversal of flow, is seen.

Systolic forward flow occurs as a result of right atrial relaxation and the descent of the tricuspid annulus toward the cardiac apex with ventricular systole. Flow is directed away from the transducer, and therefore, is displayed below the zero baseline. **Diastolic forward flow** occurs during the rapid filling phase of diastole when the tricuspid valve is open. Diastolic forward flow is usually of a lesser velocity compared with systolic forward flow. Flow is directed away from the transducer and, therefore, is displayed below the zero baseline. **Atrial flow reversal** refers to the retrograde flow of blood back into the superior vena cava secondary to atrial contraction. Normally, these velocities are very small. Flow is directed toward the transducer, and therefore, appears above the baseline.

Ventricular flow reversal refers to the retrograde flow of blood back into the SVC occurring in late systole corresponding to the atrial V wave on the right atrial pressure curve. Ventricular flow reversal is usually absent in the normal individual except with expiration [13].

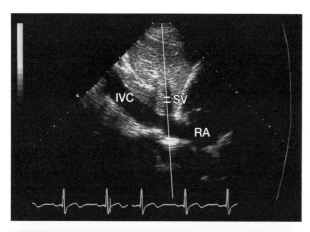

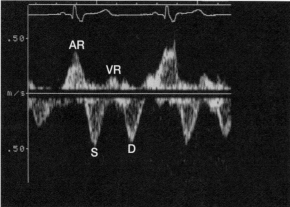

Figure 6.10: The Spectral Doppler Examination of the Right Hepatic Vein from the Subcostal View.
Top, Imaging plane and sample volume position.
Bottom, Spectral Doppler display.
Abbreviations: AR = atrial reversal; **D** = diastolic forward flow; **S** = systolic forward flow; **SV** = sample volume; **VR** = ventricular reversal.

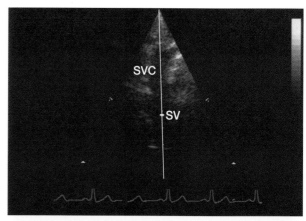

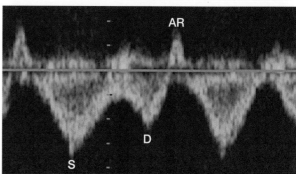

Figure 6.11: The Spectral Doppler Examination of the Superior Vena Cava from the Suprasternal View.
A. Imaging plane and sample volume position.
B. Spectral Doppler display.
Abbreviations: AR = atrial reversal; **D** = diastolic forward flow; **S** = systolic forward flow; **SV** = sample volume; **SVC** = superior vena cava.

13: Appleton, C.P. et al.: Journal of the American College of Cardiology 10:1032-1039,1987.

Table 6.1: Maximum Blood Flow Velocities in Normal Individuals.

	Children		Adults	
	Mean	Range	Mean	Range
Mitral inflow	1.00 m/s	0.8-1.3 m/s	0.90 ms	0.6-1.3 m/s
Tricuspid inflow	0.60 m/s	0.5-0.8 m/s	0.50 m/s	0.3-0.7 m/s
Pulmonary artery	0.90 m/s	0.7-1.1 m/s	0.75 m/s	0.6-0.9 m/s
Left ventricle	1.00 m/s	0.7- 1.2 m/s	0.90 m/s	0.7-1.1 m/s
Aorta	1.50 m/s	1.2-1.8 m/s	1.35 m/s	1.0-1.7 m/s

Source: Hatle, L. and Angelsen, B.: Doppler Ultrasound in Cardiology. 2nd edition. Lea and Febiger, pp: 93, 1985: patient population: 30 children aged 1 to 16 years; 40 adults aged 18 to 72 years.

When present, flow is directed toward the transducer and, therefore, is displayed above the zero baseline.

Observe that systolic and diastolic forward flow velocities within the superior vena cava are higher than those obtained from the hepatic veins. In contrast, reverse flow velocities of the hepatic vein are more prominent than those of the SVC. Possible explanations for this increase in hepatic venous flow reversals include variations in the pressure difference between the abdominal and chest cavities, and/or the closer proximity of the hepatic vein to the right atrium [13 & 14].

Respiratory variation of superior vena caval signals:

As for the hepatic vein, flow velocities of the SVC vary throughout respiration. During inspiration, there is an increase in the systolic and diastolic forward velocities. Upon expiration, a decrease in the atrial reversal velocity is seen and a ventricular reversal velocity may become evident.

References and Suggested Reading:

- Appleton, C.P. et al.: Superior vena cava and hepatic vein Doppler echocardiography in healthy adults. *Journal of the American College of Cardiology 10: 1032-1039, 1987.*

- Appleton, C.P. Doppler evaluation of left and right ventricular diastolic function: A technical guide for obtaining optimal flow velocity recordings. *Journal of the American Society of Echocardiography 10: 271-291, 1997.*

- Dittrich, H.C., et al.: Influence of Doppler sample volume location on the assessment of changes in mitral inflow velocity profiles. *Journal of the American Society of Echocardiography 3:303,1990.*

- Ding, Z.P., et al.: Effect of sample volume location on Doppler-derived transmitral inflow velocity values. *Journal of the American Society of Echocardiography 4:451,1991.*

- Feigenbaum, H.: Echocardiography. Chapter 2. 5th Ed. Lea & Febiger, 1994.

- Jaffe, W.M., et al.: Influence of Doppler sample volume location on ventricular filling velocities. *American Journal of Cardiology 68:550,1991.*

- Klein, A.L. et al.: Effects of age on left ventricular dimensions and filling dynamics in 117 normal persons. *Mayo Clinic Proceedings 69: 212-224, 1994.*

- Nishimura, R.A. : Doppler echocardiography: theory, instrumentation, technique and application. *Mayo Clinic Proceedings 60:321-343,1985.*

- Otto, C.M. and Pearlman, A.S.: Textbook of Clinical Echocardiography. Chapter 2. W.B. Saunders Company. 1995

- Reynolds, T., Appleton, C.P.: Doppler flow velocity patterns of the superior vena cava, inferior vena cava, hepatic vein, coronary sinus and atrial septal defect: A guide for the echocardiographer. *Journal of the American Society of Echocardiography 4: 503-512, 1990.*

- Weyman, A.: Principles and Practice of Echocardiography. Chapter 13. 2nd Ed. Lea & Febiger, 1994.

13: Appleton, C.P. et al.: Journal of the American College of Cardiology 10:1032-1039,1987. 14: Reynolds, T and Appleton, C.P.: Journal of the American Society of Echocardiography. 4:503-512,1990.

Chapter 7
Basic Principles of Colour Flow Doppler Imaging

Colour Flow Doppler Principles

Colour flow Doppler imaging (CFI) is a noninvasive PW Doppler technique that displays both anatomic and haemodynamic information on the real-time 2-D image. This is achieved by superimposing the colour Doppler blood flow pattern within the heart onto the real-time 2-D echocardiographic image.

Recall that spectral PW Doppler instruments display a spectrum of blood flow information obtained from a single sample volume site along one scan line; therefore, PW Doppler provides limited Doppler shift information from a relatively localised region of the heart. This information is then presented as a plot of Doppler shift versus time. With CFI, Doppler flow information is superimposed on top of the real-time, 2-D image. Therefore, B-mode provides the gray-scale image while Doppler provides the colour-coded velocity image.

Production of Colour Flow Doppler:

Converse to the spectral PW Doppler display, colour flow Doppler images are produced by using multiple sample gates along multiple scan lines (Figure 7.1)

The device that detects the Doppler shift frequency is the *autocorrelator* (meaning self-comparison). This device compares the Doppler shifts from a particular line of sight with previous signals acquired along the same scan line. Where Doppler shifts are detected, pixels representing those areas are designated a colour (each pixel can only have one colour). The colour of the pixel is determined by the *mean* Doppler shift detected at that site. Colour coding, relative to the transducer, is direction sensitive.

The Colour Doppler Display

Information displayed on the colour Doppler display includes: (1) blood flow direction, (2) blood flow velocity, (3) frequency aliasing, (4) and the timing of the colour Doppler signals (Figure 7.2).

Blood Flow Direction: As for spectral Doppler, blood flow toward the transducer is traditionally displayed above the zero baseline while blood flow away from the transducer is displayed below the zero baseline. Thus, blood flow toward the transducer is displayed in colours above the colour baseline, and blood flow away from the transducer is displayed in colours below the colour baseline. In echocardiography, blood flow moving toward the transducer is traditionally displayed as red while blood flow away from the transducer is displayed as blue. This system of blood flow display is also referred as the BART system (**B**lue **A**way, **R**ed **T**oward).

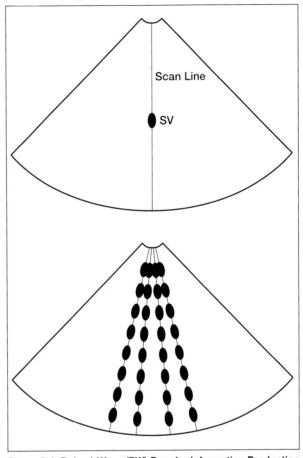

Figure 7.1: Pulsed-Wave (PW) Doppler Information Production versus Colour Flow Doppler Information Production.
Top, With PW Doppler, a whole spectrum of Doppler velocity information is obtained from a **single** sample volume placed along a **single** scan line.
Bottom, With colour flow Doppler, a single blood flow velocity (the mean velocity) is achieved from **several hundred** sample volume sites along **numerous** scan lines.

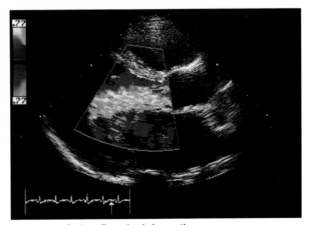

Figure 7.2: Colour Doppler Information.
Colour flow Doppler information is primarily represented on the colour bar as illustrated above. Timing of blood flow is indicated by the ECG.

Blood Flow Velocity: Blood flow velocity information is determined by the location of a colour along the colour bar. Low velocity blood flow is indicated by colours closest to the colour baseline and appears in deeper colour hues. High velocity blood flow is indicated towards the end of the colour bar and appears brighter.

As there is no angle correction in colour flow Doppler, peak velocity estimations are not possible, therefore, only the mean Doppler velocities are depicted.

Frequency Aliasing: Since colour flow imaging is a PW Doppler technique, it obeys the same principles as PW Doppler. In PW Doppler, when the blood flow velocities exceed the Nyquist limit, aliasing occurs. This same principle also applies to CFI.

Normal blood flow velocities rarely cause aliasing in PW Doppler, but frequently cause aliasing in CFI. This is because the Nyquist limit, which is equal to one-half the PRF, is lower in CFI (remember that mean velocities are detected by CFI). With CFI, aliasing appears as colour reversal.

Timing of Colour Doppler Signals: Timing of colour Doppler signals as they occur throughout the cardiac cycle are achieved by observing the colour flow Doppler image in relation to the ECG.

Other information that can be determined from CFI includes the differentiation between laminar and turbulent flow.

Laminar Versus Turbulent Flow: In normal, laminar blood flow, all the red blood cells move at about the same velocity and in the same general direction. Laminar flow is, therefore, depicted by a smooth, homogeneous pattern.

Turbulent blood flow, on the other hand, moves in many different directions and at many different velocities. Therefore, turbulent flow appears as a disorganised, mosaic pattern containing all colours on the colour bar.

References and Suggested Reading:

- Feigenbaum, H.: <u>Echocardiography.</u> Chapter 1. 5th Ed. Lea & Febiger, 1994.
- Gent, Roger. <u>Applied Physics and Technology of Diagnostic Ultrasound.</u> Milner Publishing (3 Milner Street, Prospect. South Australia 5082), 1997.
- Otto, C.M. and Pearlman, A.S.: <u>Textbook of Clinical Echocardiography.</u> Chapter 1. W.B. Saunders Company. 1995
- Weyman, A.: <u>Principles and Practice of Echocardiography.</u> Chapter 11. 2nd Ed. Lea & Febiger, 1994.

Chapter 8
The Colour Flow Doppler Examination

As mentioned, CFI is a variation of the PW Doppler technique whereby colours represent the direction and mean velocity of blood flow, and the colour box depicts the sample volume. Thus, CFI provides information pertaining to the timing, direction and velocity of blood flow, and has the ability to differentiate between laminar and turbulent flow. Since CFI is based upon the PW Doppler technique, it shares some of the advantages and disadvantages of this technique. In particular, the most important limitation of this technique is frequency aliasing.

Normal blood flow within the heart is of low velocity, smooth and laminar. Small pressure gradients exist across the normal channels of blood flow, thus, producing detectable Doppler shifts. CFI can be utilised in the investigation of the primary channels of blood flow into, out of, and within the heart. Each channel of blood flow has a characteristic pattern determined by its direction, velocity, duration, and timing of flow throughout the cardiac cycle.

Optimisation of Colour Flow Doppler Images

Optimal colour flow Doppler images are dependent upon several technical factors. Each of these factors as well as how they can be adjusted to optimise colour flow Doppler images are discussed briefly.

Frame rate:
The most important technical factor for CFI is the *frame rate* or the number of frames produced per second. In the examination of the dynamic heart, the higher the frame rate the better. Frame rate is dependent upon several factors including depth, colour sector width, and the line density. *Colour sector width* refers to the size of the colour box and defines the area on the 2-D image that will be colour encoded while *line density* refers to the spacing between each scan line. Increasing both the width of the colour box and the line density results in an increase in the processing time which, in effect, lowers the frame rate. *Depth* also affects the frame rate. As depth of interrogation increases, the time required to process the Doppler information increases resulting in a slower frame rate. Hence, the frame rate is optimised by maintaining a narrow colour box at a depth that adequately displays the region of interest.

Velocity scale:
The *velocity scale* adjusts the maximum mean velocity that can be displayed. As CFI is a form of PW Doppler, the velocity scale is limited by the Nyquist limit or pulse repetition frequency (PRF). The velocity scale should be optimised to display signals by using the highest possible velocity scale without aliasing of the signal. This can be achieved by increasing the PRF. The PRF can be increased by decreasing the depth of the colour box or using a lower frequency transducer. Occasionally, it may also be necessary to lower the velocity scale when investigating low velocity flow such as that seen within the abdominal aorta and within pseudoaneurysms.

Wall filters:
Wall filters allow the elimination of low frequency Doppler velocities which may contaminate the colour flow Doppler image. Wall filters can be either increased to exclude low velocity signals which may arise from valve or walls, or decreased to investigate low velocity signals.

Gain:
The *gain* function adjusts the degree of amplification of received Doppler signals. The gain should be adjusted to a level just below that at which background "speckling" occurs.

Angle dependency:
As for spectral Doppler, the best Doppler signals are produced when the direction of blood flow is aligned parallel to the ultrasound beam. However, with CFI, the angle between the ultrasound beam and the direction of blood flow is not as critical. This is because it is the *spatial* pattern of blood flow that is of interest rather than the absolute velocities. Furthermore, as long as there is some angle between the ultrasound beam and blood flow direction, some flow will always be detected and, therefore, displayed.

Regurgitation in the Normal Population

Regurgitant blood flow can be either low or high velocity, laminar or turbulent depending upon the cardiac output and the pressure gradient between the cardiac chambers or vessels. Normal so-called "physiological" regurgitation through the cardiac valves is commonly seen within the normal population (Table 8.1). Furthermore, the incidence of regurgitation has been reported to increase with advancing age (Table 8.2). The most important facts depicted in these two tables are: (1) very little aortic regurgitation is observed in clinically normal individuals (especially in individuals less than 50 years of age) and (2) both tricuspid and pulmonary regurgitation are quite common across all age groups.

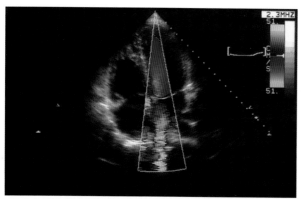

Figure 8.1: Normal Colour Flow Doppler Image of Left Atrial Inflow from the Right Upper Pulmonary Vein as seen from the Apical Four Chamber View.

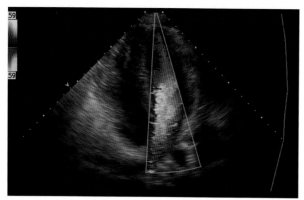

Figure 8.2: Normal Colour Flow Doppler Image of Left Ventricular Inflow as seen from the Apical Four Chamber View during Diastole.

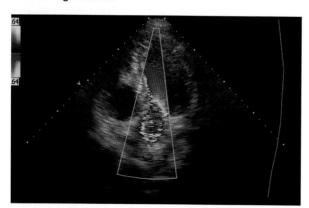

Figure 8.3: Normal Colour Flow Doppler Image of Left Ventricular Outflow Tract as seen from the Apical Five Chamber View during Systole.

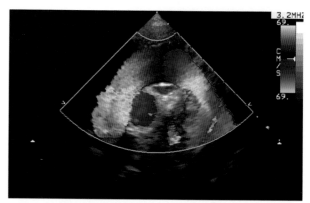

Figure 8.5: Normal Colour Flow Doppler Image of the Aortic Arch as seen from the Suprasternal View during Systole.
Observe that flow within the ascending aorta is directed toward the transducer during systole and is, therefore, encoded red. Blood flow within the descending aorta is directed away from the transducer and, therefore, is encoded blue. Also observe at the top of the aortic arch, a region devoid of colour. This region indicates zero Doppler shift because blood flow is aligned perpendicular to the ultrasound beam (not because there is no flow within this region).

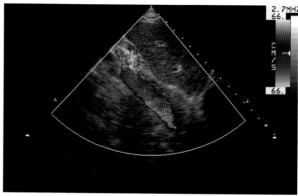

Figure 8.6: Normal Colour Flow Doppler Image of the Abdominal Aorta as seen from the Subcostal View during Systole.

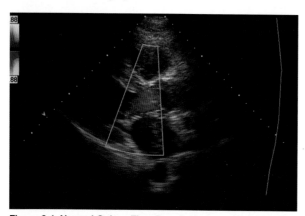

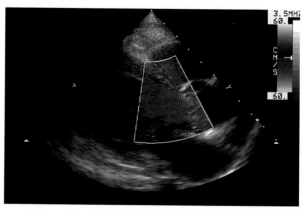

Figure 8.4: Normal Colour Flow Doppler Image of Left Ventricular Outflow Tract as seen from the Parasternal View during Systole.
Left, In this example, the LVOT is angled anteriorly toward the transducer so that blood flow is directed toward the ultrasound beam and, thus, is encoded red.
Right, In this example, the LVOT is angled posteriorly so that blood flow is directed away from the transducer and, thus, is encoded blue.

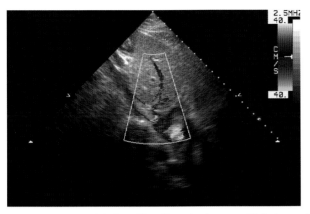 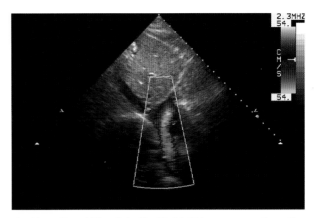

Figure 8.7: Normal Colour Flow Doppler Image of Inferior and Superior Vena Caval Flow into the Right Atrium as seen from the Subcostal View.
Left, Colour flow Doppler imaging of inferior vena caval flow into the right atrium.
Right, Colour flow Doppler imaging of superior vena caval flow into the right atrium.

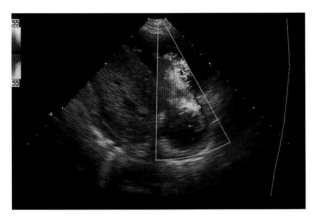 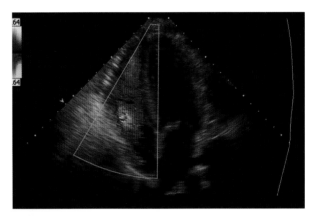

Figure 8.8: Normal Colour Flow Doppler Image of Right Ventricular Inflow.
Left, Colour flow Doppler imaging of right ventricular inflow from the parasternal long axis view during diastole.
Right, Colour flow Doppler imaging of right ventricular inflow from the apical four chamber view during diastole.

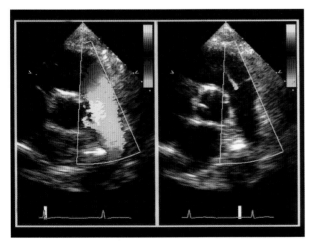

Figure 8.9: Normal Colour Flow Doppler Image of the Right Ventricular Outflow Tract (RVOT) and Pulmonary Artery as seen from the Parasternal Short Axis View.
Left, This is a systolic frame demonstrating blue flow within the RVOT and pulmonary artery. Observe colour aliasing (yellow flow) within the main pulmonary artery.
Right, This is a diastolic frame demonstrating a trivial degree of "physiological" pulmonary regurgitation which appears as a narrow red colour "flame". Remember that physiological pulmonary regurgitation is commonly seen within the normal population.

Table 8.1: Incidence of Valvular Regurgitation in the Normal Population.

First Author (Years)	MR	AR	TR	PR
Lavie et al. (1993)[1] (No. = 206)	73%	12%	68%	NS
Maciel (1991)[2] (No. = 39)	-	-	83%	93%
Klein et al. (1990)[3] (No. = 118)	48%	11%	65%	31%
Pollack et al. (1989)[4] (No. = 46)	17 - 35%	0 - 6%	24 - 93%	18 - 87%
Yoshida et al. (1988)[5] (No. = 211)	38 - 45%	0 %	17 - 77%	28 - 88%

Abbreviations: No. = number of normal individuals examined; **NS** = not stated. **AR** = aortic regurgitation; **MR** = mitral regurgitation; **PR** = pulmonary regurgitation; **TR** = tricuspid regurgitation.
Sources: (1) Lavie, C.J., et al., *Chest 103:226-231, 1993*; (2) Maciel, B.C. et al., *Journal of the American Society of Echocardiography 4: 589-597, 1991*; (3) Klein, A.L. et al., *Journal of the American Society of Echocardiography 2:54-63, 1990*; (4) Pollack, S.J. et al., *Journal of the American College of Cardiology 11:89-93,1988*; (5) Yoshida, K. et al., *Circulation 78:840-847, 1988*.

Table 8.2: Prevalence of Valvular Regurgitation in the Normal Population by Decade of Life.

Ages (years)	MR	AR	TR	PR
6 - 9 (n = 206)[1]	45%	0%	78%	88%
10 - 19 (n = 47)[1]	45%	0%	66%	64%
20-29 (n = 67)[3]	40%	0 %	57%	49%
30-39 (n = 61)[3]	41%	0 %	46%	28%
40- 49 (n = 57)[3]	40%	0%	30%	25%
50 – 59 (n = 21)[2]	48%	14%	53%	42%
60- 69 (n = 21)[2]	67%	24%	81%	31%
≥ 70 (n = 15)[2]	60%	33%	93%	50%

Sources: (1) Yoshida, K. et al., *Circulation 78:840-847, 1988;* (2) Klein, A.L. et al., *Journal of the American Society of Echocardiography 2:54-63, 1990;* (3) Combined data from sources (1) and (2).

Colour Flow Doppler Examination of Left Atrial Inflow

Blood flow into the left atrium occurs via the four pulmonary veins; that is, the right upper, right lower, left upper, and left lower pulmonary veins.

Examination Windows:

Colour Doppler interrogation of left atrial inflow is best evaluated from the apical four chamber view. From this view, three of the four pulmonary veins can be identified (the right lower pulmonary vein is not normally imaged from this view). Left atrial flow from the right upper pulmonary vein (RUPV) is easiest to identify due to its parallel alignment to the ultrasound beam.

Pulmonary venous flow into the left atrium can also be appreciated from the parasternal long and short axis views. From the parasternal long axis view, left upper and left lower pulmonary veins can be identified. From the parasternal short axis view at the level of the aorta and left atrium, RUPV flow can be seen.

Normal Flow Pattern:

Pulmonary venous flow into the left atrium is continuous throughout the cardiac cycle; that is, flow occurs during systole and diastole. From the apical and parasternal views, left atrial inflow is usually directed toward the transducer and, therefore, blood flow is encoded red (Figure 8.1). The exception to this colour flow Doppler profile occurs from the apical four chamber view whereby blood into the left atrium from the left lower pulmonary vein is directed away from the transducer and, therefore, is encoded blue.

Pulmonary venous flow is laminar and has a relatively low velocity; thus, flow is depicted in deeper shades of red or blue.

Colour Flow Doppler Examination of Left Ventricular Inflow

Left ventricular inflow normally occurs during diastole as blood flows from the left atrium, through the mitral valve, into the left ventricle.

Examination Windows:
Colour Doppler interrogation of left ventricular inflow is best evaluated from the apical four chamber view where blood flow is most parallel to the ultrasound beam. Other views that may be utilised include the apical two chamber, parasternal long axis, and the subcostal four chamber views.

Normal Flow Pattern:
Blood flow from the left atrium, through the mitral valve, into the left ventricle occurs during diastole. From the apical four chamber view, flow is directed toward the transducer and, therefore, is encoded red (Figure 8.2). High velocity flow may be observed within the centre of the jet appearing as a smooth progression from red to yellow. Flow appears biphasic in diastole corresponding to early filling and filling due to atrial contraction (the E and A waves on the spectral Doppler trace). Direct flow from the pulmonary veins into the left atrium, through the mitral valve, into the left ventricle may also be appreciated.

Colour Flow Examination of Left Ventricular Outflow Flow

Left ventricular outflow occurs during systole through the left ventricular outflow tract (LVOT) and into the aorta.

Examination Windows:
Colour Doppler interrogation of left ventricular outflow is best evaluated from the apical five and apical long axis views where blood flow is the most parallel to the ultrasound beam. LVOT flow may also be assessed from the parasternal long axis view of the left ventricle.

Normal Flow Pattern:
Blood flow through the LVOT is seen predominantly during ventricular ejection (systole). From the apical views, blood flow is encoded blue as it is directed away from the transducer (Figure 8.3). During the early ejection phase of systole, blood flow accelerates through the LVOT and almost always exceeds the Nyquist limit, resulting in colour aliasing. Therefore, during systole, colour within the LVOT changes from blue to red.
From the parasternal long axis view of the left ventricle, blood flow through the LVOT may be directed either toward the transducer or away from the transducer depending of the orientation of the LVOT to the ultrasound beam (Figure 8.4). When the LVOT is angled anteriorly toward the transducer, blood flow is directed toward the transducer and, therefore, will appear red. Conversely, when the LVOT is directed posteriorly, blood flow will appear blue as flow is directed away from the transducer.

Little or no blood flow is seen during diastole. When flow is absent, no colour is seen (depicted as black). When a small amount of normal flow is present during diastole, the velocity will be low and, therefore, flow will appear in deeper shades of red or blue (depending upon the angle between LVOT flow and the ultrasound beam).

Colour Flow Doppler Examination of Aortic Flow

Examination Windows:
Colour Doppler interrogation of **ascending aorta** can be performed from the parasternal long axis view of the left ventricle, the apical five chamber and apical long axis views, the right parasternal window, and from the suprasternal long axis view.
Colour Doppler interrogation of the **aortic arch** and **descending thoracic aorta** is typically performed from the suprasternal long axis view. Examination of flow within the descending aorta can also be achieved from the apical two chamber view when the descending aorta is opened out into its long axis.
Colour Doppler interrogation of the **abdominal aorta** can be performed from the subcostal short axis view with the transducer directed towards the patients' left clavicle.

Normal Flow Pattern:
Blood flow through the aortic valve into the aorta, around the aortic arch, and into the descending and abdominal aorta occurs during systole.

Parasternal long axis view of the left ventricle:
As for the LVOT, blood flow within the ascending aorta may be directed either toward the transducer or away from the transducer depending of the orientation of the ascending aorta to the ultrasound beam (Figure 8.4). When the aorta is angled anteriorly, blood flow is directed toward the transducer and, therefore, will appear red. Conversely, when the aorta is directed posteriorly, blood flow will appear blue as flow is directed away from the transducer.

Apical views:
From the apical views, blood flow within the ascending aorta is encoded blue as it is directed away from the transducer (Figure 8.3).

Aortic arch:
From the suprasternal long axis view, blood flow within the **ascending aorta** and the **anterior segment of the aortic arch** is directed toward the transducer and, therefore, is encoded red. Arising from the top of the aortic arch, the three head and neck vessels may be seen. Blood flow within these vessels is directed toward the transducer and, therefore, is also encoded red. Blood flow within the **posterior section of the aortic arch** and the **descending aorta** is directed away from the transducer and, therefore, is encoded blue. Blood flow around the inside of the aortic arch travels at a higher velocity than the flow around the outside of the arch.
Flow velocities within these regions often exceed the Nyquist limit resulting in colour aliasing. Hence, colour

Doppler flow around the inside of the anterior segment of the **aortic arch** changes from red to blue while colour Doppler flow around the inside of the posterior section of the aortic arch changes from blue to red. At the top and in the centre of the aorta arch, there is a black region. This region of "no flow" occurs when the direction of blood flow is directly perpendicular to the ultrasound beam so there is no detectable Doppler shift. Figure 8.5 demonstrates the normal colour flow Doppler pattern within the aortic arch.

During *early diastole*, low velocity retrograde flow can be identified within the ascending and descending aorta due to the elastic recoil of the vessel. When present, early diastolic flow reversal within the ascending aorta is directed away from the transducer and, therefore, is encoded blue while flow reversal within the descending aorta is directed toward the transducer and, therefore, is encoded red. Note that this normal reversal of flow occurs only during early diastole and does not occupy the entire vessel lumen.

Subcostal view:
From the subcostal short axis view, the abdominal aorta can be opened out into its long axis. Blood flow within the abdominal aorta is directed toward the transducer (remember that the sector orientation is such that the top of the image represents the inferior aspect of the body while the bottom of the sector depicts the superior aspect). As flow is toward the transducer, it is encoded red (Figure 8.6).

Colour Flow Doppler Examination of Right Atrial Inflow

Blood flow into the right atrium occurs via the inferior vena cava (IVC), superior vena cava (SVC), and the coronary sinus. Coronary sinus flow into the right atrium can not be easily identified by colour flow imaging due to the relatively small volume of flow and the difficulty in aligning the ultrasound beam parallel to the blood flow direction. IVC and SVC flow, as for all veins, is continuous throughout the cardiac cycle.

Examination Windows:
Colour Doppler interrogation of IVC flow into the right atrium can achieved from the parasternal long axis view of the right ventricular inflow tract, the parasternal short axis view at the level of the aorta and left atrium, the apical four chamber view, and from the subcostal views.
Colour Doppler interrogation of SVC flow into the right atrium can be achieved from the subcostal short axis view, the suprasternal short axis view, and from the right supraclavicular window.

Normal Flow Pattern:
Vena caval flow into the right atrium is continuous throughout the cardiac cycle; that is, flow occurs during systole and diastole.

Inferior vena caval flow:
From the parasternal and apical views, blood flow from the IVC into the right atrium is directed toward the transducer and is, therefore, encoded red.
From the subcostal views, blood flow from the IVC into the right atrium is predominantly directed away from the transducer and, therefore, is encoded blue. A brief phase of colour flow reversal within the proximal portion of the IVC can be observed with atrial contraction. When seen, flow appears red as flow is directed toward the transducer.
Hepatic venous flow into the IVC can also be seen from the subcostal views. Blood flow is continuous and is directed away from the transducer and, therefore, is encoded blue.

Superior vena caval flow:
From the subcostal short axis view, blood flow from the SVC into the right atrium is directed toward the transducer and, therefore, is encoded red.
From the suprasternal short axis view and the right supraclavicular window, blood flow within the SVC is directed away from the transducer and, therefore, is encoded blue.
Figure 8.7 demonstrates the normal colour flow Doppler pattern seen in the IVC and SVC from the subcostal view.

Colour Flow Doppler Examination of Right Ventricular Inflow

Right ventricular inflow occurs during diastole as blood flows into the right ventricle from the right atrium via the tricuspid valve.

Examination Windows:
Colour Doppler interrogation of right ventricular inflow is best evaluated from the apical four chamber view where blood flow is the most parallel to the ultrasound beam. Other views that may be utilised include the parasternal long axis view of right ventricular inflow tract, the parasternal short axis view at the level of the aortic valve and left atrium, and the subcostal views.

Normal Flow Pattern:
Blood flow into the right ventricle via the tricuspid valve, from all views, is directed toward the transducer and, therefore, is encoded red. The diastolic flow pattern of right ventricular inflow resembles that of the left ventricular inflow such that flow appears biphasic corresponding to early filling and filling due to atrial contraction (the E and A waves on the spectral Doppler trace). Direct flow from the IVC into the right atrium, through the tricuspid valve, into the right ventricle may also be appreciated from each of these views. Blood flow velocities are slightly less than those seen on the left side of the heart and, therefore, appear in deeper shades of red (Figure 8.8).

Colour Flow Doppler Examination of the Right Ventricular Outflow Tract and the Pulmonary Artery

Blood flow into the right ventricular outflow tract (RVOT) and within the pulmonary artery occurs during systole.

Examination Windows:

Colour Doppler interrogation of right ventricular outflow and pulmonary artery are best evaluated from the parasternal long axis view of the RVOT, the parasternal short axis views (at the level of the aorta and left atrium, and pulmonary artery bifurcation), and from the subcostal views.

Normal Flow Pattern:

Blood flow through the RVOT and the pulmonary artery occurs during ventricular ejection (systole). From the parasternal and subcostal views, blood flow is directed away from the transducer and, therefore, is encoded blue. Blood flow velocities within the pulmonary artery are lower than those seen within the aorta, therefore, flow through these regions is seen in deeper shades. Colour aliasing may occur within the centre of the pulmonary artery trunk when the Nyquist limit is exceeded.

Normally, a trivial degree of "physiological" pulmonary regurgitation is commonly seen (see Tables 8.1 and 8.2). When present, pulmonary regurgitation is encoded red as flow is directed toward the transducer (Figure 8.9).

References and Suggested Reading:

- Feigenbaum, H.: Echocardiography. Chapter 2. 5th Ed. Lea & Febiger, 1994.
- Klein, A.L. et al.: Age-related prevalence of valvular regurgitation in normal subjects: a comprehensive color flow examination of 118 volunteers. *Journal of the American Society of Echocardiography 2:54-63, 1990.*
- Lavie, C.J., et al.: Prevalence and severity of Doppler-detected valvular regurgitation and estimation of right-sided cardiac pressures in patients with normal two-dimensional echocardiograms. *Chest 103:226-231, 1993*
- Maciel, B. et al.: Color flow Doppler mapping studies of "physiologic" pulmonary and tricuspid regurgitation: evidence for true regurgitation as opposed to a valve closing volume. *Journal of the American Society of Echocardiography 4:589-597, 1991.*
- Otto, C.M. and Pearlman, A.S.: Textbook of Clinical Echocardiography. Chapter 2. W.B. Saunders Company. 1995
- Pollack, S.J. et al.: Cardiac evaluation of women distance runners by echocardiographic color Doppler flow mapping. *Journal of the American College of Cardiology 11:89-93,1988.*
- Weyman, A.: Principles and Practice of Echocardiography. Chapter 13. 2nd Ed. Lea & Febiger, 1994.
- Yoshida, K. et al.: Color Doppler evaluation of valvular regurgitation in normal subjects. *Circulation 78:840-847, 1988.*

Chapter 9
Two-Dimensional Echocardiographic Measurements and Calculations

The two-dimensional (2-D) echocardiographic technique permits the real-time and spatial display of cardiac structures. In addition, calculations used in the assessment of systolic function and left ventricular mass can also be performed. Table 9.1 lists the measurements that can be made by 2-D echocardiography.

Several factors influence the accuracy of 2-D measurements and calculations. These factors include:

(1) *image quality* which is primarily dependent upon ultrasonic instrumentation and settings such as the transducer frequency, focal depth and the resolution of the equipment. Accuracy is optimised when the highest frequency transducer that allows adequate penetration is used and when the focal depth is adjusted to the centre of the region or structure of interest;

(2) *technical factors* such as gain settings and gray scale should be optimised to improve accuracy especially when assessing the left ventricle. Too much gain will result in "blooming" of the endocardial echoes while too little gain may result in drop-out along the endocardial borders;

(3) *depth settings* can also affect the precision of 2-D measurements. Measurements should be made at the shallowest depth possible so that the structure or region of interest is "magnified". Further magnification can also be achieved by "zooming" in on the structure to be measured;

(4) *anatomic variables:* accuracy of measurements is dependent upon the correct orientation of imaging planes which is highly dependent upon the recognition of internal landmarks;

(5) *endocardial definition* also affects the accuracy of measurements. In particular, the sonographer must be aware that the endocardium of the ventricles is not smooth-walled but is indented by trabeculations and papillary muscles.

Measurement standards have been outlined and recommended by the American Society of Echocardiography (ASE) to promote uniformity of 2-D measurements [15].

The ASE recommended method for measuring structures by 2-D echocardiography is the *inner edge to inner edge* technique. This society also recommends that end-diastolic and end-systolic measurements be made by reference to the simultaneously recorded mitral valve whenever possible. *End-diastolic* measurements are performed at the frame marking the initial coaptation of the mitral leaflets, or at the frame immediately prior to initial coaptation of the leaflets. *End-systolic* measurements are made at the frame preceding initial early diastolic mitral valve opening.

If the mitral valve is not seen, then end-systole is identified as the smallest visible ventricular cavity size and end-diastole is identified at the Q wave of the ECG.

Linear Dimensional Measurements

M-Mode (motion-mode) echocardiography is generally the method of choice for the measurement of intracardiac chamber dimensions and structures due to its superior temporal and axial resolution as well as its greater interface definition. However, there are instances where 2-D echocardiography is employed in the measurement of certain structures due to particular limitations of the M-Mode technique. These limitations include: (1) the one-dimensional nature of M-mode, (2) its lack of spatial resolution, (3) the fact that structures to

Table 9.1: Two-Dimensional Echocardiographic Measurements.

Linear dimensional measurements	• intracardiac chambers • great vessels (aorta, pulmonary artery, inferior vena cava, hepatic veins) • valve annuli
Area measurements	• annular areas • chamber areas • valve areas
Volume measurements	• left ventricular volumes • right ventricular volumes • atrial volumes
Assessment of left ventricular systolic function	• global systolic function • regional systolic function
Left ventricular mass calculations	• area-length method • truncated ellipse method

15: Schiller, N.B. et al.: Journal of the American Society of Echocardiography 2 (No. 5): 358-367, 1989.

be measured must lie in the axial scan plane, and (4) structures must also be aligned perpendicular to the M-mode cursor. For these reasons, 2-D echocardiographic measurements are used when:

- the spatial orientation for measurements is important (for example, the measurements of the LVOT diameter),
- the structure(s) of interest cannot be aligned perpendicular to the ultrasound beam or do not lie within the axial plane of the ultrasound beam (for example, the pulmonary valve annulus which lies in the lateral scan plane), and
- assessing left ventricular systolic function in the presence of regional wall motion abnormalities (the M-Mode technique identifies the function of the basal segments of two regions only).

It should also be mentioned at this point that the measurement technique for 2-D measurements varies to the M-mode method. While M-mode measurements are traditionally made using the leading edge to leading edge technique, 2-D measurements are performed from the inner edge to the inner edge. M-mode measurements are discussed further in Chapter 10.

Measurement of Intracardiac Chambers:

Intracardiac chambers can be measured in the various planes and from multiple views (see Figure 9.1 and Table 9.2). The normal measurements for intracardiac chambers dimensions are listed in Table 9.3 and 9.4.

Measurements of the Left Ventricle:

The **major axis or long axis of the left ventricle** can be measured, in the superior-inferior plane, from the apical four chamber view . This measurement is made from apical endocardium to the middle of the mitral valve annulus (Figure 9.1.a). Note that the parasternal long axis rarely shows true cardiac apex; hence, the major axis of the left ventricle should not be measured from this view.

The **minor axis or short axis of the left ventricle** can be measured from the apical four chamber view and from various parasternal views. From the apical four chamber view, the minor axis of the left ventricle can be measured in the lateral-medial plane. This measurement is made perpendicular to the hypothetical long axis of

the ventricle from a point one-third the length of this axis as measured from the mitral valve annulus (Figure 9.1.a).

The minor axis of the left ventricle can also be measured from the parasternal long axis view of the left ventricle and from the parasternal short axis views at the level of the papillary muscle level. From these views, the minor axis of the left ventricle is measured in the anterior-posterior plane (Figure 9.1.b and 9.1.c).

A variation in the measurement of the minor axis of the left ventricle, from the parasternal long axis view of the left ventricle, in both diastole and systole has also been described . From this view, the minor axis is measured perpendicular to the long axis of the left ventricle at the level of the chordal-mitral valve junction or at the tips of the mitral leaflets. In this instance, an anatomical landmark, rather than a proportion of the major axis measurement, is used to determine the correct level for this measurement. This is because the minor axis changes location from diastole to systole as the base of the heart moves toward the apex with systolic contraction (Figure 9.2). Observe that the normal values for the minor axis by this method (Table 9.3) are smaller than those reported in Table 9.4 since these measurements are obtained from a more proximal or basal portion of the ventricle.

Table 9.3: Linear normal values for the left ventricle measured by 2-D echocardiography from the parasternal long axis of the left ventricle at the level of the chordal-mitral valve junction or at the tips of the mitral leaflets.

Measurement	Range (cm)	Range Indexed (cm/m²)
LVEDD	3.6 - 5.2	2.0 - 2.8
LVESD	2.3 - 3.9	1.3 - 2.1

Abbreviations: LVEDD = left ventricular end-diastolic dimension; **LVESD** = left ventricular end-systolic dimension.
Source: Feigenbaum, H. Echocardiography. 5th Edition. Lea and Febiger, pp: 669, 1994: patient population: 50 subjects aged 19 to 63 years.

Table 9.2: Measurements Of Intracardiac Chambers: Views and Planes.

Views	Planes
Parasternal long axis (left ventricle)	superior-inferior anterior-posterior lateral-medial
Parasternal short axis view (aorta and left atrium)	anterior-posterior
Parasternal short axis (papillary muscles)	anterior-posterior
Parasternal short axis (chordae tendineae)	anterior-posterior
Apical four chamber	superior-inferior lateral-medial

Measurement of the Right Ventricle:

The **major axis or long axis of the right ventricle** can be measured in the superior-inferior plane from the apical four chamber view . This measurement is made from the apical endocardium to middle of tricuspid valve annulus.

The **minor axis or short axis of the right ventricle** can be measured from either the parasternal long axis view or the apical four chamber view. From the apical four chamber view, the minor axis of the right ventricle can be measured in the lateral-medial plane. This measurement is made perpendicular to the major axis from a point one-third the length of this axis from tricuspid valve annulus (Figure 9.1.a). From the parasternal long axis of the left ventricle, the minor axis of the right ventricle can be measured in the anterior-posterior plane (Figure 9.1.c). Note that this measurement is variable as the position of the right ventricle may change with patient positioning.

Measurement of Left and Right Atrial Dimensions:

The **major or long axes of the left and right atria** can be measured in the superior-inferior plane from the apical four chamber view . This measurement is made from the middle of the atrioventricular valve annulus to the superior wall of the atrium (Figure 9.1.a).

The **minor or short axes of the right atrium** can be measured from the apical four chamber view. From this view, the minor axis of the atrium can be measured in the lateral-medial plane. This measurement is made from the point that is one-half the length of the major axis of the atrium (Figure 9.1.a).

The **minor or short axes of the left atrium** can be measured from the parasternal long and short views or from the apical four chamber view. From the apical four chamber view, the minor axis of the atrium can be measured in the lateral-medial plane. This measurement is made from the point that is one-half the length of the major axis of the atrium (Figure 9.1.a). From the parasternal long axis of the left ventricle or the parasternal short axis view at the level of aorta and left atrium, the minor axis of the left atrium can be measured in the anterior-posterior plane (Figure 9.1.c and 9.1.d). This measurement is made from posterior aortic wall to posterior left atrial wall.

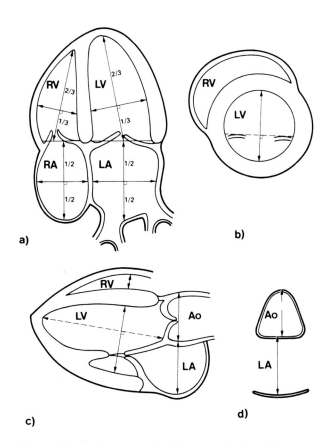

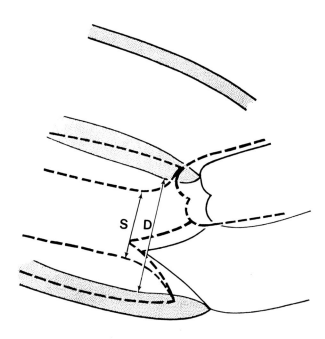

Figure 9.1: Methods used to Measure Cardiac Chamber Dimensions from the Two-Dimensional Image.

Intracardiac dimensions can be obtained from five different echocardiographic views: the apical four chamber view (**a**), the parasternal short axis view at the level of the chordae tendineae (**b**) and at the papillary muscle level (not illustrated), the parasternal long axis view (**c**), and the parasternal short axis view at the level of the aorta (**d**). The various minor and major axes are indicated by the arrows (see text for details).

Abbreviations: AO = aorta; **LA** = left atrium; **LV** = left ventricle; **RA** = right atrium; **RV** = right ventricle.

From Schittger, I. et al.: Standardized intracardiac measurements of two-dimensional echocardiography. *Journal of the American College of Cardiology 2:935,1983.* Reproduced with permission from the American College of Cardiology.

Figure 9.2: Variation of the Linear Measurement of the Minor Axis of the Left Ventricle from the Parasternal Long Axis View.

Using this method, the minor axis dimensions of the left ventricle during systole (S) and diastole (D) are determined by an anatomical landmark rather than a proportion of the long axis (as illustrated in Figure 9.1). This is because the location of the systolic dimensions varies from the diastolic dimension as the heart moves toward the apex with systolic contraction. Observe that the systolic measurement is made closer toward the apex than the diastolic measurement.

From Schiller, N.B. et al.: Recommendations from quantitation of the left ventricle by two-dimensional echocardiography. *Journal of the American Society of Echocardiography 2:362,1989.* Reproduced with permission from Mosby, Inc., St. Louis, MO, USA

Table 9.4: Normal Values for Cardiac Chambers Measured by 2-D Echocardiography.

Two-dimensional View	Normal range (cm) [mean ± 2 SD]	Mean Value (cm)	Indexed Normal Range (cm/m²)	Absolute Range (cm)
Apical Four-Chamber				
LVED major	6.9 - 10.3	8.6	4.1 - 5.7	7.2 - 10.3
LVED minor	3.3 - 6.1	4.7	2.2 - 3.1	3.8 - 6.2
LVES minor	1.9 - 3.7	2.8	1.3 - 2.0	2.1 - 3.9
RV major	6.5 - 9.5	8.0	3.8 - 5.3	6.3 - 9.3
RV minor	2.2 - 4.4	3.3	1.0 - 2.8	2.2 - 4.5
LA major	4.1 - 6.1	5.1	2.3 - 3.5	4.2 - 6.1
LA minor	2.8 - 4.3	3.5	1.6 - 2.4	2.9 - 4.3
RA major	3.5 - 5.5	4.5	2.0 - 3.1	3.4 - 5.7
RA minor	2.5 - 4.9	3.7	1.7 - 2.5	2.6 - 5.0
Minor Axis Dimensions				
Parasternal Long-Axis				
LVED	3.5 - 6.0	4.8	2.3 - 3.1	3.8 - 5.8
LVES	2.1 - 4.0	3.1	1.4 - 2.1	2.3 - 3.9
RV	1.9 - 3.8	2.8	1.2 - 2.0	1.9 - 3.9
LA	2.7 - 4.5	3.6	1.6 - 2.4	2.8 - 4.4
Ao	2.2 - 3.6	2.9	1.4 - 2.0	2.3 - 3.7
Parasternal Short-Axis (Aorta)				
LA	2.6 - 4.5	3.6	1.6 - 2.4	2.7 - 4.5
Ao	2.3 - 3.7	3.0	1.6 - 2.4	2.7 - 4.5
Parasternal Short-Axis (Chordae)				
LVED	3.5 - 6.2	4.8	2.3 - 3.2	3.8 - 6.1
LVES	2.3 - 4.0	3.2	1.5 - 2.2	2.6 - 4.2
Parasternal Short-Axis (Papillary Muscles)				
LVED	3.5 - 5.8	4.7	2.2 - 3.1	3.9 - 5.8
LVES	2.2 - 4.0	3.1	1.4 - 2.2	2.5 - 4.1

Abbreviations: Ao = aorta; **LA** = left atrium; **LVED** = left ventricle end-diastole; **LVES** = left ventricle end-systole; **RA** = right atrium; **RV** = right ventricle.

Source: Schittger, I. et al., *Journal of the American College of Cardiology* 2:934,1983: patient population: 35 subjects: 19 men and 16 women, aged 18 to 60 years.

Technical Consideration:
The body surface area (BSA) has a direct effect on the absolute measurements; hence, the comparison of absolute measurements without BSA correction can lead to significant errors. Therefore, it is recommended that all absolute measurements be corrected for the BSA.

Measurements of the Great Vessels:
The great vessels which can be measured by 2-D echocardiography include various levels of the aorta, the pulmonary artery and its branches, the inferior vena cava, and the hepatic veins. The normal ranges for great vessel dimensions are listed in Table 9.5.

Aortic Dimensions:
The various levels of the aorta that can be measured include the aortic annulus, the transaortic sinus, the sino-tubular junction, the aortic arch, and the descending aorta. The **aortic annulus, transaortic sinus,** and the **sino-tubular junction** diameters can be measured from the parasternal long axis of the left ventricle in the anterior-posterior plane (Figure 9.3). The transaortic sinus can also be measured in the anterior-posterior plane from

the parasternal short axis view at the level of aorta and left atrium . All measurements are made from the anterior aortic wall to the posterior aortic wall.

The **aortic arch** and **descending aortic** dimensions can be measured from the suprasternal long axis of the aortic arch. The aortic arch is measured in the superior-inferior dimension while the descending aorta (distal to the left subclavian artery) is measured in the anterior-posterior plane (Figure 9.4).

Pulmonary Artery Dimensions:
The pulmonary annulus, main pulmonary artery, and the left and right pulmonary artery branch diameters can be measured from the parasternal long axis of the RVOT. These dimensions can also be measured from the parasternal short axis view at the level of the pulmonary artery bifurcation in the lateral-medial plane (Figure 9.5).

Inferior Vena Cava and Hepatic Vein Dimensions:
The inferior vena cava (IVC) and hepatic veins can be measured from the subcostal short axis of the long axis of the IVC (Figure 9.6). The IVC is measured proximal to its entrance into the right atrium and the hepatic vein is measured proximal to its entrance into the IVC.

? aneurysm

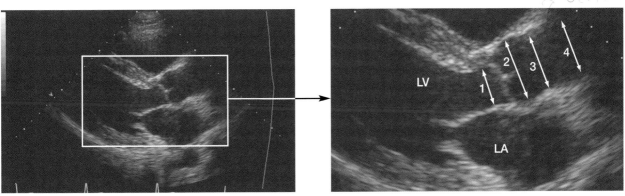

Figure 9.3: Measurements of the Various Levels of the Aorta from the Parasternal Long Axis View:
1. aortic annulus   **2.** trans-sinus   **3.** sinotubular junction   **4.** ascending aorta
Abbreviations: LV = Left Ventricle; **LA** = Left Atrium.

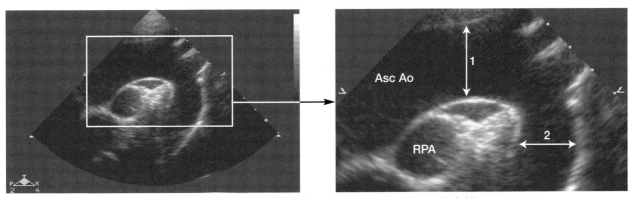

Figure 9.4: Measurements of the Various Levels of the Aorta from the Suprasternal Long Axis View:
1. aortic arch   **2.** descending aorta
Abbreviations: Asc Ao = ascending aorta; **RPA** = right pulmonary artery.

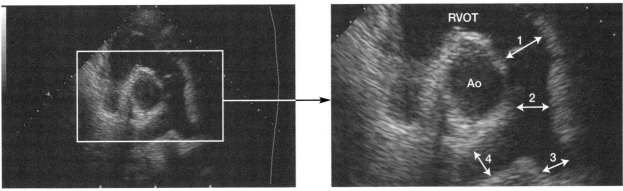

Figure 9.5: Measurements of the Various Levels of the Pulmonary Artery from the Parasternal Short Axis View.
1. pulmonary annulus   **2.** main pulmonary artery trunk   **3.** left pulmonary artery   **4.** right pulmonary artery
Abbreviations: Ao = aorta; **RVOT** = right ventricular outflow tract.

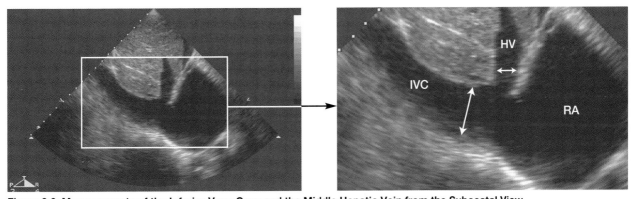

Figure 9.6: Measurements of the Inferior Vena Cava and the Middle Hepatic Vein from the Subcostal View.
1. inferior vena cava   **2.** hepatic vein
Abbreviations: HV = hepatic vein; **IVC =** inferior vena cava; **RA** = right atrium.

Table 9.5: Normal 2-D Measurements for the Great Vessels.

Cardiac Structures	Patient Population	Normal Dimensions (cm) [mean ± 1 Standard Deviation]	Range (cm)
Aortic Dimensions (end-diastolic):			
- aortic annulus	68	1.9 ± 0.2	1.4 - 2.6
- trans-sinus	68	2.8 ± 0.3	2.1 - 3.5
- sino-tubular	64	2.4 ± 0.4	1.7 - 3.4
- ascending aorta	44	2.6 ± 0.3	2.1 - 3.4
- aortic arch	42	2.7 ± 0.3	2.0 - 3.6
Pulmonary Artery Dimensions (end-diastolic):			
- pulmonary annulus	51	1.5 ± 0.3	1.0 - 2.2
- main pulmonary artery trunk	48	1.8 ± 0.3	0.9 - 2.9
- right pulmonary artery	39	1.2 ± 0.2	0.7 - 1.7
- left pulmonary artery	11	1.2 ± 0.2	0.6 - 1.4
Inferior Vena Cava	52	1.7 ± 0.3	1.2 - 2.3
Hepatic Vein	12	0.8 ± 0.2	0.5 - 1.1

Abbreviations: LPA = left pulmonary artery; **PA** = pulmonary artery; **Pt. Pop.** = patient population; **RPA** = right pulmonary artery; **SD** = standard deviation.
Source: Triulzi, M. et al., *Echocardiography 1 (no. 4): 403-426, 1984.*

Measurements of Annular Diameters:

Measurements of the annular diameters for all four cardiac valves can be made using the inner edge to inner edge method. Annulus diameters can be measured during both systole and diastole. Annulus diameters used for volumetric flow calculations are typically measured during the normal flow period through each valve. The normal ranges for valve annular dimensions are listed in Table 9.6.

Left Ventricular Outflow Tract (LVOT):

Measurements of the LVOT can be made from the parasternal long axis of the left ventricle during systole. This measurement is made from the inner edge of the junction between the anterior aortic wall and the interventricular septum to the inner edge of the junction between the posterior aortic wall and the anterior leaflet of the mitral valve (Figure 9.7).

Right Ventricular Outflow Tract (RVOT):

Measurements of the RVOT can be made from the parasternal long axis of the RVOT and from the parasternal short axis view (at the level of aorta and left atrium during systole). This measurement is made just proximal to the pulmonary valve leaflets (Figure 9.8).

Mitral Valve Annulus:

Measurements of the mitral annulus can be made from the apical four chamber view and from the apical two chamber view during mid-diastole (Figure 9.9).

Tricuspid Valve Annulus:

Measurements of the tricuspid annulus can be made from the apical four chamber view during mid-diastole (Figure 9.9).

Table 9.6: Normal 2-D Values for Annular Dimensions.

Cardiac Structures	Normal Dimensions [Range] (cm)	
	Diastole [1]	Systole [2]
LVOT	1.4 - 2.6	1.8 – 2.2
RVOT	1.8 – 3.4	…
Mitral annulus	3.0 – 3.5	1.8 – 3.1
Tricuspid annulus	…	1.3 – 2.8

Abbreviations: LVOT = left ventricular outflow tract; **RVOT** = right ventricular outflow tract.
Sources: (1) Triulzi, M. et al., *Echocardiography 1 (no. 4): 403-426, 1984;* (2) Reynolds, T.: <u>The Echocardiographer's Pocket Reference.</u> Arizona Heart Institute Foundation, pp: 144, 1993.

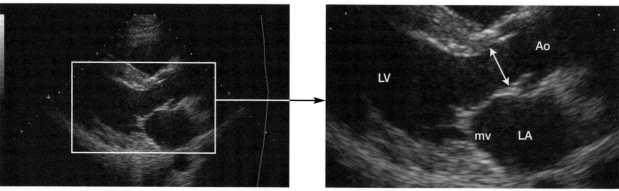

Figure 9.7: Measurement of the Left Ventricular Outflow Tract from the Parasternal Long Axis View of the Left Ventricle
Abbreviations: Ao = aorta; **LA** = left atrium; **LV** = left ventricle; **mv** = mitral valve.

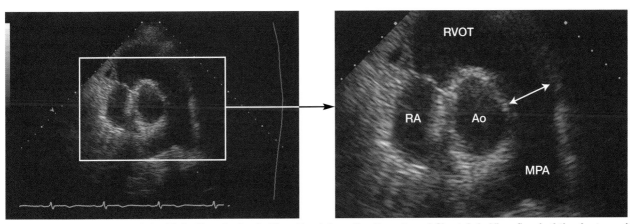

Figure 9.8: Measurement of the Right Ventricular Outflow Tract from the Parasternal Short Axis View (level of the Aorta and Left Atrium)
Abbreviations: **Ao** = aorta; **MPA** = main pulmonary artery; **RA** = right atrium; **RVOT** = right ventricular outflow tract.

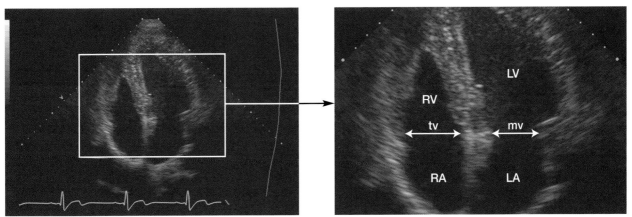

Figure 9.9: Measurement of the Mitral Valve Annulus and the Tricuspid Valve Annulus from the Apical Four Chamber View.
Abbreviations: **LA** = left atrium; **LV** = left ventricle; **mv** = mitral valve; **RA** = right atrium; **RV** = right ventricle; **tv** = tricuspid valve.

Area Calculations

The areas that can be calculated by 2-D echocardiography include annular areas, chamber areas, and valve areas.

Measurement of Annular and Chamber Areas:

The echocardiographic views used to calculate valve annular diameters have been described above. The echocardiographic view preferable for obtaining chamber area, is the apical four chamber view. 2-D echocardiographic areas are calculated based on the standard mathematical calculations where the area can be derived from: (1) the radius, (2) the diameter, or (3) the circumference. The normal values for chamber areas are listed in Table 9.7.

1. Areas from the Radius:

Annular areas can be calculated by application of the standard mathematical formula using the radius (r):

(Equation 9.1)

$$Area = \pi r^2$$

2. Areas from the Diameter:

Since valve annular diameters rather than radii are measured by 2-D echocardiography, area calculations derived from the diameter can also be employed:

(Equation 9.2)

$$Area = 0.785 \times D^2$$

Technical Consideration:
As the radius is simply the diameter divided by 2, the area using the diameter is calculated as follows:

$$Area = \pi \times \left(\frac{D}{2}\right)^2$$

$$= \pi \times \frac{D^2}{2^2}$$

$$= \pi \times \frac{D^2}{4}$$

$$= \frac{\pi}{4} \times D^2$$

$$= 0.785 \times D^2$$

---

ef normal range
wall thickness — LV. RV, Septum. Aortic root

3. Areas from the Circumference:

Chamber areas can be measured from the apical four chamber view by tracing the chamber circumference and using the following equation:

(Equation 9.3)

$$Area = \left(\frac{1}{2}\right) \sum_{i=1}^{N-1} X_i \, (Y_i - Y_{i-1}) - Y_i \, (X_i - X_{i-1})$$

Measurement of Valve Areas:

By tracing the circumference of a stenotic valve orifice, it is also possible to measure stenotic valve areas. Valve areas can be measured by direct 2-D planimetry of the valve orifice from the short axis view of the valve.

The mitral valve area (MVA) is most commonly planimetered and while it is theoretically possible to planimeter the aortic valve area (AVA), this is rarely done in routine clinical practice (see below). The tricuspid and pulmonary valves are not usually seen in a true short axis plane and, therefore, cannot be planimetered by 2-D echocardiography.

Mitral Valve Area by Direct Planimetry:

When the mitral valve is displayed in its short axis, the valve area can be planimetered and calculated from the circumference (equation 9.3). In fact, direct 2-D planimetry of the MVA is now regarded as the most accurate, noninvasive method in the quantification of mitral stenosis [16+17].

The principal advantages of 2-D echocardiography in the direct planimetry of the MVA in mitral stenosis include: (1) its ability, as a non-invasive technique, to provide a direct measurement of the actual anatomical mitral valve orifice, (2) the reported strong relationship of the planimetered MVA with other proven and accepted techniques, and (3) the reported high feasibility of this technique.

The reliability and accuracy of 2-D echocardiography in the direct planimetry of the MVA is dependent upon: (1) the ability to clearly delineate the mitral valve orifice, (2) measurement of the orifice at the correct level, (3) gain settings, and (4) the skill and experience of the operator.

Limitations: Probably the most important technical factor which affects the accuracy of direct planimetry of the MVA is the ability of the operator to identify the true valve orifice. In mitral stenosis, there is fusion and tethering of the leaflet tips of the valve resulting in a funnel-shaped orifice. Therefore, it is crucial that the valve orifice is measured at the leaflet tips and not at the base of the valve otherwise a falsely large valve area will be measured (Figure 9.10). The recommended scanning technique that should be adopted to correctly locate the stenotic mitral orifice is also outlined over (boxed).

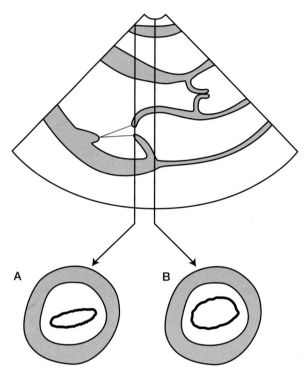

Figure 9.10: 2-D Planimetry of the Mitral Valve Area at Various Levels.
This schematic illustrates the effect of measuring the mitral valve area (MVA) from various levels. With mitral valve stenosis, there is tethering at the leaflet tips with doming of the anterior leaflet during diastole. Therefore, there is a marked difference between the area of the mitral valve orifice measured at the tips of the mitral leaflets **(A)** compared with the MVA measured through the body of the leaflets **(B)**. The correct level for planimetry of the MVA is at level A.

Table 9.7: Normal 2-D Area Measurements for the Cardiac Chambers.

Cardiac Chamber	Pt. Pop.	Normal Dimensions (cm²) [mean ± 1 SD]	Range (cm²)
Left ventricle:			
- end-diastole	62	33.2 ± 7.7	17.7 - 47.3
- end-systole	62	17.6 ± 5.2	7. - 31.5
Right ventricle:			
- end-diastole	41	20.1 ± 4.0	10.7 - 35.5
- end-systole	41	10.9 ± 2.9	4.5 - 20
Left atrium (systole)	68	14.2 ± 3.0	8.8 - 23.4
Right atrium (systole)	67	13.5 ± 2.0	8.3 - 19.5

Source: Triulzi, M. et al., *Echocardiography 1 (no. 4): 403-426, 1984.*

16. Feigenbaum, H.: Echocardiography. 5th Edition. USA: Lea and Febiger, pp: 241, 24, 1994. 17. Weyman, A.E.: Principles and Practice of Echocardiography. 2nd Edition. USA: Lea and Febiger, pp: 420, 1994.

Method for Determining the Correct Level for Planimetry of the Mitral Valve Area by 2-D Echo.
Step 1: direct the scan plane inferiorly toward the left ventricular cavity to the level of the papillary muscles;
Step 2: angle the transducer slightly medially and tilt superiorly until the tips of the mitral leaflets are identified (this should correspond to the smallest MVA);
Step 3: freeze the image in early diastole;
Step 4: trace the MVA along the inner margins of the leaflets.

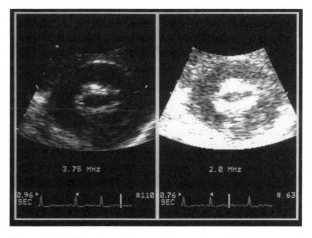

Figure 9.11: The importance of transducer frequency and gain settings on the resolution of the 2-D echocardiographic image in the measurement of the mitral valve area.
These two images illustrate the importance of image resolution on the accuracy of measuring the MVA by 2-D echocardiography. Resolution is primarily dependent on transducer frequency such that the higher the transducer frequency the better the resolution. Resolution is also dependent upon gain.
Left, This image demonstrates the MVA using a 3.75 MHz transducer frequency with minimal gain settings. This image is considered the optimal image from which the MVA can be accurately measured.
Right, This image demonstrates the MVA, from the same patient, using a lower frequency transducer (2.0 MHz) with increased gain settings. Observe that the MVA appears much smaller as a direct result of poor image resolution. Measurement of the MVA using this image will lead to a signifcant underestimation of the true MVA.

Other limitations which may prevent the clear delineation of the true mitral valve orifice include dense fibrosis or calcification along the margins of leaflets and excessive image gain. As well as distorting the valve orifice, intense reflections from calcification may cause the leaflet to appear thicker and the orifice to appear smaller resulting in an underestimation of the true orifice area. Instrument factors may also have a significant affect on the accuracy of the MVA measurement by 2-D echocardiography. Increased gain settings ("over-gain") may produce a "blooming" effect resulting in an underestimation of the true MVA due to the encroachment of artifactual echoes into the lumen of the mitral valve orifice. Furthermore, the resolution of the instrument may also significantly affect the accuracy of this technique. Resolution (axial or lateral) is defined as the ability of ultrasound to distinguish or identify two objects that lie in close proximity. Lateral resolution refers to the ability to differentiate two objects that lie side by side and is determined primarily by transducer frequency. Decreasing the transducer frequency, decreases the lateral resolution. This reduction in resolution may lead to the "drop-out" of echoes in the lateral margins of the mitral valve orifice producing a false extension of the lateral and medial commissures of the valve leading to an overestimation of the MVA. Therefore, when attempting to measure the MVA by 2-D echocardiography, careful attention to the selection of the optimal transducer frequency and the gain settings is required. Figure 9.11 demonstrates the importance of transducer frequency and gain settings in the measurement of the MVA.

Significant limitations of 2-D echocardiography in the measurement of the mitral valve orifice have also been reported following commissurotomy. The difficulty experienced in the measurement of the MVA by 2-D echocardiography in these patients occurs due a combination of distortion of the mitral valve orifice as well as extensive thickening of the valve leaflets.

However, despite these limitations described above, in the hands of a skilled operator, direct planimetry of the MVA by 2-D echocardiography remains the procedure of choice in the assessment of the severity of mitral stenosis.

Aortic Valve Area by Direct Planimetry:
As mentioned, the direct assessment of the anatomical valve area provides the most precise evaluation of the true valve area. However, although direct planimetry of the AVA by 2-D echocardiography is possible, the feasibility of performing this technique by transthoracic echocardiography is quite poor.

Direct planimetry of the AVA by 2-D echocardiography is less successful than the planimetry of the MVA for several reasons:
(1) rarely are all three leaflets of the aortic valve sufficiently imaged perpendicular to the ultrasound beam to allow adequate delineation of the entire perimeter of the orifice area in systole,
(2) the triangular-shape of the aortic orifice and the eccentricity of this trileaflet valve creates a greater potential for measurement error,
(3) structural deformities and irregularities of the stenotic aortic valve further exacerbate the difficulty of this measurement,
(4) the aortic valve moves rapidly in a superior-inferior direction during systole. Therefore, the valve orifice passes rapidly through the scan plane making the localisation of the true aortic valve orifice more difficult, and
(5) a value of only 0.25 cm² separates mild aortic

stenosis (AVA > 1.0 cm²) from severe aortic stenosis (AVA < 0.75 cm²), therefore, any small measurement error may significantly overestimate or underestimate the severity of this lesion.

Therefore, because of these significant limitations described above, direct 2-D planimetry of the AVA by transthoracic echocardiography is not recommended.

Cardiac Chamber Volumes

Cardiac chamber volumes that can be calculated by 2-D echocardiography include the left ventricular systolic and diastolic volumes, and the left and right atrial volumes (usually calculated during systole).

Left Ventricular Volume Calculations:

The ASE recommends that left ventricular volumes are calculated from the dimensional and area measurements obtained from the apical four chamber and apical two chamber views as these two views are nearly orthogonal (60 to 90 degrees) to each other. Two methods have been recommended for the calculation of left ventricular volumes: (1) the modified Simpson's biplane method and (2) the single plane area-length method.

The normal values for the left ventricular volumes calculated by each method are listed in Table 9.8.

1. The Modified Simpson's Biplane Rule:

The ASE recommended algorithm for calculation of ventricular volumes is based on the method of discs or the disc summation method (Figure 9.12). This algorithm is also known as the modified Simpson's rule and, when paired apical views are measured, it is referred to as the modified Simpson's biplane method. The primary advantage of this method is that it treats the ventricle as a series of discs and, therefore, is independent of the geometrical shape of the ventricle. Furthermore, volumes derived from this algorithm closely approximate angiographic volumes. Calculation of ventricular volumes by this algorithm is complex and, therefore, cannot be easily measured manually. Calculations are readily computed by most state-of-the-art ultrasound equipment. The formula for the method of discs divides the ventricular length (L) into 20 equal sections and is expressed by the following equation:

(Equation 9.4)

$$Volume = \frac{\pi}{4} \sum_{i=1}^{20} a_i b_i \frac{L}{20}$$

where a = diameter in plane 1 (cm)
b = diameter in plane 2 (cm)
L = length (cm)

The accuracy of ventricular volume calculations by this method is dependent upon the apical four chamber length and apical two chamber length being nearly equal. It is recommended that when the difference in length between these two views is greater than 20%, volume analysis should be disregarded.

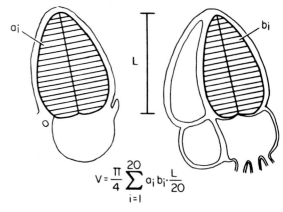

$$V = \frac{\pi}{4} \sum_{i=1}^{20} a_i b_i \cdot \frac{L}{20}$$

Figure 9.12: Calculation of Ventricular Volumes by the Simpson's Biplane Method.

Calculation of the volumes from this method results from the summation of discs (equation 9.4). The discs are derived from the length and the diameters of the disc. The length of each disc is apportioned by dividing the longest length of the left ventricle into 20 equal segments. The diameters of the disc (ai and bi) are measured from two orthogonal planes. The biplane method recommended by the ASE requires that volumes are calculated from two orthogonal planes (apical four chamber and apical two chamber views) with nearly equal long axes.

From Schiller, N.B. et al.: Recommendations from quantitation of the left ventricle by two-dimensional echocardiography. *Journal of the American Society of Echocardiography* 2:362,1989. Reproduced with permission from Mosby Inc., St. Louis, MO, USA

Table 9.8: Normal left ventricular volumes calculated from the area length and Simpson's biplane methods.

Method & Measurement	Men (No. = 29)	Women (No. = 23)
Four-chamber area-length:		
EDV - mean ± SD (cc)	112 ± 27	89 ± 20
EDV - range (cc)	65 - 193	59 - 136
EDV indexed - mean (cc/m²)	58	50
ESV - mean ± SD (cc)	35 ± 16	33 ± 12
ESV - range (cc)	13 - 86	13 - 59
ESV indexed - mean (cc/m²)	18	18
Two-chamber area-length:		
EDV - mean ± SD (cc)	130 ± 27	92 ± 19
EDV - range (cc)	73 - 201	53 - 146
EDV indexed - mean (cc/m²)	68	37
ESV - mean ± SD (cc)	40 ± 14	31 ± 11
ESV - range (cc)	17 - 74	11 - 53
ESV indexed - mean (cc/m²)	21	19
Biplane disc summation (modified Simpson's rule)		
EDV - mean ± SD (cc)	111 ± 22	80 ± 12
EDV - range (cc)	62 - 170	55 - 101
EDV indexed - mean (cc/m²)	58	50
ESV - mean ± SD (cc)	34 ± 12	29 ± 10
ESV - range (cc)	14 - 76	13 - 60
ESV indexed - mean (cc/m²)	18	18

Abbreviations: EDV = end-diastolic volume; **ESV** = end-systolic volume; **No.** = patient numbers; **SD** = standard deviation.

Source: Wahr, D.W. et al., *Journal of the American College of Cardiology* 1:863-868,1983.

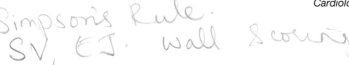

2. Single Plane Area-Length Method:
This method for ventricular volume calculations is used when only one apical view is able to be assessed and when the ventricle is considered symmetrical (Figure 9.13). The formula for calculation of ventricular volumes by this method is expressed by the following equation:

(Equation 9.5)

$$Volume = 0.85 \frac{A^2}{L}$$

where A = area of the ventricle from either the apical two or four chamber view (cm²)
  L = long axis length of the ventricle from the above view (cm)

Atrial Volume Calculations:
Left and right atrial volume calculations can be measured during ventricular systole when the volumes of the atria are at their largest. The echocardiographic views which may be utilised for left atrial volume calculations include the parasternal long axis of the left ventricle, the parasternal short axis view (at the level of aorta and left atrium), the apical four chamber view, and the apical two chamber view. Right atrial volume calculations can be measured from the apical four chamber view. The normal values for atrial volumes are listed in Table 9.9. Three methods have been described for the calculation of atrial volumes: (1) the single plane area-length method, (2) the single plane diameter-length method, and (3) the method of discs.

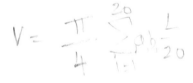

BY SINGLE PLANE AREA LENGTH

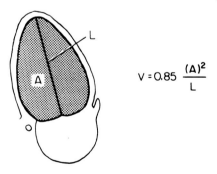

Figure 9.13: Calculation of Ventricular Volumes by the Single Plane Area Length Method.
This method for ventricular volume calculations can only be used when the ventricle is symmetrical and when only one apical view is obtainable. Volume is calculated from the area (A) of the ventricle *(shaded area)* and from the long axis length (L) of the ventricle.
From Schiller, N.B. et al.: Recommendations from quantitation of the left ventricle by two-dimensional echocardiography. *Journal of the American Society of Echocardiography* 2:362,1989. Reproduced with permission from Mosby Inc., St. Louis, MO, USA

1. Single Plane Area-Length Method:
The atrial volumes can be calculated using the area and the long axis length of the atrium (Figure 9.14 - *top*):

(Equation 9.5)

$$Volume = 0.85 \frac{A^2}{L}$$

where A = area of atrium in any view (cm²)
  L = long axis length of atrium from above view (cm)

2. Single Plane Diameter-Length Method:
The atrial volumes can also be calculated using the diameter and the long axis length of the atrium from the same view (Figure 9.14 - *middle*):

(Equation 9.6)

$$Volume = \frac{\pi D^2 L}{6}$$

where D = minor axis in any view (cm)
  L = major or long axis in the same view (cm)

3. Method of Discs:
The method of discs or Simpson's rule can also be used to calculate atrial volumes (Figure 9.14 - *bottom*). Calculation of volumes by this algorithm is based on division of the atrial length (L) into an equal number of sections (n) and is expressed by the following equation:

(Equation 9.7)

$$Volume = \frac{\pi}{4} \sum_{i=1}^{n} a_i \frac{L}{n}$$

Table 9.9: Normal Values for Left and Right Atrial Volumes.

Method & Measurement	Men (No. = 23)	Women (No. = 25)
Four Chamber Area-Length:		
LAV - Mean ± SD (cc)	38 ± 10	34 ± 12
LAV - Range (cc)	24 - 56	15 - 56
LAV - Indexed - mean ± SD (cc/m²)	20 ± 6	21 ± 8
LAV - Indexed - range (cc/m²)	11 - 31	10 - 36
RAV - Mean ± SD (cc)	39 ± 12	27 ± 7
RAV - Range (cc)	15 - 58	14 - 44
RAV - Indexed - mean ± SD (cc/m²)	21 ± 6	17 ± 4
RAV - Indexed - range (cc/m²)	8 - 33	8 - 27
Two Chamber Area-Length:		
LAV - Mean ± SD (cc)	46 ± 14	36 ± 11
LAV - Range (cc)	25 - 77	13 - 59
LAV - Indexed - mean ± SD (cc/m²)	24 ± 8	22 ± 7
LAV - Indexed - range (cc/m²)	12 - 48	8 - 23
Biplane disc summation (modified Simpson's rule)		
LAV - Mean ± SD (cc)	38 ± 10	32 ± 10
LAV - Range (cc)	20 - 57	15 - 46
LAV - Indexed - mean ± SD (cc/m²)	20 ± 6	20 ± 8
LAV - Indexed - range (cc/m²)	10 - 31	10 - 31

Abbreviations: LAV = left atrial volume; **RAV** = right atrial volume; **SD** = standard deviation.
Source: Wang, Y. et al., *Chest 86:595-601,1984.*

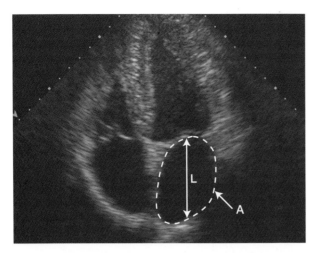

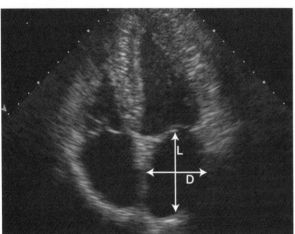

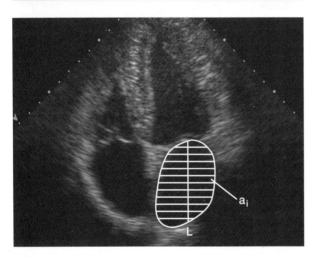

Figure 9.14: Calculation of atrial volumes by three methods.
These figures illustrate calculation of the left atrial volume from the apical four chamber view by three methods: the single plane area-length method (*top*), the single plane diameter-length method (*middle*), and the method of discs (*bottom*).
Top, The left atrial volume can be calculated by tracing the area (**A**) of the atrium and by measuring the long axis (**L**) of the atrium in the superior-inferior plane. The volume is then calculated using equation 9.5.
Middle, The atrial volume can be calculated by measuring the diameter (**D**) of the atrium in the lateral-medial plane and by measuring the long axis (**L**) of the atrium in the superior-inferior plane. The volume is then calculated using equation 9.6.
Bottom, The atrial volume can be calculated using the method of discs whereby the length (**L**) of the atria is divided into equal sections and the area, ai, of *n* number of discs of equal height are summed. The volume is calculated using equation 9.7.

Right Ventricular Volume Calculations:
Despite numerous attempts to calculate right ventricular volumes, the techniques that have been developed so far are complicated. The complexities of measuring right ventricular volumes arise from the irregular geometry of the right ventricle, the inability to visualise the entire ventricle in any one plane, and movement of the right ventricle with patient positioning. Therefore, no technique has been inaugurated into the routine echocardiographic examination for the calculation of this volume.

Left Ventricular Systolic Function
Several 2-D echocardiographic methods can be employed in the assessment of left ventricular global and regional systolic function.

Assessment of Global Left Ventricular Systolic Function:
From the 2-D measurement of left ventricular end-diastolic and end-systolic dimensions, and calculation of left ventricular end-diastolic and end-systolic volumes, it is possible to assess left ventricular systolic performance. Methods for assessing global systolic function of the left ventricle include calculation of the: (1) fractional shortening, (2) ejection fraction, and (3) stroke volume, cardiac output and cardiac index. The normal values for these calculations are listed in Table 9.10.

Fraction Shortening
Fractional shortening is the percentage of change in the left ventricular cavity dimension with systole. The standard measurements of the left ventricle required for this calculation include the left ventricular end-diastolic dimension (LVEDD) and the left ventricular end-systolic dimension (LVESD).
The percentage fractional shortening (FS%) is calculated from the following equation:

(Equation 9.8)

$$FS(\%) = \frac{LVEDD - LVESD}{LVEDD} \times 100$$

Ejection Fraction
The ejection fraction is the percentage of the left ventricular diastolic volume that is ejected with systole; that is, the ejection fraction is the ratio of the stroke volume to the end-diastolic volume. The left ventricular end-diastolic volume (LVEDV) and the left ventricular end-systolic volume (LVESV) can be measured by either the Simpson's biplane method or the area-length method. The ejection fraction (EF %) can be calculated using the following equation:

(Equation 9.9)

$$EF(\%) = \frac{LVEDV - LVESV}{LVEDV} \times 100$$

Table 9.10: Normal values for left ventricular systolic function indices by 2-D echocardiography.

Measurement of LV Systolic Function	Range	Pt. Pop.
Fractional Shortening: [1]		35
- apical 4 chamber view	27 - 50 %	
- parasternal long axis (LV)	25 - 46 %	
- parasternal short axis (chordae)	27 - 42 %	
- parasternal short axis (papillary muscles)	25 - 43 %	
Ejection Fraction [2]	70 ± 7 % (male)	44
	65 ± 10 % (female)	40
Stroke Volume [3]	75 - 100 (cc)	-
Cardiac Output [3]	4 - 8 L/min	-
Cardiac Index [3]	2.4 - 4.2 L/min/m2	-

Sources: (1) Schittger, I. et al., *Journal of the American College of Cardiology 2:934,1983*; **(2)** Mickelson, J.K. et al., *American Heart Journal.* 112: 1251-1256, 1986; **(3)** Schlant, R. and Alexander R.W.: Hurst's. The Heart. 8th Edition. McGraw-Hill, Inc. pp: 141 and 503, 1994.

Stroke Volume, Cardiac Output, and Cardiac Index

Stroke volume (SV) refers to the amount of blood pumped by the heart on each single beat. The cardiac output (CO) is the volume of blood pumped by the heart per minute and the cardiac index (CI) is the cardiac output divided by the body surface area (BSA). These variables can be calculated using the LVEDV and LVESV by either the Simpson's biplane method or the area-length method:

(Equation 9.10)

$$SV = LVEDV - LVESV$$

(Equation 9.11)

$$CO = \frac{SV \times HR}{1000}$$

(Equation 9.12)

$$CI = \frac{CO}{BSA}$$

where SV = stroke volume (cc)
CO = cardiac output (L/min)
CI = cardiac index (L/min/m²)
BSA = body surface area (m²)
LVEDV = left ventricular end-diastolic volume (cc)
LVESV = left ventricular end-systolic volume (cc)
HR = heart rate (bpm)
1000 = conversion of cc to litres

Assessment of Regional Wall Motion Abnormalities

The ASE has recommended the use of the 16-segment model in the assessment of regional wall motion abnormalities for the following reasons: (1) anatomic logic, (2) easy identification of each segment by anatomical landmarks, (3) the relationship of each segment to coronary artery blood distribution, and (4) to develop a uniform scoring system for grading the severity of segmental dysfunction.

The 16-Segment Model for the Assessment of Regional Wall Motion Abnormalities:

The 16 segment model of the left ventricle is derived by dividing the ventricle into three levels that are the further subdivided to produce a total of 16 segments. The three levels of the ventricle are divided into three equal lengths using the papillary muscles as anatomical landmarks (Figure 9.15). The *basal level* is identified from the mitral valve annulus to the tips of the papillary muscles, the *mid level* is delineated from the tips of the papillary muscles to the base of the papillary muscles, and the *apical level* is defined as the level from the base of the papillary muscles to the apex of the left ventricle. The *basal* and *mid* levels are divided into six equal segments while the *apical* level is divided into four equal segments (Figure 9.16).

Regional Wall Motion Scoring System:

Recognition of the coronary blood supply to each individual segment of the 16-segment left ventricle aids in the identification of myocardial ischaemia. Each myocardial segment can be classified by three coronary artery distributions (anterior, inferior, and lateral). Coronary artery distribution to the 16-segment model of the left ventricle is illustrated in Figure 9.17. When using coronary artery distribution to predict the site and extent of coronary artery disease, the sonographer should be aware that this distribution may vary depending on coronary artery dominance and variable vasculature supply (especially to the apex). The regional wall motion scoring system is based on the contractility of individual segments. The recommended numerical scoring system for wall segment contractility follows:

1 = normal contractility (systolic increase in free wall thickness greater than 50%),
2 = hypokinesis (an increase in systolic wall thickness less than 40%),
3 = akinesis (an increase in systolic wall thickness less than 10%),
4 = dyskinesis (outward movement of wall during systole with associated systolic wall thinning),
5 = aneurysmal (dilatation and outward movement of wall during systole with associated systolic wall thinning and diastolic deformation).

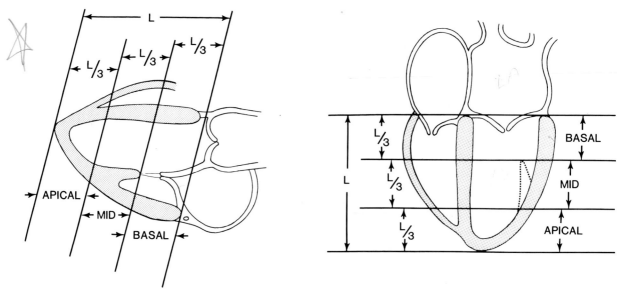

Figure 9.15: Division of the Left Ventricle into the Basal, Mid and Apical levels from the Parasternal Long Axis and the Apical Four Chamber Views.

Left, This schematic illustrates the method of subdivision of the myocardial walls along the long axis (L) into three equal lengths using the left ventricular papillary muscles as landmarks from the parasternal long axis view .

Right, This schematic illustrates the method of subdivision of the myocardial walls along the long axis (L) into three equal lengths using the left ventricular papillary muscles as landmarks from the apical four chamber view .

From Henry, W.L. et al.: Report of the American Society of Echocardiography, Committee on Nomenclature and Standards: Identification of myocardial wall segments. *American Society of Echocardiography, Raleigh, N.C., Nov., 1982.* Reproduced with permission from Mosby Inc., St. Louis, MO, USA

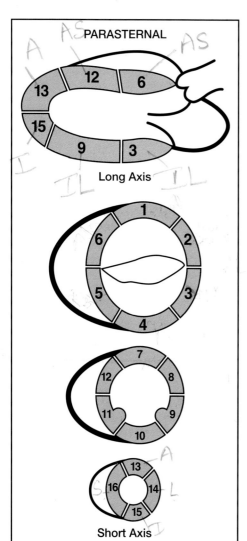

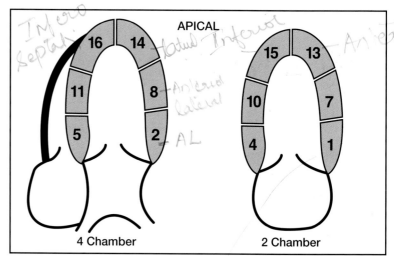

LEVEL	SEGMENT No.	SEGMENT
BASAL	1	Anterior
	2	Anterolateral
	3	Inferolateral
	4	Inferior
	5	Inferoseptal
	6	Anteroseptal
MID	7	Anterior
	8	Anterolateral
	9	Inferolateral
	10	Inferior
	11	Inferoseptal
	12	Anteroseptal
APEX	13	Anterior
	14	Lateral
	15	Inferior
	16	Septal

Figure 9.16: The 16-Segment Model of the Left Ventricle.

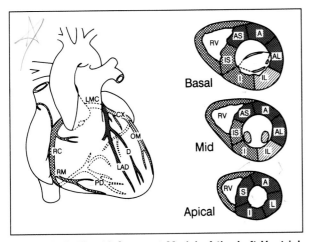

Figure 9.17: The 16-Segment Model of the Left Ventricle and the Coronary Artery Supply to each Region.
Left, Coronary arteries and branches: **CX** = circumflex; **D** = diagonal; **LAD** = left anterior descending; **LMC** = left main coronary artery; **OM** = obtuse marginal; **PD** = posterior descending; **RC** = right coronary; **RM** = right marginal.
Right, Parasternal short axis views of the left ventricle: **A** = anterior; **AL** = anterolateral; **AS** = anteroseptal; **I** = inferior; **IS** = inferoseptal; **L** = lateral; **RV** = right ventricle; **S** = septal.
From Roger, V.L. et al.: Stress echocardiography. Part 1. Exercise echocardiography: Techniques, implementation, clinical applications and correlations. *Mayo Clinic Proceedings 70:8, 1995.* Reproduced with permission from the Mayo Clinic Proceedings.

Regional Wall Motion Score Index:
A wall motion score index (WMSI) is derived from the sum of the wall motion score divided by the number of segments visualised:

(Equation 9.13)

$$WMSI = \frac{\sum wall\ motion\ scores}{No.\ segments\ visualised}$$

A normal WMSI equals 1. The WMSI increases with larger myocardial infarctions and with more extensive regional wall motion abnormalities.

Left Ventricular Mass

Left ventricular mass measurements can be measured by M-mode and 2-D echocardiography. The 2-D method is the preferred method due to the one-dimensional limitations of the M-mode technique which does not account for asymmetric hypertrophy or alterations in ventricular geometry, and is relatively insensitive for detecting serial changes in individuals.
The left ventricular mass is determined from the left ventricular muscle volume and the specific gravity of muscle. Left ventricular muscle volume is equal to the total ventricular volume contained within the epicardial boundaries of the ventricle minus the chamber volume contained by the endocardial surfaces (Figure 9.18). Both the total epicardial volume and the chamber volume can be derived by 2-D echocardiographic

measurements of left ventricular area, length and wall thickness. Left ventricular mass is then calculated by multiplying the left ventricular muscle volume by the specific gravity of muscle (1.04 g/ml). The normal values for left ventricular mass are listed in Table 9.11. There are two methods recommended by the American Society of Echocardiography for the calculation of left ventricular mass by 2-D echocardiography: (1) the area-length method and (2) the truncated ellipse method.

Area-Length Method
Using the area-length method, the volume of the left ventricular myocardium is calculated from the myocardial area, the average myocardial wall thickness and the ventricular length at end-diastole (Figure 9.19). From these measurements, the left ventricular mass is calculated using the following equation:

(Equation 9.14)

$$LVmass = 1.05 \left[\frac{5}{6} A_1(L+t) \right] - \left[\frac{5}{6} A_2 L \right]$$

where A_1 = epicardial area (cm²)
A_2 = endocardial area (cm²)
L = ventricular length (cm)
t = average wall thickness (cm)
1.05 = specific gravity of muscle (g/ml)

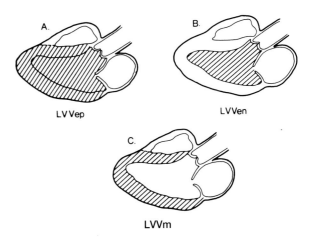

Figure 9.18: Calculation of Left Ventricular Mass.
The left ventricular muscle volume (LVVm - C) is calculated by subtracting the left ventricular endocardial or chamber volume (LVVen - B) from the left ventricular epicardial volume (LVVep - A). The left ventricular mass is then derived by multiplying the LVVm by the specific gravity of muscle (1.05 g/ml).
From Salcedo, E.: *Atlas of Echocardiography.* 2nd Edition. W.B. Saunders Company pp: 211, 1985. Reproduced with permission from W.B. Saunders Company.

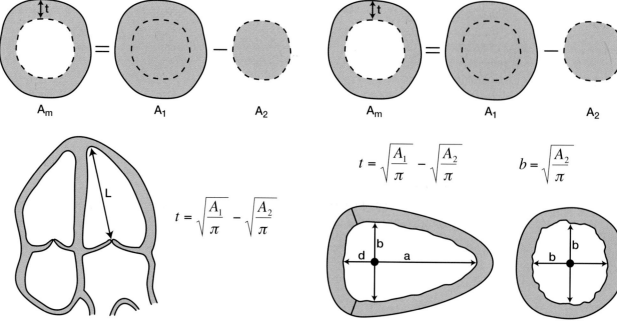

Figure 9.19: The Area-Length Method for Determination of Left Ventricular Mass.
From the parasternal short axis view at the level of the papillary muscles, the myocardial area (A_m) is calculated by subtraction of the endocardial area (A_2) from the epicardial area (A_1). Assuming that the short axis view of the left ventricle is circular, the average wall thickness **(t)** is calculated from the difference between the radii of the endocardial (A_2) and epicardial (A_1) areas. The maximal ventricular length **(L)** is determined by measuring the major or long axis of the ventricle from either the apical four chamber or from the apical two chamber view.

Figure 9.20: The Truncated-Ellipse method for determination of left ventricular mass.
From the parasternal short axis view at the level of the papillary muscles, the myocardial area (A_m) is calculated by subtraction of the endocardial area (A_2) from the epicardial area (A_1). Assuming that the short axis of the left ventricle is circular, the average wall thickness **(t)** is calculated from the difference between the radii of the endocardial (A_2) and epicardial (A_1) areas. Furthermore, assuming that the left ventricle is shaped as a truncated ellipse, the major axis of the ventricle is divided into a semimajor axis **(a)** and a truncated semimajor axis **(d)** at the level of the short axis radius **(b)** which is derived from the parasternal short axis view

Truncated-Ellipse Method

Using this method, the volume of the left ventricular myocardium is calculated from the myocardial area, the average myocardial wall thickness, the semimajor axis, and the truncated semimajor axis at end-diastole (Figure 9.20). From these measurements, the left ventricular mass is calculated using the following equation:

(Equation 9.15)

$$LVmass = 1.05\pi \ (b+t)^2\left[\frac{2}{3}(a+t)+d-\frac{d^3}{3(a+t)^2}\right]-b^2\left[\frac{2}{3}a+d-\frac{d^3}{3a^2}\right]$$

where   a   = semimajor axis length (cm)
       b   = short axis radius (cm)
       d   = truncated semimajor axis length (cm)
       t   = average wall thickness (cm)
       1.05   = specific gravity of muscle (g/ml)

Table 9.11: Normal Values for Left Ventricular Mass by the Truncated Ellipse Method.

	Males (No. = 44)	Females (No. = 40)
LV Mass (g)	148 ± 26	108 ± 21
LV Mass index (g/m²)	76 ± 13	66 ± 11

Mean ± one standard deviation
Source: Byrd, B.F. et al., *Journal of the American College of Cardiology 6: 1021-1025, 1985.*

Method for Calculation of the Left Ventricular Mass:
Below is a "step-by-step" method for the calculation of the left ventricular mass by 2-D echocardiography.

Method for Calculating Left Ventricular Mass by 2-D Echocardiography

Step 1: **Obtain an end-diastolic frame of the left ventricle:**
- from the parasternal short axis view of the left ventricle at the level of the papillary muscles

Step 2: **Calculate the left ventricular epicardial short axis area - area 1 (A_1):**
- trace the epicardial circumference of the heart from the short axis view

Step 3: **Calculate the left ventricular endocardial short axis area - area 2 (A_2):**
- trace the endocardial circumference of the heart from the short axis view (excluding the papillary muscles)

Step 4: **Calculate the myocardial area (Am):**

- $A_m = A_1 - A_2$

Step 5: **Calculate the cavity short axis radius and mean wall thickness:**
- assuming a circular cross-section:
- cavity short axis radius (b) is derived by:

$$b = \sqrt{\frac{A_2}{\pi}}$$

- mean wall thickness (t) is derived by

$$t = \sqrt{\frac{A_1}{\pi}} - b$$

Step 6: **Determine the length(s) of the left ventricle:**
- from the apical four or two chamber views at end-diastole
- length(s) measured depends on the method employed (area-length or truncated ellipse)
- *area-length method:* length (L) is measured from the apex to the base
- *truncated ellipse method:* the long axis of the ventricle in divided into 2 parts at the level of the widest minor axis (b). The major axis (a) is measured from the apex to point (b), the truncated semi-major axis (d) is measured from point (b) to the base (see Figure 9.20)

Step 7: **Calculate the left ventricular mass:**
- *area-length method:*

$$LVmass = 1.05 \left[\frac{5}{6} A_1 (L + t) \right] - \left[\frac{5}{6} A_2 L \right]$$

- *truncated-ellipse method:*

$$LVmass = 1.05\pi \ (b + t)^2 \left[\frac{2}{3}(a + t) + d - \frac{d^3}{3(a+t)^2} \right] - b^2 \left[\frac{2}{3}a + d - \frac{d^3}{3a^2} \right]$$

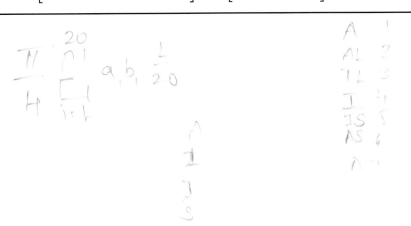

References and Suggested Reading:

General References:
- Feigenbaum, H.: Echocardiography. Chapter 1. 5th Ed. Lea & Febiger, 1994.
- Otto, C.M. and Pearlman, A.S.: Textbook of Clinical Echocardiography. Chapter 1. W.B. Saunders Company. 1995
- Weyman, A.: Principles and Practice of Echocardiography. 2nd ed. Lea & Febiger,1994.

Linear Dimensional Measurements, Area Calculations, Cardiac Chamber Volumes:
- Reynolds, T.: Echocardiographer's Pocket Reference. Arizona Heart Institute Foundation.1993.
- Schiller, N.B. et al.: Recommendations from quantitation of the left ventricle by two-dimensional echocardiography. *Journal of the American Society of Echocardiography 2:358-367,1989*
- Schittger, I. et al.: Standardized intracardiac measurements of two-dimensional echocardiography. *Journal of the American College of Cardiology 2:934-938,1983*
- Triulzi, M. et al.: Normal adult cross-sectional echocardiographic values: linear dimensions and chamber areas. *Echocardiography 1: 403-426, 1984.*
- Wahr, D.W. et al.: Left ventricular volumes determined by two-dimensional echocardiography in a normal adult population. *Journal of the American College of Cardiology 1:863-868,1983.*
- Wang, Y. et al: Atrial volumes in a normal adult population by two-dimensional echocardiography. *Chest 86:595-601,1984.*

Left Ventricular Systolic Function:
- Henry, W.L. et al.: Report of the American Society of Echocardiography, Committee on Nomenclature and Standards: Identification of myocardial wall segments. *American Society of Echocardiography, Raleigh,N.C.,Nov., 1982.*

- Mickelson, J. K. et al.: Left ventricular dimensions and mechanics in distance runners. *American Heart Journal 112: 1251-1256, 1986*
- Roger, V.L. et al.: Stress echocardiography. Part 1. Exercise echocardiography: Techniques, implementation, clinical applications and correlations. *Mayo Clinic Proceedings 70:8, 1995.*
- Schiller, N.B. et al.: Recommendations from quantitation of the left ventricle by two-dimensional echocardiography. *Journal of the American Society of Echocardiography 2:358-367,1989*
- Schittger, I. et al.: Standardized intracardiac measurements of two-dimensional echocardiography. *Journal of the American College of Cardiology 2:934-938,1983*
- Shiina, A. et al.: Prognostic significance of regional wall motion abnormality in patients with prior myocardial infarction: a prospective correlative study by two-dimensional echocardiography and angiography. *Mayo Clinic Proceedings 61:254-262,1986.*

Left Ventricular Mass Calculations:
- Byrd, B.F. et al.: Left ventricular mass and volume/mass ratio determined by two-dimensional echocardiography in normal adults. *Journal of the American College of Cardiology 6: 1021-1025, 1985.*
- Reick, N. et al.: Anatomic validation of left ventricular mass estimates from clinical two-dimensional echocardiography: initial results. *Circulation 67: 348-352, 1983.*
- Schiller, N.B. et al.: Recommendations from quantitation of the left ventricle by two-dimensional echocardiography. *Journal of the American Society of Echocardiography 2:358-367,1989*

Chapter 10
M-Mode Echocardiographic Measurements and Calculations

As for 2-D measurements, several factors also influence the accuracy of M-mode measurements. These include:

(1) *theoretical resolution* of the ultrasonic equipment which depends on the transducer frequency and the inherent axial and lateral resolution of the imaging equipment;

(2) *overall technical quality* of the derived M-mode trace such as the clarity of interface delineation;

(3) *inconsistency in measurements* because of inter-operator variability in the selection of measured interfaces and the specific timing of measurements.

The most important of these factors is the inter-operator variability. For this reason the American Society of Echocardiography (ASE) has developed a set of guidelines outlining standardised measurement criteria that allow accurate and reproducible measurements and calculations [18]. The ASE recommended method for measuring structures by M-mode is the *leading edge to leading edge* technique following the most continuous echo line. The ASE also recommends that *end-diastolic* measurements be made from the onset of QRS complex while *end-systolic* measurements of the left ventricle should be performed based on the motion of the interventricular septum. When the motion of the interventricular septum is normal, the end-systolic measurement is taken from the lowest posterior point of the septum; when septal motion is abnormal, this measurement is taken from the peak anterior point of the posterior wall. Figure 10.1 illustrates the recommended method for the measurement of M-Mode dimensions. Table 10.1 lists the measurements that can be made by M-mode echocardiography.

Cardiac Chamber Dimensions

Measurement methodology for cardiac structures by M-mode is described below. The normal values for these measurements, including measurements indexed for body surface area, are listed in Table 10.2.

Measurements of Aorta and Left Atrium: (Figure 10.2)

The **aortic root (Ao)** is measured in the anterior-posterior plane at end-diastole (Q wave on the ECG) from the leading edge of the aortic anterior wall to the leading edge of posterior aortic wall.

The **left atrium (LA)** is measured in the anterior-posterior plane at end-systole (end of T wave on ECG) from the leading edge of the posterior wall of the aorta to the leading edge of the posterior wall of the left atrium.

Measurements of the Left Ventricle: (Figure 10.3)

The **end-diastolic dimension of the left ventricle (LVEDD)** is measured at the Q wave on the ECG from the posterior endocardial surface of the interventricular septum to the endocardial surface of the posterior wall.

The **end-systolic dimension of the left ventricle (LVEDS)** is measured from the peak posterior endocardial surface of the septum to the posterior wall of the left ventricle.

The **interventricular septal thickness (IVST)** is measured at end-diastole (onset of the QRS complex) or end-systole between the anterior and posterior endocardial surfaces of the interventricular septum.

The **posterior wall thickness (PWT)** is measured at end-diastole (Q wave of the ECG) or end-systole from endocardial surface to epicardial surface of the posterior wall of the left ventricle.

Table 10.1: M-Mode Echocardiographic Measurements.

Cardiac chamber dimensions	• aorta and left atrium • left ventricle • right ventricle
Left ventricular systolic function	• fractional shortening • ejection fraction • mean circumferential fibre shortening • stroke volume and cardiac output • systolic time intervals of the aortic valve • mitral E point-septal separation
Left ventricular mass	• Penn convention • ASE method
Assessment of valvular stenosis	• maximal aortic cusp separation (aortic valve stenosis) • mitral EF slope (mitral valve stenosis) • pulmonary a wave amplitude (pulmonary valve stenosis)
Assessment of left ventricular outflow tract obstruction	• systolic anterior motion of mitral valve leaflet(s) • premature (mid-systolic) closure of the aortic valve
Intracardiac pressure estimation	• pulmonary hypertension • elevated left ventricular end-diastolic pressure

18: Sahn, D.J., et al.: Circulation 58 (No. 6): 1072-1083, 1978.

METHODS OF MEASUREMENT

NORMAL DATA

EKG

ST(D)
(A.S.E.)
ST(S)

} VENTRICULAR
SEPTUM

LVD(D)
(A.S.E.)

LEFT
VENTRICULAR
DIMENSIONS

LVD(S)
(A.S.E.)

CHORDAE TENDINEAE
ENDOCARDIUM

LV POSTERIOR
FREE WALL

EPICARDIUM

PWT(D)
(A.S.E.)

PWT(S)

ANTERIOR WALL
OF AORTA

AORTIC ROOT
AND
LEFT ATRIAL
DIMENSIONS

AO
(A.S.E.)

AORTIC VALVE

POSTERIOR WALL
OF AORTA

LA
(A.S.E.)

POSTERIOR WALL
OF LEFT ATRIUM

Figure 10.1: Method Recommended by the American Society of Echocardiography for the Measurement of Cardiac Dimensions.
From Feigenbaum, H. Echocardiography. 5th Ed. Lea & Febiger, pp 660,1994. Reproduced with permission from Lippincott, Williams & Wilkins and from the author.

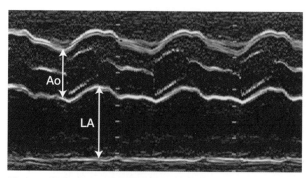

Figure 10.2: M-mode Measurements of the Aorta and Left Atrium.
Both the aorta and left atrium are measured in the anterior-posterior plane. The **aortic root (Ao)** is measured at end-diastole (Q wave on the ECG) from the leading edge of the anterior aortic wall to the leading edge of posterior aortic wall. The **left atrium (LA)** is measured at end-systole (end of T wave on ECG) from the leading edge of the posterior wall of the aorta to the leading edge of the posterior wall of the left atrium.

Measurements of the Right Ventricle: (Figure 10.3)
The **anterior right ventricular wall** measurement is often difficult due to poor resolution between the chest wall and the epicardial surface of the right ventricle. When resolved, this measurement may be taken at end-diastole from the epicardial surface to the endocardial surface.

The **right ventricular cavity (RV)** is measured at end-diastole (Q wave on the ECG) from the endocardial surface of the anterior right ventricular wall to the anterior endocardial surface of the interventricular septum. This measurement is an estimation only and is often unreliable due to the variable position of the right ventricle between patients and because of the inconsistent orientation of the M-mode cursor through the right ventricle.

Technical Consideration:
In order to compare measurements between individuals of different sizes, measurement of cardiac structures are often expressed in terms of square meters of the body surface area (BSA) or the "index". For example, the left ventricular cavity index is simply the left ventricular cavity dimension divided by the BSA.

Table 10.2: Normal Values for Cardiac Structures.

M-Mode Parameter	Normal Values	
	Mean	Range
Aortic Root	2.7 cm	2.2 - 3.7 cm
Aortic Root Index	1.6 cm/m²	1.3 - 2.4 cm/m²
Left Atrium	3.2 cm	2.5 - 4.0 cm
Left Atrium Index	-	1.2 - 2.1 cm/m²
Left Ventricular Cavity - Diastole	4.5 cm	4.0 - 5.6 cm
Left Ventricular Cavity Index - Diastole	2.5 cm/m²	2.0 - 2.9 cm/m²
Left Ventricular Cavity - Systole	3.1 cm	2.0 - 3.8 cm
Left Ventricular Cavity Index - Systole	1.6 cm/m²	1.3 - 1.9 cm/m²
Interventricular Septum - Diastole	0.9 cm	0.70 - 1.1 cm
Posterior Wall - Diastole	0.9 cm	0.70 - 1.1 cm

Source: Reynolds, T: The Echocardiographer's Pocket Reference. Arizona Heart Institute, pp: 164, 1994.

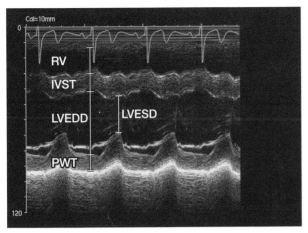

Figure 10.3: M-mode Measurements of the Left and Right Ventricles.
All end-diastolic measurements are performed at the Q wave of the ECG while end-systolic measurements are performed at the point marking the peak posterior deflection of the interventricular septum. The end-diastolic dimension of the **right ventricular cavity (RV)** is measured from endocardial surface of anterior right ventricular wall to the anterior endocardial surface of the interventricular septum. The **end-diastolic dimension of the left ventricle (LVEDD)** is from the posterior endocardial surface of the interventricular septum to the endocardial surface of the posterior wall. The **end-systolic dimension of the left ventricle (LVESD)** is measured from the peak posterior endocardial surface of septum to the posterior wall of the left ventricle. The **interventricular septal thickness (IVST)** is measured at end-diastole and end-systole between the anterior and posterior endocardial surface of interventricular septum. The **posterior wall thickness (PWT)** is measured at end-diastole and end-systole from endocardial surface to epicardial surface of the posterior wall of the left ventricle.

Left Ventricular Systolic Function

From the measurement of the left ventricular end-diastolic and end-systolic dimensions (LVEDD and LVESD), several indices can be derived for the assessment of left ventricular systolic function. These parameters are described below and the normal values for each of these indices are listed in Table 10.3.

Other M-mode measurements which can be employed in the evaluation of left ventricular systolic function include the mitral-septal separation and left ventricular systolic time intervals. These M-mode calculations are also described below.

Fractional Shortening

Fractional shortening is the percentage of change in the left ventricular cavity dimension with systole. The standard measurements of the left ventricle required for this calculation includes the LVEDD and the ventricular LVESD (see Figure 10.3).

The percentage fractional shortening (FS%) is calculated from the equation:

(Equation 10.1)

$$FS\% = \frac{LVEDD - LVESD}{LVEDD} \times 100$$

Ejection Fraction

The ejection fraction is the percentage of the left ventricular diastolic volume that is ejected with systole; that is, the ejection fraction is the ratio of the stroke volume to the end-diastolic volume. End-diastolic and end-systolic volumes can be estimated using the standard M-Mode measurements of the left ventricular dimensions taken in diastole and systole (Figure 10.3). Two methods of ejection can be calculated: (1) the uncorrected ejection fraction, and (2) the corrected ejection fraction.

1. Uncorrected Ejection Fraction:
The "uncorrected" ejection fraction (EF%) provides a global assessment of left ventricular systolic performance and can be estimated by the following equation:

(Equation 10.2)

$$EF\% = \frac{LVEDD^2 - LVESD^2}{LVEDD^2} \times 100$$

2. Corrected Ejection Fraction:
One of the principal limitations of the "uncorrected" ejection fraction is the fact that it accounts for only two walls of the left ventricle. To overcome this problem, an alternative method has been described in which the fractional shortening of the square of the minor axis and the fractional shortening of the long axis of the left ventricle are incorporated.

The fractional shortening of the square of the minor axis is simply the uncorrected ejection fraction (equation 10.2) while the fractional shortening of the long axis of the left ventricle refers to the contractility of the apex of the left ventricle. Although this method was described using 2-D imaging, it can also be performed using a combination of M-mode and 2-D imaging.

Hence, the "corrected" ejection fraction (EFc %) be calculated by the following equation:

(Equation 10.3)

$$EF_c\% = \left[\left(1 - \%D^2\right)\%\Delta L\right] + \%D^2$$

where $\%D^2$ = fractional shortening of the square of the minor axis (equation 10.2)
  $\%\Delta L$ = contractility of the left ventricular apex, where:
  - 15% normal
  - 5% hypokinetic
  - 0% akinetic
  - -5% dyskinetic
  - -10% frankly dyskinetic (aneurysmal)

19: Quinones, M.A. et al.: Circulation 64 (No. 4): 744-753, 1981.

Circumferential Fibre Shortening

As well as measuring the extent of shortening, the rate of shortening of the left ventricle can also be calculated. This index of systolic function is determined by the mean velocity of circumferential fibre shortening (mean Vcf) which is expressed in units of circumferences/second (circ/s). This measurement reflects the mean velocity of ventricular shortening of the minor axis of the left ventricle and is calculated from the following equation

(Equation 10.4)

$$Mean\ Vcf = \frac{LVEDD - LVESD}{LVEDD \times LVET}\ or\ \frac{FS}{LVET}$$

where LVEDD = left ventricular end-diastolic dimension (cm)
LVESD = left ventricular end-systolic dimension (cm)
LVET = left ventricular ejection time (seconds)
FS   = fractional shortening (no units)

Technical Consideration:

Units are important in the calculation of this parameter. Observe that the units for the LVEDD and LVESD are in cm and the units for the LVET are in seconds. Furthermore, when calculating the Vcf by the simplified version; that is, the fractional shortening divided by the LVET, the fractional shortening used is not the percentage fractional shortening (not multiplied by 100). The LVET is measured from the aortic valve M-mode trace (see "Systolic Time Intervals" on page 110).

Stroke Volume, Cardiac Output, and Cardiac Index

Stroke volume refers to the amount of blood pumped by the heart on each single beat. The cardiac output is the volume of blood pumped by the heart per minute. Both the cardiac output and stroke volume can be calculated using the end-diastolic and end-systolic volumes which can be derived from the M-Mode recording of the left ventricle. In order to compare measurements between individuals of different sizes, measurement of the cardiac output is often expressed in terms of the cardiac index which is simply the cardiac output divided by the body surface area (BSA).

Left ventricular volume calculations are based on the assumption that the left ventricle is shaped like a prolate ellipse (Figure 10.4). This structure has two minor axes (D_1 and D_2) and a major axis (L). The equation that calculates the volume (V) of a prolate ellipsoid structure is as follows:

(Equation 10.5)

$$V = \frac{4}{3}\pi \left(\frac{D_1}{2}\right)\left(\frac{D_2}{2}\right)\left(\frac{L}{2}\right)$$

This ellipsoid model when applied to the calculation of left ventricular volumes is known as the **cubed** or

D^3 method. The basic assumption of this method is that the left ventricle dilates primarily along the minor axis. In addition, this method also assumes that: (1) the left ventricular internal diameter (short axis) is equal to one of the minor axes of the ellipse (D_1), (2) both minor axes are equal ($D_1 = D_2$), and (3) the major axis to minor axis ratio is 2:1 ($L = 2 D_1$). Therefore, left ventricular volumes (LVV) can be determined by:

(Equation 10.6)

$$LVV = \frac{4}{3}\pi \left(\frac{D_1}{2}\right)\left(\frac{D_1}{2}\right)\left(\frac{2 D_1}{2}\right)$$

$$= \frac{\pi}{3} \times D^3$$

$$= 1.047 \times D^3$$

$$= D^3$$

However, because the left ventricle becomes more spherical as it dilates, the relationship between the major and minor axes changes. Therefore, a regression formula was devised to correct for this change in ventricular shape [20]:

(Equation 10.7)

$$LVV = \left(\frac{7.0}{2.4 + D}\right) \times D^3$$

Using this equation, the left ventricular end-diastolic and end-systolic volumes can be estimated using a single minor axis dimension of the left ventricle which can be obtained from the standard M-Mode assessment of the left ventricle.

Stroke Volume (SV), **Cardiac Output** (CO), and **Cardiac Index** (CI) can, thus, be calculated using these M-mode derived left ventricular volumes:

(Equation 10.8)

$$SV = LVEDV - LVESV$$

(Equation 10.9)

$$CO = \frac{SV \times HR}{1000}$$

(Equation 10.10)

$$CI = \frac{CO}{BSA}$$

where SV   = stroke volume (cc)
CO   = cardiac output (L/min)
CI   = cardiac index (L/min/m²)
LVEDV = end diastolic volume (cc)
LVESV = end systolic volume (cc)
HR   = heart rate (bpm)
1000 = conversion of cc to litres
BSA   = body surface area (m²)

20: Teicholz, L.E. et al.: American Journal of Cardiology 37: 7-11, 1976.

Mitral E-Point-Septal Separation

The mitral E-point-septal separation (EPSS) is a measure of the perpendicular distance between the most posterior point of the interventricular septum during systole and the E point of the anterior mitral valve leaflet in the same cardiac cycle (Figure 10.5). With impairment of left ventricular systolic function, this distance increases due to a combination of: (1) the anterior displacement of the interventricular septum as the ventricle dilates, and (2) reduced opening of the mitral valve because of decreased transmitral flow into the left ventricle [21].

The principal advantage of this technique is that this measurement is independent of left ventricular geometry, size and abnormal wall motion. In addition, the EPSS has a reasonable correlation with the angiographic ejection fraction. The primary limitation of this technique is the assumption that there is **normal** mitral valve motion and **unimpeded** left ventricular inflow. Hence, this measurement is inaccurate in the presence of aortic regurgitation where the motion of the mitral valve may be affected by the aortic regurgitant jet, and in mitral stenosis where the flow from the left atrium to the left ventricle is "slowed". Furthermore, it has been shown that this measurement is less specific for patients with inferior myocardial infarction. In this subset of patients, the motion of the posterior mitral leaflet may be reduced because of papillary muscle dysfunction. This causes a subsequent decrease in the displacement of the anterior mitral leaflet and, therefore, falsely increases the EPSS. The normal values for the EPSS as well as the relationship of the EPSS to the left ventricular ejection fraction (EF) are listed in Table 10.4.

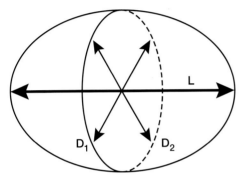

Figure 10.4: A Prolate Ellipse demonstrating the Major or Long Axis (L) and the Two Minor Axes or Dimensions (D_1 and D_2).

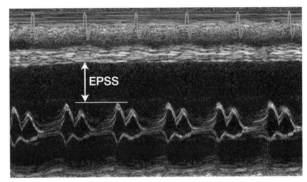

Figure 10.5: Measurement of the Mitral E-Point-Septal Separation (EPSS).
The EPSS is measured as the perpendicular distance between a line drawn between the most posterior point of the interventricular septum during systole and the E point of the anterior mitral valve leaflet in the same cardiac cycle.

Table 10.3: Normal Values for Left Ventricular Systolic Function Indices by M-mode Echocardiography.

Parameter	Normal Range	Pt. Pop.
Fractional Shortening (%) [1]	28 - 44 (mean 36)	208
Ejection Fraction (%) [1]	64 - 83 (mean 74)	208
Mean Circumferential Fibre Shortening (circ/s) [2]	1.12 - 1.24 (mean 1.18)	62
Stroke Volume (cc) [3]	75 - 100	...
Cardiac Output (L/min) [3]	4 - 8	...
Cardiac Index (L/min/m2) [3]	2.8 - 4.2 (mean 3.4)	...

Sources: (1) Henry, W.L. et al., *Circulation 62 (Vol. 5): 1054-1061, 1980*; (2) Remes, J. et al., *Cardiology 78: 267-277, 1991*; (3) Schlant, R. and Alexander R.W.: Hurst's. The Heart. 8th Edition McGraw-Hill, Inc. pp: 141 and 503, 1994.

Table 10.4: Clinical Significance of the Mitral EPSS.

	EPSS	Pt. Pop.	Sensitivity	Specificity
Normal EPSS [1]	≤ 5.5 mm	30	-	-
Ejection fraction < 50% [2]	> 7 mm	85	87%	75%
Ejection fraction ≤ 35% [2]	≥ 13 mm	85	87%	84%

Sources: (1) Lew, W. et al., American Journal of Cardiology 41: 836-845, 1978; (2) Ahmadpour, H. et al., American Heart Journal 106:21-28,1983: patient population: 37 patients = EF < 50%; 48 patients = EF > 50% [23/37 patients = EF, 35%].

21: Lew, W. et al.: American Journal of Cardiology 41: 836-845, 1978.

Systolic Time Intervals

Systolic time intervals can also be used as indicators of left ventricular performance. The most commonly measured systolic time intervals include left ventricular pre-ejection period, the left ventricular ejection period, and the ratio between these two variables (Figure 10.6).

The **left ventricular pre-ejection period (LVPEP)** is measured from the Q wave on the ECG to the onset of aortic valve opening while the **left ventricular ejection period (LVET)** is measured from aortic valve opening to aortic valve closure. Both these intervals vary with the heart rate with intervals decreasing with increasing heart rate. The **LVPEP/LVET** is the ratio of pre-ejection period divided by the ejection time of the left ventricle. This ratio is unrelated to heart rate and, therefore, provides a simple and uncomplicated method for the assessment of left ventricular systolic function.

When there is left ventricular systolic dysfunction, the left ventricular systolic time intervals vary from normal such that the LVPEP is prolonged and the LVET is shortened, resulting in an overall increase in the LVPEP/LVET ratio [22]. This ratio has been found to correlate with the ejection fraction [EF] (see Table 10.5).

Left Ventricular Mass

The left ventricular mass is determined from the left ventricular muscle volume and the specific gravity of muscle. Left ventricular muscle volume is equal to the total ventricular volume contained within the epicardial boundaries of the ventricle minus the chamber volume contained by the endocardial surfaces (Figure 10.7). Both the total epicardial volume and the chamber volume can be derived by M-mode echocardiographic measurements of the left ventricular internal diameter and wall thickness. **Left ventricular mass** is then calculated by multiplying the left ventricular muscle volume by the specific gravity of muscle (1.04 g/ml). The normal values for left ventricular mass are listed in Table 10.6.

Volumes can be determined by the D^3 method which assumes that the shape of the left ventricle approximates a prolate ellipse with a long-axis to short-axis ratio of 2:1. Based on this cube function formula, volume is equal to diameter cubed.

Hence, by measuring the left ventricular internal dimension (LVID), interventricular septal thickness (IVST), and posterior wall thickness (PWT), and by using the D^3 method for the calculation of volume, left ventricular mass can be determined.

The two most commonly employed measurements for the determination of left ventricular mass by M-mode include: (1) the Penn-cube method and (2) the ASE-cube method.

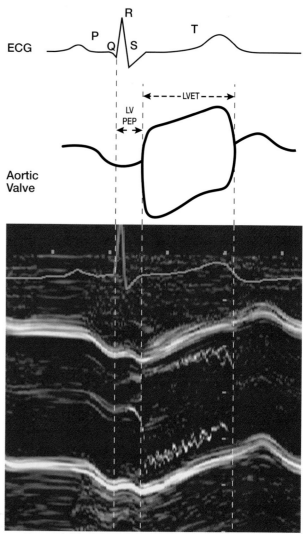

Figure 10.6: Systolic Time Intervals measured from the Aortic Valve M-Mode Trace.
The left ventricular pre-ejection period **(LVPEP)** is measured from the Q wave on the ECG to the onset of aortic valve opening. The left ventricular ejection period (LVET) is measured from aortic valve opening to aortic valve closure. The **LVPEP/LVET** is simply derived by dividing the LVPEP by the LVET.

Table 10.5: The Relationship between the LVPEP/LVET Ratio and the Ejection Fraction.

	LVPEP/LVET	Pt. Pop.	Sensitivity	Specificity
Normal (EF ≥ 55 %) [1]	< 0.35	-	24%	100 %
Ejection fraction < 55 % [2]	≥ 0.35	68	100%	72 %
Ejection fraction ≤ 30 % [2]	≥ 0.65		89%	89 %

Sources: (1) Weissler, A.M. et al.: Systolic time intervals in heart failure in man. *Circulation 37:149-159,1968.* **(2)** Garrard, C.L. et al., *Circulation 42:455-462, 1970*: patient population: 21 patients = EF ≥ 55%; 47 patients = EF < 55% [18/47 patients = EF ≤ 30%] [23].

22: Garrard, C.L. et al.: Circulation 42:455-462, 1970. 23: Note systolic time intervals were derived from simultaneous recordings of the ECG, phonocardiogram and carotid arterial pulse; the ejection fractions were determined at cardiac catheterisation.

1. The Penn-Cube Method: [24]

By the Penn convention, left ventricular measurements are made during diastole just below the tips of the mitral valve. This method excludes the thickness of endocardial echoes from measurements of the interventricular septum and posterior wall and includes the thickness of the endocardial echoes from the left side of the septum and the posterior wall endocardium in the measurement of the left ventricular internal dimension (Figure 10.8). Furthermore, there is no myocardium over the mitral and aortic orifices. Therefore, a constant of 13.6 is subtracted to correct for the absence of cardiac muscle over the base of the heart. Therefore, by the Penn convention, left ventricular mass is equal to:

(Equation 10.11)

$$LV\ mass = 1.04\ [(LVID + IVST + PWT)^3 - (LVID)^3] - 13.6$$

where 1.04 = specific gravity of the myocardium (g/ml)
LVID = left ventricular internal dimension (cm)
PWT = posterior wall thickness (cm)
IVST = interventricular septal thickness (cm)

2. The ASE Method:

Most M-mode measurements are performed using the recommendations by the American Society of Echocardiography (ASE); that is, the leading edge to leading edge methodology. However, calculation of left ventricular mass using the ASE method and the D^3

method (equation 10.11) has been found to overestimate left ventricular mass by approximately 25% [25]. Therefore, a regression equation has been derived for the calculation of left ventricular mass using the measurements performed based on the ASE convention (Figure 10.8):

(Equation 10.12)

$$LVmass = 1.04\left(\left[LVID + PWT + IVST\right]^3 - LVID^3\right) \times 0.8 + 0.6$$

where 1.04 = specific gravity of the myocardium (g/ml)
LVID = left ventricular internal dimension (cm)
PWT = posterior wall thickness (cm)
IVST = interventricular septal thickness (cm)

Left ventricular mass has been shown to correlate with body surface area and is significantly different between men and women. Therefore, left ventricular mass should be indexed for the body surface area (BSA) by simply dividing the calculated left ventricular mass by the BSA. Furthermore, for women, but not men, left ventricular mass has also been found to increase with advancing age (Figure 10.9) [26].

The normal values for left ventricular mass as listed in Table 10.6.

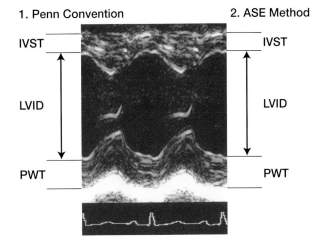

Figure 10.8: Measurements for Left Ventricular Mass calculations.

1. The Penn Convention:
By this method, the thickness of endocardial echoes from measurements of the interventricular septum (IVST) and posterior wall (PWT) are *excluded* while the thickness of the endocardial echoes from the left side of the septum and the posterior wall endocardium are *included* in the measurement of the left ventricular internal dimension (LVID). Therefore, the value for the LVID is larger, and the values for the PWT and IVST are smaller, than the measurements for the ASE method.

2. The ASE Method:
By this method, M-mode measurements (IVST, LVID, and PWT) are performed using the recommendations by the American Society of Echocardiography; that is, using the leading edge to leading edge technique.

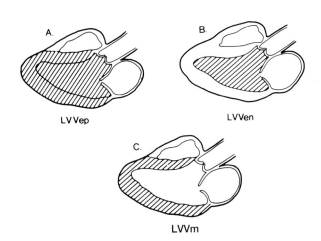

Figure 10.7: Calculation of Left Ventricular Mass.
The left ventricular muscle volume (LVVm - C) is calculated by subtracting the left ventricular endocardial or chamber volume (LVVen - B) from the left ventricular epicardial volume (LVVep - A). The left ventricular mass is then derived by multiplying the LVVm by the specific gravity of muscle (1.040 g/ml).
From Salcedo, E.: Atlas of Echocardiography. 2nd Edition. W.B. Saunders Company pp: 211, 1985. Reproduced with permission from W.B. Saunders Company.

24: Devereux, R.B. et al.: Circulation 55: 613-618, 1977. 25: Devereux, R.B. et al.: American Journal of Cardiology 57: 450-458, 1986. 26: Shub, C. et al.: Mayo Clinic Proceedings 69: 205-211, 1994.

Method for Calculating Left Ventricular Mass by M-Mode Echocardiography:
Below is a "step-by-step" method for the calculation of the left ventricular mass by M-mode echocardiography using the Penn method and the ASE method.

Method for Calculating Left Ventricular Mass by M-Mode

Step 1: Measure the following parameters from the left ventricular M-mode trace:
- left ventricular internal dimension (LVID)
- interventricular septal thickness (IVST)
- posterior wall thickness (PWT)

    - Penn method : the IVST and PWT are measured by excluding the endocardial echoes
                   : the LVID measurement includes the thickness of the endocardial echoes from the septum
                     and posterior wall

    - ASE method   : using the leading edge to leading edge method

Step 2: Calculate the total left ventricular epicardial volume (LVVep):

$$LVVep = (LVID + IVST + PWT)^3$$

Step 3: Calculate the left ventricular endocardial or chamber volume (LVVen):

$$LVVen = (LVID)^3$$

Step 4: Determine the left ventricular muscle volume (LVVm):

$$LVVm = LVVep - LVVen$$
or
$$LVVm = (LVID + IVST + PWT)^3 - (LVID)^3$$

Step 5: Calculate the left ventricular mass (LV mass):

- Penn method:

$$LV\ mass\ (g) = (1.04 \times LVVm) - 13.6$$

- ASE method:

$$LV\ mass\ (g) = (1.04 \times LVVm) \times 0.8 + 0.6$$

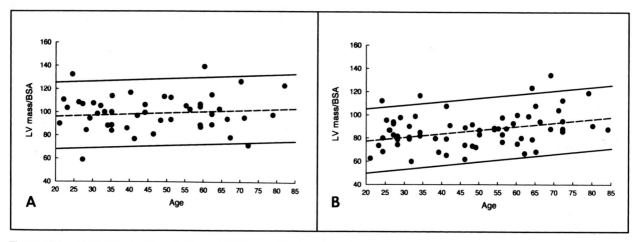

Figure 10.9: Left Ventricular Mass in Normal Subjects of Various Ages (normalised for body surface area).
A. Men; B. Women.
Solid lines = 95% confidence limits; dashed lines = mean values.
From Shub. C. et al.: Determination of left ventricular mass by echocardiography in a normal population: Effect of age and sex in addition to body size. *Mayo Clinic Proceedings 69: 205-211, 1994.* Reproduced with permission from the Mayo Clinic Proceedings.

Table 10.6: Normal ranges of Left Ventricular Mass.

	Males	Females
Penn Method: [1]	No. = 78	No. = 55
LV Mass (g)	181 ± 44	128 ± 42
LV Mass index (g/m²)	93 ± 22	76 ± 18
ASE Method:		
Children/young adults: [2]	No. = 167	No. = 167
LV Mass (g)	99.7 ± 42.6	80.9 ± 24.7
LV Mass index (g/m²)	70.4 ± 16.3	67.7 ± 11.8
Adults: [3]	No. = 47	No. = 64
LV Mass index (g/m²)	99 ± 15	88 ± 15

Sources: (1) Devereux, R.B. et al., *Journal of the American College of Cardiology 4: 1222-1230, 1984*: patient age range = 18 to 69 years, mean age of 44 ± 22 years; **(2)** Daniels, S.R. et al.: *Journal of the American College of Cardiology 12: 703-708, 1983*: patient age range = 12.6 ± 4.0 years [male] and 12.7 ± 4.4 years [females]; **(3)** Shub, C. et al., *Mayo Clinic Proceedings 69: 205-211, 1994*: patient age range = 21 to 82 years, mean age of 48 ± 17 years.

Technical Consideration:

Left ventricular mass calculations using M-mode echocardiography are most accurate using the Penn convention when the length of the left ventricle is twice its diameter at the papillary muscle level. However, the accuracy of this method is significantly affected by: (1) alterations or distortion in left ventricular shape such as that which may occur with chronic severe right or left ventricular volume overload, (2) massive myocardial infarction or ventricular aneurysm, or (3) asymmetric septal hypertrophy. In these instances, the 2-D estimation of left ventricular mass (see Chapter 9 - "Left Ventricular Mass") is considered to be more accurate than the M-mode estimate as the 2-D estimate accounts for alteration in left ventricular geometry.

Valvular Stenosis

Various M-mode measurements attempting to quantitate the severity of valvular stenosis have been investigated in the past. Although these measurements have since been superseded by 2-D and Doppler echocardiographic calculations, M-mode data can occasionally provide additional information that may support both the 2-D and Doppler findings.

Maximal Aortic Cusp Separation

The severity of aortic stenosis can be estimated by observation of restricted leaflet motion and measurement of the **maximal aortic cusp separation** (MACS). The MACS is the vertical distance between the right coronary cusp and the non-coronary cusp of the aortic valve measured during systole (Figure 10.10). Reduced flow across the restricted or stenotic aortic valve results in a reduction of the MACS. This measurement has been found to roughly correlate with the AVA allowing differentiation between severe and mild aortic stenosis. The relationship between the MACS and the AVA is tabulated in Table 10.7.

Limitations: There are several limitations of this measurement in the evaluation of aortic stenosis. Firstly, this measurement is obtained through one dimension and, therefore, assumes that the MACS occurs perpendicular to the ultrasound beam. Secondly, this single measurement reflects the overall geometry of the valve area and, therefore, does not account for asymmetric involvement of the leaflets, eccentric orifices, or severe distortion of the valve. Thirdly, extensive calcification or thickening of the valve leaflets results in the display of multiple echoes sometimes making the identification of valve leaflet opening impossible. Fourthly, this measurement assumes that leaflets are maximally distended which may not be true when there is a marked reduction in left ventricular systolic function, low cardiac output states, or sub-aortic obstruction. Finally, the accuracy of this measurement requires that the MACS be measured at the site of maximal obstruction.

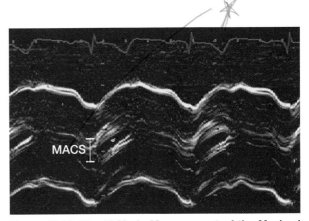

Figure 10.10: The M-Mode Measurement of the Maximal Aortic Cusp Separation (MACS).
The MACS is the vertical distance between the anterior and posterior cusps of the aortic valve measured during systole.

Table 10.7: The Relationship between the MACS and the Aortic Valve Area.

Aortic Valve Area (AVA)	MACS Measurement	Pt. Pop.	Predictive Value
Normal AVA (> 2 cm²)	Normal MACS > 15 mm	17	100%
AVA < 0.75 cm²	MACS < 8 mm	81	97%
AVA > 1.0 cm²	MACS > 12 mm		96%
"gray area" **	MACS 8 - 12 mm		...

** The "gray area" constitutes an overlap between mild, moderate, and severe aortic stenosis.
Source: DeMaria, A.N. et al., *Circulation (Suppl II) 58: 232, 1978*; (+) Godley, R.W., et al., *Chest 79:657-662,1981*: patient population: 37 patients = severe aortic stenosis [AVA < 0.75 cm²]; 28 patients = moderate aortic stenosis [AVA = 0.75 - 1.0 cm²]; 16 patients = mild aortic stenosis [AVA > 1.0 cm²].

Mitral Valve EF Slope

The severity of mitral stenosis can be estimated by observation of the mitral **EF slope**. A prolongation of the EF slope is a characteristic feature of mitral valve stenosis (Figure 10.11). The mitral E-F slope is the measurement of the slope of the anterior mitral leaflet during its partial closure in early diastole. This slope is a function of the rate of left atrial emptying and left ventricular filling. Therefore, in mitral stenosis, the EF slope is prolonged due to a prolongation of left atrial emptying. The rate of this slope has been found to correlate with the mitral valve area (MVA) - see Table 10.8.

Limitations: There are several important factors that affect the reliability of measurement of the EF slope in the evaluation of mitral stenosis. Firstly, there is a poor correlation of this measurement compared with the catheter-derived MVA due to the fact that other variables besides mitral stenosis can affect the EF slope. For example, cycle length (the variable R-R interval with atrial fibrillation is a problem), and valvular calcification. Secondly, prolongation of the EF slope is affected by other conditions that alter the diastolic properties of the left ventricle, such as diminished left ventricular compliance, which also reduces EF slope in the *absence* of mitral stenosis. Finally, the one-dimensional nature of M-Mode focuses on only one point of the long anterior leaflet; therefore, if the ultrasound beam is not aligned at the tips of the restricted leaflet, a normal EF slope may be erroneously recorded.

Pulmonary Valve "*a*" Wave Amplitude

The severity of pulmonary stenosis can be estimated by observation of an increase in the pulmonary *a* **wave amplitude**. The *a* wave amplitude is the depth of the posterior deflection of pulmonary valve observed immediately following atrial contraction. The depth of the *a* wave has been found to correlate with the peak pressure gradient across the pulmonary valve (see Table 10.9). The postulated mechanism for this increase in the pulmonary *a* wave amplitude is depicted in Figure 10.12.

Limitations: Two important conditions are known to affect the reliability of this measurement in the evaluation of pulmonary stenosis. Firstly, in patients with atrial fibrillation there is no effective atrial contraction so there is no *a* wave; hence, this measurement cannot be performed in these patients. Secondly, this measurement is only valid in patients with normal heart rates. Patients with slow heart rates will yield an increased inspiratory *a* wave in the absence of pulmonary stenosis. An additional limitation of this measurement is the frequency of false positive and false negative results.

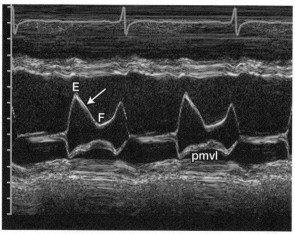

Normal Mitral Valve Motion

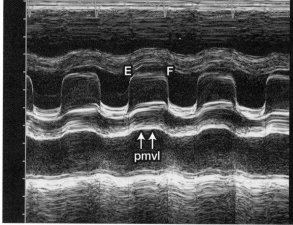

Severe Mitral Valve Stenosis

Figure 10.11: Mitral EF Slope on the Mitral M-Mode Trace: Normal and with Mitral Stenosis.
Left, This is an example of normal mitral valve motion. Observe the rapid decline of the EF slope (arrow) in early diastole as well as the posterior motion of the posterior mitral leaflet.
Right, This is an M-mode example of severe mitral stenosis. Marked prolongation of the EF slope is evident. Also observe anterior motion of the posterior mitral leaflet which results due to commissural fusion and "pulling" of the posterior leaflet by the larger anterior leaflet (double arrows).

Table 10.8: The Relationship between the Mitral EF Slope and the Mitral Valve Area.

Mitral Valve Area (MVA)	EF Slope	Pt. Pop.	Sensitivity	Specificity
Normal MVA (4 - 6 cm²)	> 80 mm/s	NS	….	….
MVA < 1.3 cm²	< 15 mm/s	427	30%	55.6%
MVA > 1.8 cm²	> 35 mm/s		60.5%	75%

Abbreviations: NS = not stated; **Pt. Pop.** = patient population.
Source: Cope, G.D., et al., *Circulation 52:664-670,1975.* Data obtained from composite results from numerous studies. Patient population: 210 patients = severe mitral stenosis [MVA < 1.3 cm²]; 112 patients = moderate mitral stenosis [MVA = 1.3 - 1.8 cm²]; 105 patients = mild mitral stenosis [MVA > 1.8 cm²].

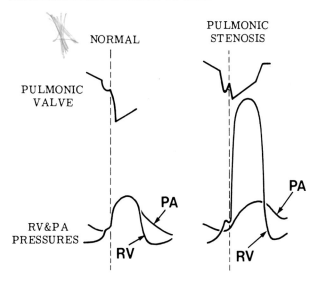

Figure 10.12: The Relationship between the Pulmonary *a* Wave and Pulmonary Stenosis.

Left, Normally, there is minimal difference between the right ventricular end-diastolic pressure (RVEDP) and pulmonary artery end-diastolic pressure (PAEDP). Therefore, even a small increase in the RVEDP, such as that which occurs following atrial contraction, is transmitted to the pulmonary valve resulting in a small deflection or opening motion of the valve - the *a* wave.

Right, In pulmonary stenosis, the pressure relationship across the pulmonary valve prior to ventricular systole indicates that forceful right atrial contraction causes the RVEDP to exceed the PAEDP. This ***positive*** pressure gradient causes the valve to dome as it is "pushed" open ***prior*** to ventricular systole. This opening or doming motion of the fused pulmonary leaflets is reflected on the M-mode trace by a marked increase in the *a* wave depth.

From Feigenbaum, H. Echocardiography. 5th Edition Lea and Febiger pp: 204, 1994. Reproduced with permission from Lippincott, Williams & Wilkins and from the author.

Table 10.9: The Relationship between the Pulmonary *a* Wave and the Peak Pulmonary Gradient.

Pulmonary valve Pressure Gradient (mmHg)	*a wave* Amplitude Range
No gradient	2 - 7 mm (Normal)
≤ 50 mmHg	2 - 10 mm (average 6 mm)
> 50 mmHg	6 - 18 mm (average 9.9 mm)

Source: Weyman, A.E., *American Journal of Medicine* 62:843-855,1977: patient population = 122: 50 patients = normal; 41 patients = pulmonary hypertension; 14 patients = mild pulmonary stenosis [gradient ≤ 50 mm Hg]; 17 patients = moderate to severe pulmonary stenosis [gradient > 50 mm Hg].

Left Ventricular Outflow Tract Obstruction

Left ventricular outflow tract (LVOT) obstruction is typically caused by three conditions: (1) hypertrophic obstructive cardiomyopathy (HOCM), (2) subaortic stenosis, and (3) hyperdynamic left ventricular systolic function with basal septal hypertrophy as seen in the elderly.

Two important M-mode findings have been identified which are characteristic of LVOT obstruction: (1) systolic anterior motion of the anterior mitral leaflet, and (2) premature closure of the aortic valve.

Systolic Anterior Motion of Mitral Valve Leaflets

Systolic anterior motion (SAM) of the anterior mitral valve leaflet refers to the marked and abnormal forward movement of the anterior mitral leaflet toward the LVOT in systole (Figure 10.13). This abnormal mitral valve motion occurs due to the Venturi effect or suction of the mitral valve apparatus into the LVOT. In patients with HOCM, anterior displacement of the papillary muscles toward each other has also been found to contribute to this phenomenon.

Although this finding is considered very specific for hypertrophic obstructive cardiomyopathy, the mere presence of SAM of the anterior mitral leaflet is not a reliable indicator of a coexistent LVOT gradient. In fact, it is the pattern of SAM of the anterior mitral leaflet that predicts the degree of obstruction. The magnitude of the LVOT pressure gradient is dependent upon three important variables: (1) the closeness of the anterior mitral leaflet to the interventricular septum, (2) the onset of SAM to the onset of SAM-septal contact, and (3) the duration of SAM-septal contact (Figure 10.14) [27].

Hence, low pressure gradients occur when SAM of the anterior mitral leaflet does not contact the interventricular septum, or when SAM-septal contact occurs late in systole and is of short duration.

Conversely, high pressure gradients occur when there is septal contact of the anterior mitral leaflet, when the SAM-septal contact occurs early in systole, and when the duration of contact is long.

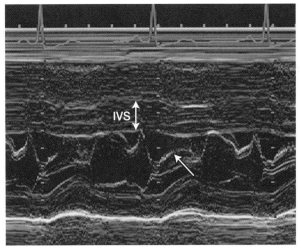

Figure 10.13: Systolic Anterior Motion (SAM) of the Anterior Mitral Valve Leaflet in Hypertrophic Obstructive Cardiomyopathy (HOCM).

This example illustrates systolic anterior motion of the anterior mitral leaflet (arrows). Also observe the asymmetric hypertrophy of the interventricular septum (IVS).

27: Pollick, M.B. et al.: Circulation 69 (No. 1): 43-49, 1984.

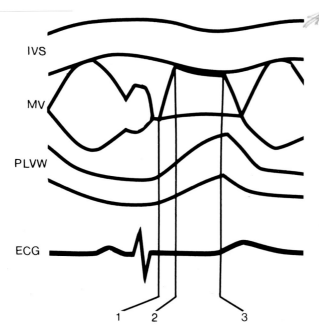

Figure 10.14: Variables affecting the Degree of Left Ventricular Outflow Tract Obstruction in Hypertrophic Obstructive Cardiomyopathy.

Numbers refer to points of measurement: 1 = onset of SAM of the anterior mitral leaflet; 2 = onset of SAM-septal contact; 3 = end of SAM-septal contact. The duration of SAM-septal contact is measured from point 2 to point 3. The period of onset of SAM to the onset of SAM-septal contact is measured from point 1 to point 2.

Abbreviations: ECG = electrocardiogram; **IVS** = interventricular septum; **MV** = mitral valve; **PLVW** = posterior left ventricular wall.

From Pollick, et al.: Muscular subaortic stenosis: The quantitative relationship between systolic anterior motion and the pressure gradient. *Circulation 69 (No. 1): 44,1984*. Reproduced with permission from Lippincott, Williams & Wilkins.

Premature (Mid-Systolic) Closure of Aortic Valve

Premature closure of the aortic valve occurs due to mid-systolic obstruction to blood flow through the valve. LVOT obstruction reduces the flow through the aortic valve such that the aortic valve begins to close, the aortic leaflets re-open once the obstruction is overcome (Figure 10.15).

While premature closure of the aortic valve is considered to be of great diagnostic value in the detection of LVOT obstruction, the mere presence of this echocardiographic sign *does not quantify* the severity of obstruction. Table 10.10 lists the reported sensitivities and specificities of the presence of mid systolic closure of the aortic valve in the identification of patients with LVOT obstruction

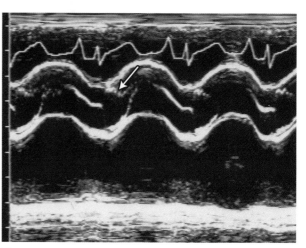

Figure 10.15: Premature (Mid-Systolic) Closure of the Aortic Valve in the presence of Left Ventricular Outflow Tract Obstruction.

This example illustrates premature closure of the aortic valve *(arrows)*. Also observe the coarse fluttering of the aortic leaflets.

Table 10.10: Sensitivities and Specificities of the Presence of Mid Systolic Closure of the Aortic Valve as an Indicator of Left Ventricular Outflow Tract Obstruction.

First Author (Year)	Pt. Pop.	Sensitivity (%)	Specificity (%)
Krajcer et al. (1978) [1]	Pre-operative - 40	100	100
	Post-operative - 18	75	64
Chahine et al. (1979) [2]	15	83	90
Krueger et al. (1979) [3]	243	95	96
Doi et al. (1980) [4]	84	77	93

Sources: (1) Krajcer, Z. et al., *American Journal of Cardiology 41: 823-829, 1978*: patient population: 9 patients = discrete subaortic stenosis with a resting gradient; 22 patients = idiopathic hypertrophic subaortic stenosis with a resting gradient; 9 patients = idiopathic hypertrophic subaortic stenosis without a resting gradient; **(2)** Chahine, R.A. et al., *American Journal of Cardiology 43: 17-23, 1979*: patient population: 15 patients = hypertrophic cardiomyopathy [8 with LVOT obstruction]; **(3)** Krueger, S.K. et al., *Circulation 59: 506-513, 1979*: patient population: 234 = normal subjects; 41 patients = aortic valve stenosis; 22 patients = discrete subaortic stenosis; **(4)** Doi, Y.L. et al., *American Journal of Cardiology 45: 6-14, 1980*: patient population: 70 patients = hypertrophic cardiomyopathy [27 patients = LVOT obstruction at rest; 21 patients = LVOT gradient with provocation; 22 patients = no LVOT obstruction at rest or with provocation].

Intracardiac Pressure Estimation

M-mode findings for increases in pulmonary artery pressures and left ventricular end-diastolic pressure (LVEDP) have been described with many of these findings being highly specific for the elevation of these pressures. Although these measurements have since been superseded by Doppler echocardiographic methods, the M-mode signs may occasionally provide the important supporting evidence as to the elevation of these pressures.

Pulmonary Hypertension

Three abnormalities of the pulmonary valve can be appreciated on the M-mode examination in cases of pulmonary hypertension: (1) absent or diminished *a* wave, (2) midsystolic notching or closure of the pulmonary valve, and (3) increased right ventricular pre-ejection period to right ventricular ejection time (RVPEP/RVET) ratio.

1. Absent or Diminished a wave Amplitude:

The *a* wave amplitude is the depth of the posterior deflection of pulmonary valve observed immediately following atrial contraction normally measuring 2 to 7 mm. An absent or diminished *a* wave has been proven useful in the differentiation of those patients with pulmonary hypertension (mean pulmonary artery pressure ≥ 20 mm Hg) from individuals with normal pulmonary

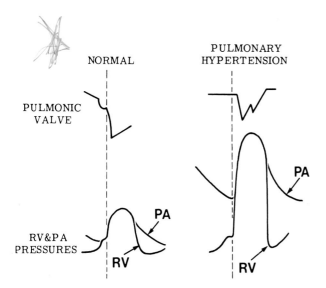

Figure 10.16: The Relationship between the Pulmonary *a Wave* and Pulmonary Hypertension.
Left, Normally, there is minimal difference between the right ventricular end-diastolic pressure (RVEDP) and pulmonary artery end-diastolic pressure (PAEDP). Therefore, even a small increase in the RVEDP, such as that which occurs following atrial contraction, is transmitted to the pulmonary valve resulting in a deflection or opening motion of the valve - the *a wave*.
Right, In pulmonary hypertension, the increase in PAEDP is much greater than the RVEDP. Therefore, even with the additional increase in the RVEDP following atrial contraction, the RVEDP still fails to approach the PAEDP, resulting in little or no movement of the valve.
From Feigenbaum, H. Echocardiography. 5th Edition Lea and Febiger pp: 204, 1994. Reproduced with permission from Lippincott, Williams & Wilkins and from the author.

artery pressures. The postulated mechanism for this reduction in the pulmonary a wave amplitude is depicted in Figure 10.16. The sensitivities and specificities of a reduced a wave amplitude as an indication of pulmonary hypertension are listed in Table 10.11.

Limitations: The most obvious limitation of this finding occurs in patients with atrial fibrillation when there is no effective atrial contraction and, therefore, there is no *a* wave. Also "normalisation" of the *a* wave amplitude may occur in those patients with pulmonary hypertension and coexistent severe right ventricular failure [28+29].

Furthermore, despite a high specificity of this sign in the identification of patients with pulmonary hypertension, there is no correlation between the *a* wave amplitude and actual pulmonary artery pressure.

2. Mid-systolic Closure or Notching of the Pulmonary Valve:

Mid-systolic closure or notching of the pulmonary valve M-mode trace produces a characteristic "W-shaped" pattern (Figure 10.17). This distinctive finding is considered the most valuable sign of pulmonary hypertension. The sensitivities and specificities of mid-systolic notching of the pulmonary valve as an indicator of pulmonary hypertension are listed in Table 10.12.

Limitations: As for an absent or diminished *a* wave and despite a high specificity of this sign in the identification of patients with pulmonary hypertension, there is no correlation between mid-systolic notching and actual pulmonary artery pressure.

3. Increased RVPEP/RVET ratio:

Right ventricular systolic time intervals have been used in the past to indirectly assess pulmonary hypertension in children. Commonly measured systolic time intervals include the right ventricular pre-ejection period (RVPEP), the right ventricular ejection time (RVET), and the ratio between these two variables (Figure 10.18). The **right ventricular pre-ejection period**

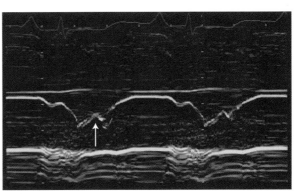

Figure 10.17: Mid-systolic Notching on the Pulmonary Valve M-Mode with Pulmonary Hypertension.
This example illustrates mid-systolic notching of the pulmonary valve in a patient with pulmonary hypertension *(arrow)*.

28: Nanda, N.C. et al.: Circulation 50: 575-581, 1974. 29: Weyman, A.E. et al.: Circulation 50: 905-910, 1974.

Table 10.11: Sensitivity and Specificity of a decreased *a* wave Amplitude (≤ 2 mm) as an indicator of Pulmonary Hypertension (mean pulmonary artery pressure ≥ 20 mm Hg).

First Author (Year)	Pt. Pop.	Pt. Pop.	Sensitivity	Specificity
Nanda (1974) [1]	63	NS	88%	95%
Weyman (1974) [2]	56	427	79%	100%
Lew (1979) [3]	48		69%	100%
Haddard (1981) [4]	64		94%	100%

Sources: (1) Nanda, N.C. et al., *Circulation 50: 575-581, 1974*: patient population: 22 patients = normal; 41 patients = pulmonary hypertension; **(2)** Weyman, A.E. et al., *Circulation 50: 905-910, 1974*: patient population: 24 patients = normal; 32 patients = pulmonary hypertension; **(3)** Lew, W. et al., *British Heart Journal 42: 147-161, 1979*: patient population: 20 patients = normal; 28 patients = pulmonary hypertension; **(4)** Haddard, K.A. et al., *Acta Cardiologica 36: 21-34, 1981*: patient population: 40 patients = normal; 24 patients = pulmonary hypertension.

Table 10.12: Sensitivity and Specificity of Mid-Systolic Notching of the Pulmonary Valve M-Mode as an indicator of Pulmonary Hypertension (mean pulmonary artery pressure ≥ 20 mm Hg.).

First Author (Year)	Pt. Pop.	Sensitivity	Specificity
Nanda et al. (1974) [1]	63	88 %	100 %
Weyman et al. (1974) [2]	56	90 %	100 %
Lew et al. (1979) [3]	39	69 %	100 %
Haddard et al. (1981) [4]	64	42 %	100 %

Sources: (1) Nanda, N.C. et al., *Circulation 50: 575-581, 1974*: patient population: 22 patients = normal; 41 patients = pulmonary hypertension; **(2)** Weyman, A.E. et al., *Circulation 50: 905-910, 1974*: patient population: 24 patients = normal; 32 patients = pulmonary hypertension; **(3)** Lew, W. et al., *British Heart Journal 42: 147-161, 1979*: patient population: 20 patients = normal; 28 patients = pulmonary hypertension; **(4)** Haddard, K.A. et al., *Acta Cardiologica 36: 21-34, 1981*: patient population: 40 patients = normal; 24 patients = pulmonary hypertension.

(RVPEP) is measured from the Q wave of the ECG to the onset of valve opening while the **right ventricular ejection time (RVET)** is the interval in which the valve remains open (b-e points). Both of these intervals are affected by the heart rate (interval decreases with increasing heart rate) while the RVET is also affected by the age of the patient (interval increases with advancing age). The **RVPEP/RVET ratio** is simply derived by dividing the RVPEP by the RVET. This interval is not significantly affected by either heart rate or age and, therefore, provides a simple and uncomplicated method for the assessment of pulmonary hypertension.

With pulmonary hypertension, right ventricular systolic time intervals vary from normal such that the RVET shortens with early closure of the pulmonary valve and the RVPEP lengthens, resulting in an overall increase in the RVPEP/RVET ratio [30 + 31].

The RVPEP/RVET ratio has been found to correlate best with the pulmonary artery end-diastolic pressure (see Table 10.13).

Limitations: Although the RVPEP/RVET ratio may be useful in the estimation of pulmonary artery end-diastolic pressure, it is not sufficiently sensitive or specific to be considered diagnostic and has since been superseded by Doppler echocardiography. Furthermore, it is often difficult to adequately record opening and closure of the pulmonary valve and, therefore,

measurement accuracy is compromised. Measurement accuracy is crucial as any small measurement error may lead to large errors in the calculation of this ratio. Another limitation of this technique is conduction defects such as right bundle branch block which alter the pre-ejection period (the RVPEP is increased with complete right bundle branch block). Finally, in patients with congestive cardiomyopathies, the RVPEP/RVET ratio reflects the right ventricular dysfunction rather than the pulmonary artery end-diastolic pressure.

Table 10.13: The Relationship between the RVPEP/RVET and the Pulmonary Artery End-Diastolic Pressure (PAEDP).

PAEDP	RVPEP/RVET
Normal (PAEDP 10 - 15 mm Hg)	≤ 0.30
Pulmonary Hypertension (PAEDP > 20 mm Hg)	> 0.35
"gray area" *	0.30 - 0.35

* The "gray area" constitutes an overlap between normal and elevated pulmonary artery end-diastolic pressures (from 6 to 50 mm Hg).
Source: Riggs, T. et al., *Circulation 57:939-947,1978*: patient population: 85 patients = normal; 140 patients = PAEDP < 20 mm Hg; 65 patients = PAEDP ≥ 20 mm Hg.

30: Riggs, T. et al.: Circulation 57:939-947,1978. 31: Hirschfeld, S. et al.: Circulation 52: 642-650, 1975.

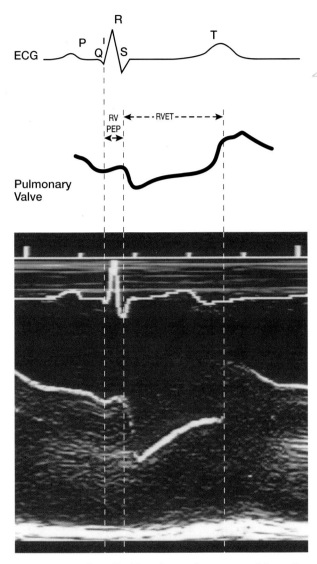

Figure 10.18: Systolic Time Intervals measured from the Pulmonary Valve M-Mode Trace.
The **RVPEP** is measured from the Q wave of the ECG to the onset of valve opening. The **RVET** is interval in which the valve remains open (*b-e* points). The **RVPEP/RVET** is simply derived by dividing the RVPEP by the RVET.

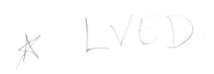

Elevated Left Ventricular End-Diastolic Pressure

A reasonably reliable indicator for elevation of the left ventricular end-diastolic pressure is the presence of a "B-notch" interrupting the AC slope of the anterior mitral leaflet M-mode trace (Figure 10.19). The basis of this finding is delineated in Figure 10.20. The sensitivities and specificities of the "B-notch" on the mitral M-mode trace as an indicator for an elevated left ventricular end-diastolic pressure are listed in Table 10.14.

Limitations: The primary limitation of this finding is that it is not very sensitive. Furthermore, false positive results may occur with first degree heart block (particularly, when the PR interval is greater than 0.20 seconds), and with left bundle branch block due to prolongation of the AC interval itself.

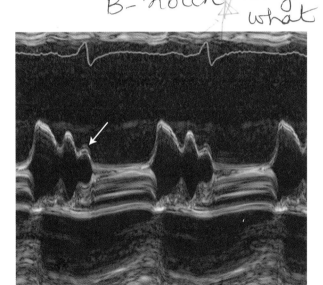

Figure 10.19: Mitral valve B-notch.
The presence of a B-notch (arrow) on the M-mode trace of the anterior mitral valve is a very specific sign indicating an elevation of the left ventricular end-diastlic pressure (> 20 mm Hg).

Table 10.14: Sensitivity and Specificity of a "B-notch" on the Mitral Valve M-Mode Trace as an indicator of Elevated Left Ventricular End-diastolic Pressure.

First Author (Year)	Pt. Pop.	Sensitivity	Specificity
Konecke et al. (1973) [1]	36	79 %	-
Ambrose et al. (1979) [2]	24	29 %	100 %
D'Cruz et al. (1990) [3]	50	39 % (70 % *)	78.6 %

* When patients with a normal left ventricular ejection fraction (> 55%) and an LVEDP > 15 mm Hg were excluded.
Sources: (1) Konecke, L.L. et al., *Circulation 47: 989-996, 1973*: patient population: 19 patients = LVEDP < 20 mm Hg; 17 patients = LVEDP ≥ 20 mm Hg; **(2)** Ambrose, J.A. et al., *Circulation 60: 510-519, 1979*: patient population: 10 patients = LVEDP < 20 mm Hg; 14 patients = LVEDP ≥ 20 mm Hg; **(3)** D'Cruz, I.A. et al., *Echocardiography 7: 69-75, 1990*: patient population: 19 patients = LVEDP < 15 mm Hg and LVEF > 55%; 18 patients = LVEDP < 15 mm Hg and LVEF < 55%; 3 patients = LVEDP > 15 mm Hg and LVEF < 55%; 10 patients = LVEDP > 15 mm Hg and LVEF < 55%.

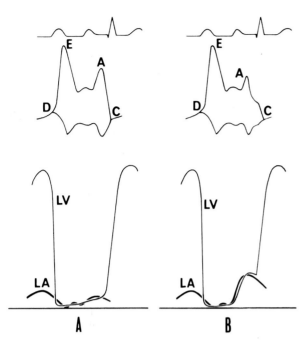

Figure 10.20: Schematic M-mode Trace of the Mitral Valve Reflecting Changes in the Left Atrial and Left Ventricular Pressure Recordings.
A. Normal Left Ventricular End-Diastolic Pressures.
In the normal individual, the left ventricular diastolic pressure is relatively low with an initial or early diastolic pressure around 0 mmHg. Due to the relatively large mitral valve orifice, there is minimal obstruction to the passage of blood flow from the left atrium (LA) to the left ventricle (LV) in diastole so that the LA pressure is only slightly higher than that of the LV. When the LV pressure has fallen below that of the LA, the mitral valve leaflets open abruptly and blood flows rapidly from the LA to the LV. This rapid opening of the mitral valve leaflets is represented as a steep D-E slope on the M-mode trace. Throughout diastole, as the LV continues to fill, the ventricular pressure rises slowly and gradually and the mitral valve begins to close. Following atrial contraction, there is a slight rise in the LA pressure, which re-opens the mitral valve and forces a further bolus of blood from the atrium to the ventricle. In the normal compliant LV, this additional atrial contraction is accepted with a relatively small increase in pressure (the A point of the M-mode trace corresponds to the *a* wave of the LA pressure trace). When LA pressure falls below that of the LV, the mitral valve begins to close. Following ventricular systole, there is a rapid rise in ventricular pressure, which completes mitral valve closure. Closure of the mitral valve occurs between the A and C points, the slope of the A-C interval is smooth, uninterrupted and of a short duration.
B. Increased Left Ventricular End-Diastolic Pressure.
This Figure illustrates the changes that occur on the mitral valve M-mode trace when the left ventricular end-diastolic pressure (LVEDP) is elevated. Elevation of the LVEDP occurs as a result of a marked increase in the LV pressure following atrial contraction due to diminished ventricular compliance which may occur with hypertrophy, fibrosis or coronary artery disease. With atrial contraction, the LA pressure rises rapidly as blood is forced from the atrium to the ventricle as depicted by an increase in the *a* wave on the LA pressure trace. This increase in pressure results in a parallel rapid rise in the LVEDP. The parallel increase in these two pressures results in the early cross-over of pressures subsequently leading to the premature onset of mitral valve closure as depicted by the A point occurring earlier than usual on the M-mode trace. When the atrial and ventricular pressures approach equality, closure of the mitral valve (A-C slope) may be interrupted with the appearance of a plateau or notch (B-notch). Termination of mitral valve closure may be delayed as more time is required for the LV pressure to exceed that of the elevated LA pressure. The final result of the earlier onset and delayed completion of mitral valve closure is prolongation of the A-C interval.
From Feigenbaum, H. Echocardiography. 5th Edition. USA: Lea and Febiger, pp: 199, 1994. Reproduced with permission from Lippincott, Williams & Wilkins and the author.

References and Suggested Reading:

General References:
- Feigenbaum, H.: Echocardiography. Chapter 1. 5th Ed. Lea & Febiger, 1994.
- Otto, C.M. and Pearlman, A.S.: Textbook of Clinical Echocardiography. Chapter 1. W.B. Saunders Company . 1995
- Weyman, A.: Principles and Practice of Echocardiography. 2nd ed. Lea & Febiger,1994.

Cardiac Chamber Dimensions:
- Reynolds, T.: Echocardiographer's Pocket Reference. Arizona Heart Institute Foundation.1993.

Left Ventricular Systolic Function:
Fractional Shortening, Ejection Fraction, Stroke Volume and Cardiac Output:
- Gardin, J.M. et al.: Echocardiographic measurements in normal subjects: evaluation of an adult population without clinically apparent heart disease. *Journal of Clinical Ultrasound 7: 439-447, 1979.*
- Henry, W.L. et al.: Echocardiographic measurements in normal subjects: Growth related changes that occur between infancy and early adulthood. *Circulation 57: 278-285, 1977.*
- Henry, W.L. et al.: Echocardiographic measurements in normal subjects from infancy to old age. *Circulation 62: 1054-1061, 1980.*
- Popp, R. L.: M-Mode echocardiographic assessment of left ventricular function. *American Journal of Cardiology 49: 1312-1318, 1982.*
- Quinones, M.A. et al.: A new, simplified and accurate method for determining ejection fraction with two-dimensional echocardiography. *Circulation 64: 744-753, 1981.*
- Remes, J. et al.: Usefulness of M-mode echocardiography in the diagnosis of heart failure. *Cardiology 78: 267-277, 1991.*
- Sahn, D.J. et al.: Recommendations regarding quantitation in M-mode echocardiography: Results of a survey of echocardiographic measurements. *Circulation 58: 1072-1083, 1978.*
- Schiller, N.B., Foster, E. Analysis of left ventricular systolic function. *Heart (Supplement 2): 75: 17-26, 1996.*
- Teicholz, L.E. et al.: Problems in echocardiographic volume determinations: Echocardiographic-angiographic correlations in the presence or absence of asynergy. *American Journal of Cardiology 37: 7-11, 1976.*

Mitral E-Point-Septal Separation:
- Ahmadpour, H. et al.: Mitral E point septal separation: A reliable index of left ventricular performance in coronary artery disease. *American Heart Journal 106: 21-28, 1983.*

- Child, J.S. et al.: Effect of left ventricular size on mitral E point to ventricular septal separation in assessment of cardiac performance. *American Heart Journal 101: 797-805, 1981.*
- Lew, W. et al.: Assessment of mitral valve E point-septal separation as an index of left ventricular performance in patients with acute and previous myocardial infarction. *American Journal of Cardiology 41: 836-845, 1978.*

Systolic Time Intervals:
- Garrard, C.L. et al.: The relationship of alterations in systolic time intervals to ejection fraction in patients with cardiac disease. *Circulation 42: 455-462, 1970.*
- Lewis, R.P et al.: A critical review of the systolic time intervals. *Circulation 56: 146-158, 1977.*
- Weissler, A.M. et al.: Systolic time intervals in heart failure in man. *Circulation 37: 149-159, 1968.*

Left Ventricular Mass:
- Daniels, S.R. et al.: Echocardiographically determined left ventricular mass index in normal children, adolescents and young adults. *Journal of the American College of Cardiology 12: 703-708, 1988.*
- Devereux, R.B. et al.: Echocardiographic determination of left ventricular mass in man. *Circulation 55:613-618, 1976.*
- Devereux, R. B. et al.: Standardization of M-mode echocardiographic left ventricular anatomic measurements. *Journal of the American College of Cardiology 4: 1222-1230, 1984.*
- Devereux, R.B. et al.: Echocardiographic assessment of left ventricular hypertrophy: comparison to necropsy findings. *American Journal of Cardiology 57: 450-458, 1986.*
- Shub, C. et al.: Determination of left ventricular mass by echocardiography in a normal population: effect of age and sex in addition to body size. *Mayo Clinic Proceedings 69: 05-211, 1994.*

Valvular Stenosis and Left Ventricular Outflow Tract Obstruction:
Aortic Stenosis:
- DeMaria, A. N. et al.: Sensitivity and specificity of cross-sectional echocardiography in the diagnosis and quantification of valvular aortic stenosis. *Circulation 57 (Supplement II): II-232, 1978.*
- DeMaria, A.N. et al.: Value and limitations of cross-sectional echocardiography of the aortic valve in the diagnosis and quantification of valvular aortic stenosis. *Circulation 62: 304-312, 1980.*
- Godley, R.W. et al.: Reliability of two-dimensional echocardiography in assessing the severity of valvular aortic stenosis. *Chest 79: 657-662, 1981.*

Mitral Stenosis:
- Cope, G.D. et al.: A reassessment of the echocardiogram in mitral stenosis. *Circulation 52: 664-670, 1975.*

Pulmonary Stenosis:
- Weyman, A.E. et al.: Echocardiographic patterns of pulmonary valve motion in valvular pulmonary stenosis. *American Journal of Cardiology 34: 644-651, 1974.*
- Weyman, A.E.: Pulmonary valve echo motion in clinical practice. *American Journal of Medicine 62: 843-855, 1977.*

Left Ventricular Outflow Tract Obstruction:
- Chahine, R.A. et al.: Mid systolic closure of aortic valve in hypertrophic cardiomyopathy. *American Journal of Cardiology. 43: 17-23, 1979.*
- Doi, Y.L. et al.: M-mode echocardiography in hypertrophic cardiomyopathy: diagnostic criteria and prediction of obstruction. *American Journal of Cardiology. 45: 6-14, 1980.*
- Krajcer, Z. et al.: Early systolic closure of the aortic valve in patients with hypertrophic subaortic stenosis and discrete subaortic stenosis. *American Journal of Cardiology. 41: 823-829, 1978.*
- Krueger, S.K. et al.: Echocardiography in discrete subaortic stenosis. *Circulation 59: 506-513, 1979.*
- Pollick, . et al.: Muscular subaortic stenosis: the quantitative relationship between systolic anterior motion and the pressure gradient. *Circulation 69: 43-49, 1984.*

Intracardiac Pressure Estimation:
Pulmonary Hypertension:
- Haddard, K.A. et al.: Use of echocardiography in the diagnosis of pulmonary hypertension. *Acta Cardiologica 36: 21-34, 1981.*
- Hirschfeld, S. et al.: The echocardiographic assessment of pulmonary artery pressure and pulmonary vascular resistance. *Circulation 52: 642-650, 1974.*
- Lew, W. , Karliner, J.S.: Assessment of pulmonary valve echogram in normal subjects and in patients with pulmonary arterial hypertension. *British Heart Journal 42: 147-161, 1979.*
- Nanda, N.C. et al.: Echocardiographic evaluation of pulmonary hypertension. *Circulation 50: 575-581, 1974.*
- Riggs, T. et al.: Assessment of the pulmonary vascular bed by echocardiographic right ventricular systolic time intervals. *Circulation 57: 939-947, 1978.*
- Weyman, A.E. et al.: Echocardiographic patterns of pulmonic valve motion with pulmonary hypertension. *Circulation 50: 905-910, 1974.*
- Weyman, A.E.: Pulmonary valve echo motion in clinical practice. *American Journal of Medicine 62: 843-855, 1977.*

Elevated Left Ventricular End-Diastolic Pressure:
- Ambrose, J. A. et al.: The influence of left ventricular late diastolic filling on the A wave of the left ventricular pressure trace. *Circulation 60: 510-519, 1979.*

- D'Cruz, I.A et al.: A reappraisal of the mitral B-bump (B-inflection): its relationship to left ventricular dysfunction. *Echocardiography 7: 69-75, 1990.*
- Konecke, L.L. et al.: Abnormal mitral valve motion in patients with elevated left ventricular diastolic pressures. *Circulation 47: 989-996, 1973.*

Chapter 11
Doppler Haemodynamic Calculations

As discussed in Chapter 9 (Two-Dimensional Calculations) and Chapter 10 (M-Mode Measurements), there are many measurements and calculations which can provide indirect evidence of the haemodynamic severity of cardiac lesions. In addition, 2-D and M-mode echocardiography are able to identify the secondary consequences of the primary haemodynamic pathology (see Table 11.1). However, these findings lack sensitivity and specificity in the detection of these disease processes. Because of the limitations of 2-D and M-mode echocardiography and prior to the development of Doppler echocardiography, haemodynamic information regarding the severity of valve lesions and intracardiac pressures was only achieved via invasive cardiac catheterisation. The advent of Doppler echocardiography has provided a means by which haemodynamic information such as transvalvular pressure gradients, intracardiac pressures, and stroke volumes can be obtained noninvasively. Hence, Doppler echocardiography has superseded many of the 2-D and M-mode findings and calculations tabulated below.

Most Doppler haemodynamic calculations can be classified into: (1) the volumetric flow calculations, (2) the continuity principle, and (3) the Bernoulli equation. The principles of each of these three methods are discussed in detail below. Other Doppler measurements that can be performed involve the measurement of time intervals.

Table 11.1: Examples of the 2-D and M-mode Echocardiographic Findings suggestive of Haemodynamic Abnormalities.

HAEMODYNAMIC ABNORMALITY	2-D AND M-MODE FINDINGS
Aortic regurgitation	• diastolic mitral valve flutter • diastolic flutter of the interventricular septum • reversed doming of the anterior mitral leaflet
Acute, severe aortic regurgitation	• premature closure of the mitral valve • premature opening of the aortic valve
Valvular stenosis	• reduced aortic cusp separation (aortic stenosis) • reduced EF slope (mitral stenosis) • increased pulmonary valve *a* wave amplitude (pulmonary stenosis)
Left ventricular outflow tract obstruction	• midsystolic closure of the aortic valve • coarse systolic fluttering of the aortic valve • systolic anterior motion of the anterior mitral leaflet
Pulmonary hypertension	• absent or diminished pulmonary valve *a* wave • mid systolic closure or notching of the pulmonary valve • alterations in right ventricular systolic time intervals • D-shaped left ventricle or flattening of the interventricular septum
Increased right atrial pressure	• dilated IVC with lack of respiratory collapse • persistent bowing of interatrial septum toward the left atrium
Increased left atrial pressure	• persistent bowing of interatrial septum toward the right atrium
Elevated left ventricular end-diastolic pressures	• B-notch of the anterior mitral leaflet
Cardiac tamponade	• diastolic right atrial and right ventricular collapse

Volumetric Flow Calculations

Spectral Doppler velocity measurements, in conjunction with 2-D echocardiographic imaging, can be reliably used to noninvasively measure volumetric flow at specific locations within the heart and great vessels. The clinical applications of volumetric flow calculations include: (1) the assessment of the stroke volume and cardiac output, (2) calculation of regurgitant volumes and regurgitant fractions, (3) calculation of the stenotic or prosthetic orifice areas, and (4) the calculation of intracardiac shunt ratios.

Theoretical Considerations:

The basic concepts of volumetric flow calculations have been briefly discussed in Chapter 5. Recall that calculations of volumetric flow are based on a simple hydraulic principle which states that the volumetric flow (Q) through a tube of a constant diameter is directly proportional to the cross-sectional area (CSA) of the tube and the mean velocity of fluid moving through the tube (V) providing that the CSA is fixed and the velocity is constant (Figure 11.1).

Hence, the calculation of volumetric flow is expressed

by the following equation:

(Equation 5.6)

$$Q = V \times CSA$$

where   Q   = volumetric flow rate (cc/s)
       CSA = cross-sectional area (cm²)
       V   = mean fluid flow velocity (cm/s)

Calculation of volumetric flow becomes more complex when the velocity is not constant. This is the situation within the heart where blood flow is pulsatile changing with systole and diastole as well as throughout the flow period. In this situation, volumetric flow is actually the product of the "integrated" velocity over time and the CSA (Figure 11.2). The integrated velocity over time is equal to the area under the curve (velocity [cm/s] **x** time [s]). Therefore, the area under the curve is measured in cm and hence, is a measure of the distance (D) that the column of fluid flows. Since the integrated velocity over time is equal to the distance that the column of fluid travels, calculation of the volumetric flow is analogous to the calculation of the volume of a cylinder (Figure 11.3). This simplified concept can be applied to the calculation of volumetric flow through the heart and cardiovascular system where the "fluid" is blood and the "tube" is the vessel or valve lumen through which flow is occurring.

Doppler Echocardiographic Determination of Volumetric Flow:

In the heart, the volume of blood flow through a specific region is determined from its CSA and the actual distance that the column of blood moves with each stroke or heart beat. The CSA can be readily determined from measuring the diameter of a specific location within the heart or great vessels while the stroke distance can be derived from the velocity time integral (VTI).

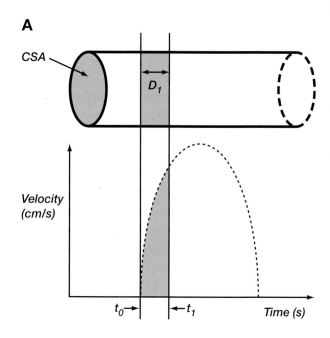

A

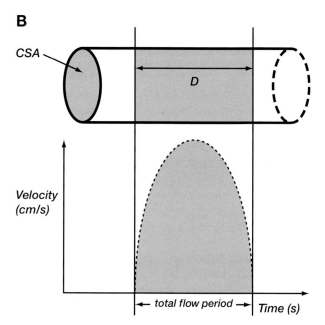

B

Figure 11.2: Calculation of Volumetric Flow (Changing Velocities). This schematic illustrates the more complex situation in which velocity is changing throughout the flow period.
A. Observe that from the time interval t_0 to t_1, the column of fluid has moved a distance of D_1.
B. By integrating the entire velocity-time curve, the total distance that blood flows during the total period of flow can be determined. This total distance is equal to the entire area under the velocity-time curve.

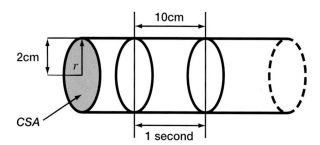

Figure 11.1: Calculation of Volumetric Flow (Constant Velocity). Volumetric flow is equal to the product of the cross-sectional area (CSA) of the tube and the velocity of flow. In this example, the column of fluid moves forward 10 cm every second, therefore, the velocity of flow (V) equates to 10 cm/s. The radius of the tube is 2 cm, therefore, using the equation to calculate the area of a circle (πr^2), the CSA equates to 12.6 cm². Hence, the volumetric flow (Q) can be calculated using equation (5.5):

$$Q = 12.5 \ cm^2 \ \times 10 \ cm/s = 126 \ cc/s$$

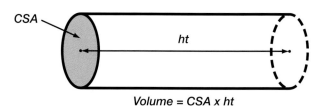

$$Volume = CSA \times ht$$

Figure 11.3: Calculation of the Volume of a Cylinder. The volume of a cylinder is the product of the cross-sectional area (CSA) of the cylinder and the height or length (ht) of the cylinder.

Cross-Sectional Area (CSA):
As outlined in Chapter 9, the CSA of valve annuli can be calculated by 2-D echocardiography from the diameter assuming a circular geometry:

(Equation 9.2)

$$Area = 0.785 \times D^2$$

Since the stroke volume is a measure of the blood flow through a specific region with each heart beat, determination of the CSA must be performed during the flow period. Therefore, when calculating the stroke volume from the LVOT, the diameter is measured during systole. Conversely, when calculating the stroke volume from the mitral annulus, the diameter is measured during diastole.

Velocity Time Integral (VTI):
As mentioned, measurement of changing velocity over the flow period is determined by integrating the area under the velocity-time curve. In Doppler echocardiography, this velocity-time integral (VTI) is obtained by measuring the area under the Doppler curve by tracing either the leading edge of the velocity spectrum (aortic and pulmonary velocities) or the modal velocity (mitral and tricuspid velocities). The modal velocity reflects the dominant flow velocity at any given instant in time and is identified as the darkest velocity signal on the spectral Doppler display. Because the Doppler signal represents velocity (cm/s) versus time (s), the area under the Doppler curve is equal to distance (cm). Thus, the VTI is sometimes also referred to as the "stroke distance" which is the distance that a column of blood travels with each heart beat.

Calculation of Volumetric Flow:
Volumetric flow or the stroke volume is calculated from the following equation:

(Equation 11.1)

$$SV = CSA \times VTI$$

where SV = stroke volume (cc)
      VTI = distance a column of blood travels with each stroke (cm)
      CSA = cross-sectional area (cm²)

Limitations to Volumetric Flow Calculations:
Assumptions of Volumetric Flow Calculations:
As described above, volumetric flow calculations are based on a simple hydraulic formula that determines the volumetric flow rate through a cylindrical tube under steady flow conditions. Therefore, in applying this concept to the heart, the following assumptions are made: (1) flow is occurring in a rigid, circular tube, (2) there is a uniform velocity across the vessel, (3) derived CSA is circular, (4) CSA remains constant throughout the period of flow, and (5) the sample volume remains in a constant position throughout the period of flow.

However, blood vessels are elastic (not rigid) and annular diameters may change throughout the period of flow. Furthermore, while the left and right ventricular outflow tracts assume a circular configuration, the same may not be said for the atrioventricular valves, which are more elliptical in shape.

Technical Consideration:
The area of an ellipse can be determined by the following equation:

(Equation 11.2)

$$area = \frac{\pi}{4} a\, b$$

where area = area of an ellipse (cm²)
      a   = diameter in one plane (cm)
      b   = diameter in plane perpendicular to a (cm)

Error in VTI Measurements:
Technical errors in the VTI measurements may also occur. Failure to optimise the Doppler velocity spectrum by inadequate beam alignment with blood flow direction (that is, a large angle θ) will lead to suboptimal Doppler signals. Other errors in the VTI measurement include failure to correctly trace the VTI. Typically, VTI measurements obtained from atrioventricular valves are traced along the modal velocity (darkest, brightest line) while VTI measurements obtained from the outflow tracts and great vessels are traced along the leading edge of the Doppler signal. Measurement of too few beats can also produce inaccuracies. For sinus rhythm it is recommended that 3 - 5 beats are measured and averaged. For atrial fibrillation, 8 - 10 beats should be measured and averaged.

Error in Diameter Measurement:
Technical errors in the diameter measurement will be reflected in the calculation of the CSA and, hence, the volumetric flow. Technical errors which may occur include: (1) measurement of the diameter during the wrong phase of the cardiac cycle (measurement of CSA must be performed at the time of flow through that site), (2) inconsistent annulus measurements, and (3) difficulty in measuring the right ventricular outflow tract (RVOT). Measurement of the RVOT in the direction of axial resolution is not possible and it is often difficult to measure the left lateral border of the RVOT due to adjacent lung tissue. Any error in the diameter measurement is magnified in the area (recall that the CSA is derived by squaring the diameter [equation 9.2]).

Evaluation of Intracardiac Shunts

Intracardiac shunt lesions can be quantified based on comparisons of flow through individual valves. In the normal heart, the stroke volume across each of the four cardiac valves is equal; thus, the stroke volume through the left and right sides of the heart is equal. Therefore, the volume of pulmonary venous flow (QP) equals the volume of systemic venous flow (QS) so that the ratio of pulmonary venous flow to systemic venous flow (QP:QS) equals 1. Studies comparing the accuracy of QP:QS calculations performed by Doppler echocardiography with those by other techniques are listed in Appendix 1.

In the presence of an intracardiac shunt, the stroke volume through one side of the heart will be greater than that through the other side. Whether flow is greater through the left or right side of the heart is dependent upon the direction of the shunt. Most commonly, because the pressures are greater in the left heart and the aorta, intracardiac shunts are typically directed from left to right. Based on this concept, the flow ratio between the pulmonary and systemic circulation can be used to indicate the size of the shunt.

Theoretical Considerations:

The theoretical principles of volumetric flow calculations have been discussed in detail at the beginning of this chapter. Recall that the calculation of volumetric flow is based on a simple hydraulic principle which states that the amount of flow (Q) through a tube of a constant diameter is directly proportional to the cross-sectional area (CSA) of the tube and the mean velocity of fluid moving through the tube (V) when the orifice CSA is fixed and the velocity is constant. In the heart, because flow is pulsatile changing with systole and diastole, volumetric flow is calculated as the product of the "integrated" velocity over time (velocity time integral) and the CSA:

(Equation 11.2)

$$Q = CSA \times VTI$$

where Q   = volumetric flow (cc)
         VTI = distance a column of blood travels with
                     each stroke (cm)
         CSA = cross-sectional area (cm^2)

Method of Measurement:

The methods used in the calculation of the volumetric flow or stroke volume through each of the cardiac valves as well as through the aorta and main pulmonary artery are discussed in detail in Chapter 14. The QP:QS is simply the ratio of pulmonary venous flow (QP) to systemic venous flow (QS):

(Equation 11.3)

$$QP:QS = \frac{SV_{pulmonary}}{SV_{systemic}}$$

where $SV_{pulmonary}$ = pulmonary venous stroke volume (cc)
       $SV_{systemic}$ = systemic stroke volume (cc)

The locations selected for the determination of flow volumes will depend upon the location of the shunt. Calculation of the QP:QS through various shunt lesions is discussed below and summarised in Table 11.2.

Atrial Septal Defects (ASD):
Calculation of QP:

QP reflects the stroke volume through the pulmonary venous circulation; that is, through the lungs. Assuming that the shunt is directed left-to-right, then QP will include both the normal forward stroke volume as well as the shunt volume. Thus, QP is calculated downstream from the shunt. In a patient with an ASD, QP can be calculated using the RVOT, the main pulmonary artery or tricuspid valve since the stroke volume through each of these regions is the same (Figure 11.4).

Calculation of QS:

QS reflects the normal stroke volume through the systemic circulation; hence, QS is calculated distal to the shunt. In a patient with an ASD, QS can be calculated using the LVOT, the ascending aorta, or the mitral valve since the stroke volume through each of these regions is the same (Figure 11.4).

Ventricular Septal Defects (ASD):
Calculation of QP:

QP reflects the stroke volume through the pulmonary venous circulation. Assuming that the shunt is directed left-to-right, then QP will include both the normal forward stroke volume as well as the shunt volume. Thus, QP is calculated downstream from the shunt. In a patient with a VSD, QP can be calculated using the RVOT, the main pulmonary artery or the mitral valve since the stroke volume through each of these regions is the same (Figure 11.5).

Calculation of QS:

QS reflects the normal stroke volume through the systemic circulation; hence, QS is calculated distal to the shunt. In a patient with a VSD, QS can be calculated using the LVOT, the ascending aorta, or the tricuspid valve (Figure 11.5).

Patent Ductus Arteriosus (PDA):
Calculation of QP:

QP reflects the stroke volume through the pulmonary venous circulation. Assuming that the shunt is directed left-to-right, then QP will include both the normal forward stroke volume as well as the shunt volume. Thus, QP is calculated downstream from the shunt. In a patient with a PDA, QP can be calculated using the LVOT, the ascending aorta, or the mitral valve since the stroke volume through each of these regions is the same (Figure 11.6).

Calculation of QS:

QS reflects the normal stroke volume through the systemic circulation; hence, QS is calculated distal to the shunt. In a patient with a PDA, QS can be calculated using the RVOT, the main pulmonary artery (proximal to the PDA) or the tricuspid valve (Figure 11.6).

Method for determining the QP:QS for an atrial septal defect (ASD) or a ventricular septal defect (VSD)

On the following page is a "step-by-step" method for calculating the QP:QS for an atrial or ventricular septal defect.

Clinical Significance of the QP:QS:

In the normal heart, the volumetric flow through the left and right sides of the heart is equal; thus, the QP:QS equals 1. A haemodynamically significant shunt occurs when the QP:QS is greater than 1.5:1.

Limitations to QP:QS Calculations:

Limitations of QP:QS calculations are essentially the same as those described for the calculation of the stroke volume (see "Limitations to Volumetric Flow Calculations").

Table 11.2 Recommended locations utilised in the determination of pulmonary venous flow (QP) and systemic venous flow (QS) in the calculation of the QP:QS ratio for intracardiac shunt lesions.

Defect	Measurement Site for QP	Measurement Site for QS
Atrial Septal Defect (ASD)	Right ventricular outflow tract Main pulmonary artery Tricuspid valve	Left ventricular outflow tract Ascending aorta Mitral valve
Ventricular Septal Defect (VSD)	Right ventricular outflow tract Main pulmonary artery Mitral valve	Left ventricular outflow tract Ascending aorta Tricuspid valve
Patent Ductus Arteriosus (PDA)	Left ventricular outflow tract Ascending aorta Mitral valve	Right ventricular outflow tract Main pulmonary artery Tricuspid valve

Note: Calculation of the QP and QS are easiest to perform using the outflow tracts. Alternative sites may be used when measurements cannot be made from the outflow tracts due to technical difficulties or when there is significant aortic/pulmonary stenosis or regurgitation.

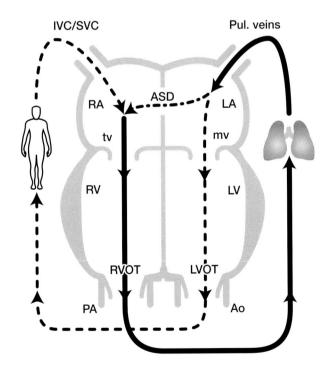

Figure 11.4: Calculation of the QP:QS in Atrial Septal Defects.
This schematic illustrates the volumetric flow through the systemic and pulmonary venous circulations in an atrial septal defect (ASD). The magnitude of volumetric flow is depicted by the width of the arrows so that the greater the stroke volume, the wider the arrow. QP (solid line) represents the volumetric flow to the lungs while QS (dashed line) represents the volumetric flow to the systematic circulation (the body).

Observe that there is shunting from the LA to the right atrium, through the ASD (dash-dot line), resulting in a greater volume of blood flow to the pulmonary circulation compared with that to the systemic circulation (QP > QS).

Also observe that the volumetric flow through the tricuspid valve (TV), right ventricular outflow tract (RVOT), and main pulmonary artery (PA) and the volumetric flow through the mitral valve (MV), left ventricular outflow tract (LVOT), and the ascending aorta (Ao) are the same. Therefore, QP can be calculated using the TV, RVOT, or MPA; while QS can be calculated using the MV, LVOT, or ascending aorta.

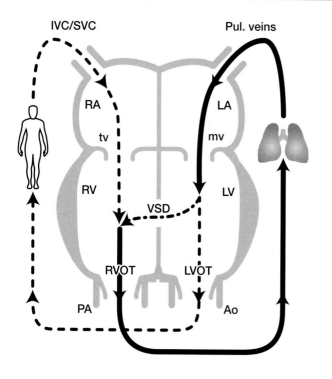

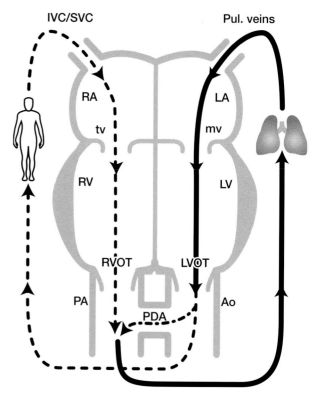

Figure 11.5: Calculation of the QP:QS in Ventricular Septal Defects.

This schematic illustrates the volumetric flow through the systemic and pulmonary venous circulations in a ventricular septal defect (VSD). The magnitude of volumetric flow is depicted by the width of the arrows so that the greater the stroke volume, the wider the arrow. QP (solid line) represents the volumetric flow to the lungs while QS (dashed line) represents the volumetric flow to the systematic circulation (the body).

Observe that there is shunting from the left ventricle to the right ventricle, through the VSD (dash-dot line), resulting in a greater volume of blood flow to the pulmonary circulation compared with that to the systemic circulation (QP > QS).

Also observe that the volumetric flow through the right ventricular outflow tract (RVOT), main pulmonary artery (PA) and mitral valve (MV) and the volumetric flow through the left ventricular outflow tract (LVOT), the ascending aorta (Ao) and tricuspid valve are the same. Therefore, QP can be calculated using the RVOT, MPA or MV while QS can be calculated using the LVOT, ascending aorta or TV.

Figure 11.6: Calculation of the QP:QS in Patent Ductus Arteriosus.

This schematic illustrates the volumetric flow through the systemic and pulmonary venous circulations in a patent ductus arteriosus (PDA). The magnitude of volumetric flow is depicted by the width of the arrows so that the greater the stroke volume, the wider the arrow. QP (solid line) represents the volumetric flow to the lungs while QS (dashed line) represents the volumetric flow to the systemic circulation (the body).

Observe that there is shunting from the aorta to the pulmonary artery, through the PDA (dash-dot line), resulting in a greater volume of blood flow to the pulmonary circulation compared with that to the systemic circulation (QP > QS).

Also observe that the volumetric flow through the left ventricular outflow tract (LVOT), ascending aorta (Ao) and mitral valve (MV) and the volumetric flow through the right ventricular outflow tract (RVOT), the main pulmonary artery (PA) and tricuspid valve are the same. Therefore, QP can be calculated using the LVOT, ascending aorta or MV while QS can be calculated using the RVOT, main pulmonary artery (proximal to the PDA) or TV.

Method for determining the QP:QS for an atrial septal defect (ASD) or ventricular septal defect (VSD)

Step 1.   **calculate the pulmonary venous stroke volume using the right ventricular outflow tract:**
   a)   measurement of RVOT diameter:
   - from the parasternal long axis or short axis view of the RVOT
   - parasternal long axis usually delineates the lateral border better
   - colour flow imaging also facilitates the lateral border identification of the RVOT
   - measured during systole
   - measured at the level of the pulmonary annulus
   - measured from the inner edge to the inner edge of pulmonary cuspal insertion

   b)   assuming a circular shape of the RVOT, the RVOT area can be calculated:
   - $CSA = 0.785 \ x \ D^2$

   c)   measurement of RVOT VTI:
   - from the same view used to measure RVOT diameter
   - P-W Doppler sample volume positioned in the centre of RVOT proximal to pulmonary valve
   - VTI is traced along the leading edge velocity

   d)   calculation of pulmonary stroke volume ($SV_{pulmonary}$):
   - $SV_{pulmonary} \ (cc) = CSA \ (cm^2) \ x \ VTI \ (cm)$

Step 2.   **calculate the systemic stroke volume using the left ventricular outflow tract:**
   a)   measurement of LVOT diameter:
   - from the parasternal long axis view of the LV during systole
   - measured at the level of the aortic annulus
   - measured from the inner edge to the inner edge of aortic cuspal insertion

   b)   assuming a circular shape of the LVOT, the LVOT area can be calculated:
   - $CSA = 0.785 \ x \ D^2$

   c)   measurement of LVOT VTI:
   - from the apical five chamber view
   - P-W Doppler sample volume is positioned in the centre of LVOT proximal to aortic valve
   - VTI is traced along the leading edge velocity

   d)   calculation of systemic stroke volume ($SV_{systemic}$):
   - $SV_{systemic} \ (cc) = CSA \ (cm^2) \ x \ VTI \ (cm)$

Step 3. determination of the shunt ratio (QP:QS):

$$QP:QS = \frac{SV_{pulmonary}}{SV_{systemic}}$$

The Continuity Principle

The continuity principle, in conjunction with volumetric flow calculations, is a fundamental concept that is extremely important in the assessment of various cardiac lesions. The clinical applications of the continuity principle include: (1) the calculation of valve areas (stenotic or prosthetic), (2) calculation of regurgitant volumes and regurgitant fractions, (3) calculation of regurgitant orifice areas, and (4) the calculation of intracardiac shunt ratios.

Theoretical Considerations:
The continuity principle is based on the ***principle of the conservation of mass*** which can be applied to any specified region of flow. This principle states that providing there is no loss of fluid from the system, whatever mass flows in must also flow out. Therefore, for steady flow in the geometry shown in Figure 11.7, the continuity principle states when the flow rate (Q) is maintained, volumetric flow on each side of the narrowing is equal ($Q_1 = Q_2$). Since the flow rate (Q) is equal to the product of the mean velocity (V) and the cross-sectional area (CSA), this relationship can be written:

(Equation 11.4)

$$CSA_1 \ x \ V_1 \ = \ CSA_2 \ x \ V_2$$

Therefore, as the CSA decreases, the mean velocity *must* increase to maintain a constant flow rate.

Since flow is pulsatile within the heart, the volumetric flow is a product of the integrated velocity over time (VTI) and the CSA; hence, the continuity equation can be expressed by:

(Equation 11.5)

$$CSA_1 \times VTI_1 \; = \; CSA_2 \times VTI_2$$

Doppler Echocardiography and the Continuity Principle:

The continuity principle is commonly used in echocardiography to calculate stenotic or prosthetic valve areas, or regurgitant orifice areas. By measuring the proximal velocity time integral (VTI_1), the proximal cross-sectional area (CSA_1), and the distal velocity time integral (VTI_2), the unknown area (CSA_2) can be derived:

(Equation 11.6)

$$CSA_2 = \frac{CSA_1 \times VTI_1}{VTI_2}$$

The principal application of stenotic valve and regurgitant orifice area calculations are discussed in further detail under "Valve Area Calculations" and "Quantification of Regurgitation".

Limitations of the Continuity Principle:
Determination of CSA:

Calculation of the CSA is derived from diameter measurements; hence, any error in this measurement will be reflected in the calculation of the CSA. Technical errors which may occur include: (1) measurement of the diameter during the wrong phase of the cardiac cycle (measurement of CSA must be performed at the time of flow through that site), (2) inconsistent annulus measurements, and (3) difficulty in measuring the RVOT. Measurement of the RVOT in the direction of axial resolution is not possible and it is often difficult to measure the left lateral border of the RVOT due to adjacent lung tissue. Any error in the diameter measurement is magnified in area (recall that the CSA is derived by squaring the diameter [equation 9.2]. Furthermore, when calculating the CSA from the diameter measurement one assumes that the valve annulus has a circular geometry and that the annular area remains constant throughout the period of flow.

Erroneous Velocity Time Integral Measurements:

Errors may also occur in the measurement of the VTI. These errors include: (1) incorrect placement of the PW sample volume for VTI measurement, (2) a significant angle θ between Doppler beam and blood flow direction, (3) incorrect gain settings (over gain = over-estimation of signal), and (4) incorrect filter settings (too high a setting may miss low velocity signals). Furthermore, measurement of too few beats can also produce inaccuracies. For sinus rhythm it is recommended that 3 - 5 beats are measured and averaged. For atrial fibrillation, 8 - 10 beats should be measured and averaged.

Error in the Calculation of CSA_2:

Other errors that may occur are related to the calculation of the unknown CSA. For example, a large angle between ultrasound beam and blood flow direction due to poor beam alignment results in underestimation of peak velocity and, therefore, an overestimation of the area. In addition, failure to obtain the highest Doppler signal from a stenotic jet may lead to an overestimation of the area.

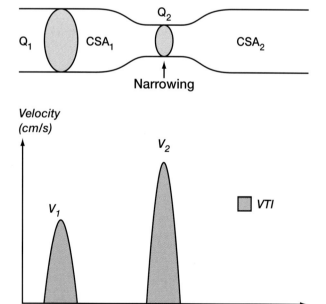

Figure 11.7: The Continuity of Flow through a Narrowing.
When flow rate (Q) is maintained, the volumetric flow on each side of the narrowing is equal ($Q_1 = Q_2$). Flow rate (Q) is equal to the product of the mean velocity (V) and the cross-sectional area (CSA). Therefore, $A_1 \times V_1 = A_2 \times V_2$. Hence, as the CSA decreases, the mean velocity *must* increase to maintain a constant flow rate.

The Bernoulli Equation

One of the most fundamental applications of Doppler echocardiography is the determination of pressure gradients using the Bernoulli equation. Clinical applications of the Bernoulli equation include: (1) the determination of the maximum and mean pressure gradients across stenotic valve lesions, (2) maximum pressure gradients across regurgitant valve lesions and abnormal "shunt" communications, and (3) intracardiac pressure estimation.

Theoretical Considerations:

The basic principles of the Bernoulli equation have been briefly covered in Chapter 5. Recall that the Bernoulli equation is based on the principle of the conservation of energy. This principle states that in the absence of applied forces, the total energy of a system remains constant so that the total energy flowing into the system is equal to the total energy flowing out. Therefore, in the presence of a narrowing, the velocity distal to the narrowing must accelerate or increase to maintain energy (Figure 11.8). Since velocity and pressure are inversely related, this means that the pressure distal to the narrowing must drop. This creates a pressure gradient between the region proximal to the narrowing and the region distal to the narrowing. This pressure difference is determined by application of the Bernoulli equation:

(Equation 5.10)

$$\Delta P = \tfrac{1}{2}\rho\,(V_2^2 - V_1^2) + \int_1^2 \frac{d\vec{v}}{dt} \times d\vec{s} + R(\vec{v})$$

$$\begin{matrix}\text{Pressure}\\\text{decrease}\end{matrix} = \begin{matrix}\text{convective}\\\text{acceleration}\end{matrix} + \begin{matrix}\text{flow}\\\text{acceleration}\end{matrix} + \begin{matrix}\text{viscous}\\\text{friction}\end{matrix}$$

where ΔP = the pressure difference between 2 points (mm Hg)

V_1 = velocity at proximal location (m/s)
V_2 = velocity at distal location (m/s)
ρ = density of fluid (g/cm³)
dv = change in velocity over the time period (dt)
ds = distance over which pressure decreases
R = viscous resistance in the vessel
V = velocity of blood flow (m/s)

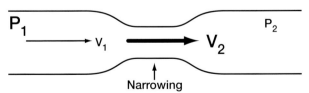

Figure 11.8: The Principle of the Bernoulli Equation.
In order to maintain energy through a narrowing, the velocity through that narrowing must accelerate or increase. Since pressure and velocity are inversely related, this means that the pressure distal to the stenosis must drop. This creates a pressure gradient between the region proximal to the narrowing and the region distal to the narrowing. This pressure difference is determined by application of the Bernoulli equation.

Doppler Echocardiographic Application of the Bernoulli Equation:

From the above equation, it can be seen that there are three important components to the Bernoulli equation: (1) *convective acceleration* which occurs whenever there is a change in the CSA of flow, (2) *flow acceleration* which refers to the pressure drop required to overcome inertial forces, and (3) *viscous friction* which is the loss of velocity due to friction between blood cells and vessel walls.

In most clinical situations, the following assumptions can be made: (1) flow acceleration can be ignored (as at peak velocities, acceleration is zero), (2) viscous friction is negligible (as losses are minimal toward the centre of the vessel where the flow profile is generally flat), (3) one-half of the mass density ($\tfrac{1}{2}\rho$) for normal blood equals 4, and (4) there is conservation of energy, that is, there is no energy transfer. Therefore, accounting for these factors, the Bernoulli equation can be modified or simplified to:

(Equation 5.11)

$$\Delta P = 4\left(V_2^2 - V_1^2\right)$$

Furthermore, flow velocity proximal to fixed orifice (V_1) is usually much lower than the peak flow (V_2), and therefore can be ignored further simplifying the Bernoulli equation to:

(Equation 5.12)

$$\Delta P = 4V^2$$

Limitations to the Simplified Bernoulli Equation:
Significant Flow Acceleration:

In most clinical situations, flow acceleration (inertial force) is usually ignored. However, under some conditions, flow acceleration becomes relevant and may significantly contribute to the overall result of the Bernoulli equation. Flow acceleration becomes important when evaluating prosthetic valves as a greater increase in the momentum of blood flow is required to open the valve. Hence, flow acceleration may significantly contribute to the derived pressure gradient and if this is not taken into consideration, the true pressure gradient will be underestimated.

Effect of Significant Viscous Forces:

As for flow acceleration, viscous friction is usually negligible in most clinical situations. However, conditions may arise in which significant viscous forces exist. Viscous forces become significant in the presence of long, tubular obstructions such as in (1) some muscular ventricular septal defects, (2) tunnel subaortic stenosis, and (3) long coarctations. Therefore, in these circumstances, the use of the simplified Bernoulli equation will lead to an underestimation of the true pressure gradient.

Effect of Angle θ:

When there is a large angle between ultrasound beam and

blood flow (or jet) direction, a significant underestimation of the true velocity occurs. This error is determined based on the Doppler equation:

(Equation 5.8)

$$V = \frac{C\,(\pm\Delta f)}{2\,f_0\,\cos\theta}$$

where   V   = peak velocity (m/s)
        Δf = frequency shift (Hz)
        c   = speed of sound in blood (m/s)
        f_0 = transmitted frequency (Hz)
        $\cos\theta$ = incident angle between ultrasound beam
                  and blood flow

From this equation, it is evident that the *recorded* velocity and actual blood flow velocity is dependant upon the angle θ which is the incident angle between the ultrasound beam and the blood flow direction. Observe in Figure 11.9 that the true velocity is obtained when the angle θ equals zero (cos θ = one); that is, when the blood flow is parallel to the ultrasound beam. Angles of less than 20° will underestimate the true velocity by less than 7%, whereas, greater angles will significantly underestimate the true velocity. It is important to note, however, that even though an angle of 20° only slightly underestimates the actual velocity, pressure is proportional to the velocity squared; thus, the error in the estimation of the pressure gradient will be much higher.

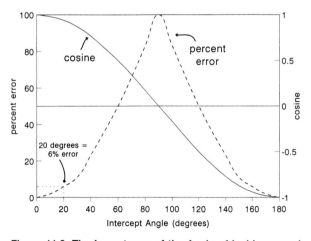

Figure 11.9: The Importance of the Angle of Incidence and the Direction of Blood Flow.
Observe that cosine (*solid* line) equals 1 when the intercept angle (*X-axis*) is either 0° or 180°; that is, when the ultrasound beam is aligned parallel to blood flow direction. In this instance, the percentage error *(dashed* line) is 0%; therefore, the true maximal velocity is determined. Observe that cosine equals 0 when the intercept angle is 90°; that is, when the ultrasound beam is aligned perpendicular to blood flow direction. In this instance, the percentage error is 100% so that no velocities are recorded. When the intercept angle between the direction of blood flow and the ultrasound beam is 20° or less, cosine approaches 1 and the percentage error is ≤ 6%.
From Otto and Pearlman: *Textbook of Clinical Echocardiography*. pp: 22, W B Saunders Company, 1995. Reproduced with permission from W.B. Saunders Company.

Therefore, to minimise error in both the velocity and pressure estimation from a large angle θ, parallel alignment of the ultrasound beam to the direction of blood flow is essential. This is accomplished by careful Doppler interrogation utilising multiple transducer positions. Colour flow imaging can be extremely valuable in determining the parallel alignment of the ultrasound beam with jet direction. This is especially true when searching for regurgitant and ventricular septal defect jets which can be quite eccentric.

Effect of Increased Proximal Velocity:
When the proximal velocity (V_1) becomes significantly elevated (> 1.2 m/s), calculation of the pressure gradient will be overestimated. In these instances, V_1 can no longer be ignored and this value should be taken into account. Hence, the pressure gradient should be "corrected" for the increased V_1 by using equation (5.11).
Situations in which V_1 is increased includes aortic stenosis with: (1) an associated high output state such as anaemia, sepsis and coexistent atriovenous fistula, (2) significant aortic regurgitation, or (3) a coexistent subvalvular obstruction (such as hypertrophic obstructive cardiomyopathy). Other situations in which V_1 may be increased include coarctation of the aorta, and stenoses in series such as long coarctations and tunnel-like ventricular septal defects.

Alterations of Blood Viscosity:
Normally, half of the mass density of blood (ρ) is equal to 4. However, the blood viscosity may be altered in the presence of severe anaemia (↓ viscosity) or polycythemia (↑ viscosity).
In these instances, it is important to recognise that the actual velocity obtained is unaffected but calculation of the pressure gradient will be incorrect. For example, in a patient with severe anaemia, 1/2 ρ may only be 2 instead of 4 leading to an overestimation of the pressure gradient.

Discrepancies between Catheter-Derived and Doppler-Derived Pressure Gradients:
Pressures gradients derived at cardiac catheterisation by direct measurement and those derived by the application of the modified Bernoulli equation may differ. Discrepancies between these two techniques may occur in the presence of aortic valve stenosis and due to a phenomenon called "pressure recovery".
In *aortic stenosis*, the catheter-derived pressure gradients differ from the Doppler-derived pressure gradients. (Figure 11.10). This can be explained by the fact that the catheter-derived pressure gradient between the left ventricle (LV) and aorta is the *peak-to-peak* gradient which is the arithmetic difference between the peak LV and the peak aortic pressure. This is a nonsimultaneous measurement as the peak aortic pressure occurs *after* the peak LV pressure and is, therefore, a nonphysiological measurement. The Doppler-derived pressure gradient, however, is the maximum *instantaneous* gradient obtained from application of the modified Bernoulli equation. The Doppler gradient is always greater than the peak-to-peak gradient because the instantaneous gradient occurs before

the peak aortic pressure. Note, however, that the calculated *mean* pressure gradients are comparable and have correlated well in comparative studies.

"*Pressure recovery*" is an important concept in the assessment of certain types of prosthetic valves. Pressure recovery is a complex hydrodynamic concept based on the conservation of energy principle which states that the pressure of fluid decreases as the velocity increases. The site of highest velocity and lowest pressure occurs at the narrowest point of the orifice (the *vena contracta*). Once flow has passed through the orifice, pressure recovers and increases toward its original value. The rate and magnitude of pressure recovery is variable (Figure 11.11). In native valves, pressure recovery is gradual and, therefore, the catheter- and Doppler-derived pressure gradients are similar. In the prosthetic valve, the extent of pressure recovery depends on the geometry of the valve. Pressure recovery is particularly important in small sized bileaflet prostheses, for example, with 19 - 21 mm St Jude prostheses where high velocities may be recorded. In these bileaflet prosthetic valves, there are three effective orifices: two large orifices to the side of the valve and one smaller, funnel-shaped central orifice. The site of the highest velocity and lowest pressure occurs at the site of the narrowest orifice (central, funnel-shaped orifice). Immediately distal to this orifice, velocity decreases and pressure increases (recovers) rapidly. Doppler-derived pressure gradients may yield higher velocities compared with the catheter-derived pressure gradients because the Doppler gradients are recorded at the smallest orifice whereas the catheter-derived pressure gradients are typically recorded downstream to the prosthetic valve orifice where the pressure has recovered.

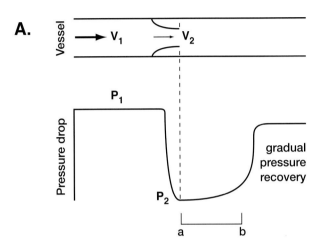

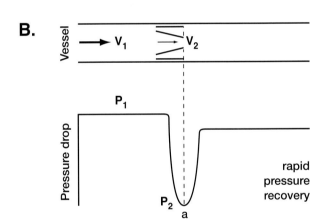

Figure 11.11: Pressure Recovery.
When flow passes through a narrowed orifice, velocity (V_2) increases and pressure (P_2) decreases. Once flow has passed through this orifice, pressure recovers and increases toward its original value. The rate and magnitude of pressure recovery is variable depending upon valvular geometry.

A. Native valves:
- Doppler velocities are recorded at the narrowest orifice (V_2) and the pressure drop is calculated from the modified Bernoulli equation ($\Delta P = 4V^2$);
- catheter-derived pressure recorded between point (a) and point (b) will yield similar results to the Doppler-derived pressure gradient due to gradual pressure recovery.

B. Bileaflet prosthetic valves:
- Doppler velocities are recorded at the narrowest orifice (V_2) and the pressure drop is calculated from the modified Bernoulli equation ($\Delta P = 4V^2$),
- catheter-derived pressure must be recorded at point (a), the vena contracta, if this value is to equate with the Doppler-derived pressure gradient. Catheter-derived pressures recorded distal to this point will be lower due to rapid pressure recovery.

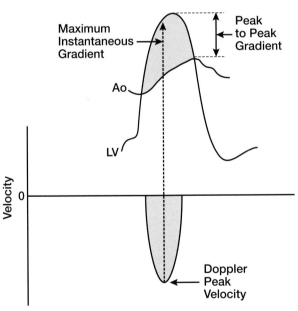

Figure 11.10: Doppler-Derived Pressure Gradient versus Catheter-Derived Pressure Gradient in Aortic Stenosis.
The peak left ventricular (LV) and peak aortic (Ao) pressures occur at different points in systole. The catheter-derived pressure gradient is a nonphysiological measurement of the difference between the peak LV and peak aortic pressures and is hence termed the "peak-to-peak" gradient. The Doppler-derived pressure gradient measures the maximal instantaneous pressure gradient between the LV and the aorta during systole. The Doppler-derived pressure gradient is **always** higher than the peak-to-peak catheter-derived gradient. Note that the calculated *mean* pressure gradients (shaded area of the catheter and Doppler traces) are comparable and have correlated well in comparative studies.
Adapted from Oh, J.K., Seward, J.B. and Tajik, A.J.: The Echo Manual. Little Brown and Company. pp 58, 1994. Reproduced with permission from the Mayo Foundation.

Doppler Haemodynamic Calculations

Based on the principles described above, semiquantitative and quantitative haemodynamic and functional information can be derived from the Doppler echocardiographic assessment. The calculations that may be employed in the assessment of cardiac function and disease are listed in Table 11.3.

Determination of Pressure Gradients

Pressure gradients that are commonly determined by Doppler echocardiography include: (1) the maximum instantaneous pressure gradient and (2) the mean pressure gradient (Figure 11.12). Pressure gradients can be used in the assessment of the severity of valvular stenosis or in the estimation of intracardiac pressures. Studies validating the accuracy of Doppler echocardiography in determination of pressure gradients are tabulated in Appendix 2. The clinical significance of transvalvular pressure gradients and the severity of valvular stenosis are listed in Table 11.4. The normal pressure gradients for prosthetic valves are tabulated in Appendix 3.

Maximum Instantaneous Pressure Gradients

The maximum instantaneous pressure gradient (MIPG) is calculated using the simplified Bernoulli equation:

(Equation 11.7)

$$MIPG = 4\,V^2$$

where MIPG = maximum instantaneous pressure
                    gradient (mm Hg)
     V   = peak velocity (m/s)

Mean Pressure Gradients

The mean pressure gradient can be determined from the calculation of the arithmetic mean of derived instantaneous pressure gradients obtained at regular intervals throughout the period of flow. Thus, the mean

pressure gradient (MPG) is calculated from the following equation:

(Equation 11.8)

$$MPG = \frac{4\left[\sum \left(V_1\right)^2 + \left(V_2\right)^2 + \left(V_3\right)^2 + \dots\dots\left(V_n\right)^2\right]}{n}$$

where MPG   = mean pressure gradient (mm Hg)
     V_1 to V_n = peak velocity measured at various
                       intervals (m/s)
     n   = number of intervals measured

Simplified Calculation of the Mean Pressure Gradient:
The mean pressure gradient can also be calculated from the maximum pressure gradient (ΔP_{max}) [32] and from the peak velocity (V_{max}) [33] in patients with native aortic valve stenosis using the following equations:

(Equation 11.9)

$$MPG = \frac{\Delta P_{max}}{1.45} + 2$$

(Equation 11.10)

$$MPG = 2.4\,\left(V_{max}\right)^2$$

Intracardiac Pressure Calculations

In the presence of regurgitant jets or shunt lesions, Doppler echocardiography can be used to noninvasively measure intracardiac pressures. The peak velocity of these jets can be converted to measure the pressure gradient between the two cardiac chambers or vessels using the modified Bernoulli equation (equation 5.12). The most commonly estimated pressures are those of the right and left sides of the heart (Table 11.5). Studies validating the accuracy and reliability of Doppler echocardiography in estimation of right and left heart pressures are tabulated

Table 11.3: Semiquantitatve and Quantitative Doppler Haemodynamic and Functional Information derived by Doppler Echocardiography.

Determination of pressure gradients	• maximum pressure gradients • mean pressure gradients • intracardiac pressure estimation
Assessment of systolic and diastolic ventricular function	• stroke volume and cardiac output • dP/dt • diastolic filling parameters • myocardial performance index
Calculation of valve areas	• pressure half-time method • continuity method • proximal isovelocity surface area (PISA) method
Quantification of regurgitant lesions	• "indirect" signs of significant regurgitation • colour Doppler jet area ratios • regurgitant volumes and regurgitant fractions • effective regurgitant orifice area
Quantification of intracardiac shunts	• QP:QS

32: Otto and Pearlman: Archives of Internal Medicine 148: 2553-2560, 1988 (n = 103, r = 0.99). 33: Otto, C.M. et al.: American Journal of Cardiology 68: 1477-1484, 1991 (n = 589, r = 0.92).

in Appendix 4. The normal intracardiac pressures are listed in Appendix 5.

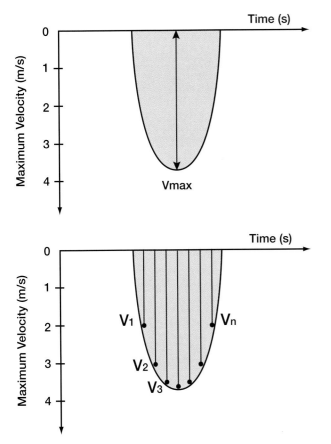

Figure 11.12: Methods of Calculating the Maximum Instantaneous and Mean Pressure Gradients using the Simplified Bernoulli Equation.

Top, This is a schematic illustration measuring the peak velocity (V_{max}). Application of equation (11.7) provides an estimation of the maximum instantaneous pressure gradient.
Bottom, This is a schematic illustration measuring the peak velocities at various intervals throughout the Doppler trace (V_1 to V_n). The mean pressure gradient is approximated by application of equation (11.8).

Estimation of Right Heart Pressures:
Systolic Right Ventricular (Pulmonary Artery) Pressure Estimation:
In the absence of RVOT obstruction or pulmonary valve stenosis, the right ventricular systolic pressure (RVSP) and pulmonary artery systolic pressure (PASP) are equal. Therefore, under these circumstances, Doppler methods used in the estimation of the RVSP can also be applied in the estimation of the PASP.

Table 11.4: Clinical Significance of Transvalvular Pressure Gradients in Valvular Stenosis.

AORTIC STENOSIS [1]	
Peak Velocity	
Mild	< 3.5 m/s
Moderate	3.5 - 4.5 m/s
Severe	> 4.5 m/s
Mean Pressure Gradient	
Mild	< 25 mm Hg
Moderate	25 - 50 mm Hg
Severe	> 50 mm Hg
MITRAL STENOSIS [2]	
Mean Pressure Gradient	
Mild	< 5 mm Hg
Moderate	5 - 10 mm Hg
Severe	> 10 mm Hg
TRICUSPID STENOSIS [3]	
Mean Pressure Gradient	
Severe	≥ 5 mm Hg
PULMONARY STENOSIS [4]	
Peak Gradient	
Mild	< 40 mm Hg
Moderate	40 – 75 mm Hg
Severe	> 75 mm Hg

Sources: (1) Oh et al., *Journal of the American College of Cardiology 11:1227-1234,1988*; **(2)** Nishimura, R.A. and Tajik, A.J., *Progress in Cardiovascular Disease 34:309-342,1994*; **(3)** Grossman, W. and Baim, D.S. Cardiac Catherization, Angiography and Interventions. 5th Edition Williams and Wilkins pp: 162, 1996; **(4)** Alexander R.W., Schlant, R.C., and Fuster, V.: Hurst's. The Heart. 9th Edition McGraw-Hill, Inc. pp: 1962, 1998.

Table 11.5: Intracardiac Pressures derived from Doppler Echocardiography.

Intracardiac Pressures	**Doppler Velocity Signals**
Right Heart Pressures: ● systolic pulmonary artery pressure	● tricuspid regurgitation (TR) ● ventricular septal defect (VSD) ● patent ductus arteriosus (PDA) ● right ventricular isovolumic relaxation time (IVRT)
● diastolic pulmonary artery pressure	● pulmonary regurgitation (PR)
● mean pulmonary artery pressure	● pulmonary regurgitation (PR) ● right ventricular acceleration time (RVA_cT)
Left Heart Pressures: ● left atrial pressure	● mitral regurgitation (MR)
● left ventricular end-diastolic pressure	● aortic regurgitation (AR)

Systolic right heart pressures can be determined from the peak systolic velocities of: (1) the tricuspid regurgitant (TR) signal, (2) the ventricular septal defect (VSD) signal, (3) the patent ductus arteriosus (PDA). The systolic pulmonary artery pressure can also be estimated using by using the right ventricular isovolumic relaxation time (RVAcT) in association with Burstin's nomogram.

1. Estimation of the RVSP (PASP) in the Presence of Tricuspid Regurgitation:

The tricuspid regurgitant Doppler signal represents the pressure difference between the right ventricle and right atrium during systole (Figure 11.13). If the right atrial pressure is estimated, then it is possible to estimate the RVSP using the following equation:

(Equation 11.11)

$$RVSP = 4\left(V_{TR}\right)^2 + RAP$$

where RVSP = right ventricular systolic pressure
                (mm Hg)
     V_{TR} = peak tricuspid regurgitation velocity (m/s)
     RAP = mean right atrial pressure (mm Hg)

As mentioned above, in the absence of RVOT obstruction, the RVSP is equal to the PASP.

2. Estimation of the RVSP (PASP) in the Presence of a Ventricular Septal Defect:

In the presence of a ventricular septal defect, the peak systolic velocity detected by Doppler echocardiography across this defect can be used to derive the pressure difference between the left and right ventricles during systole (Figure 11.14). If the left ventricular pressure is known, the RVSP can be estimated from the following equation:

(Equation 11.12)

$$RVSP = LVSP - 4\left(V_{VSD}\right)^2$$

where RVSP = right ventricular systolic pressure
              (mm Hg)
     LVSP = left ventricular systolic pressure (mm Hg)
     V_{VSD} = maximum VSD velocity (m/s)

In the absence of LVOT obstruction, the left ventricular systolic pressure is equal to the systolic arm blood pressure measured by cuff sphygmomanometer; therefore,

(Equation 11.13)

$$RVSP = BP_{systolic} - 4\left(V_{VSD}\right)^2$$

where RVSP   = right ventricular systolic pressure
                      (mm Hg)
     $BP_{(systolic)}$ = systolic arm blood pressure (mm Hg)
     V_{VSD} = maximum VSD velocity (m/s)

In the absence of RVOT obstruction, the RVSP is equal to the PASP.

3. Estimation of the PASP in the presence of a Patent Ductus Arteriosus:

In the presence of a patent ductus arteriosus, a continuous pressure gradient usually exists between the aorta and pulmonary artery. The systolic component of this signal represents the systolic pressure gradient between these two vessels (Figure 11.15). If the systolic aortic pressure is known, the PASP can be estimated from the following equation:

(Equation 11.14)

$$PASP = AoSP - 4\left(V_{PDA}\right)^2$$

where PASP = pulmonary artery systolic pressure
               (mm Hg)
     AoSP = aortic systolic pressure (mm Hg)
     V_{PDA} = peak systolic PDA velocity gradient (m/s)

In the absence of coarctation of the aorta, the aortic systolic pressure is equal to the systolic arm blood pressure measured by cuff sphygmomanometer; therefore:

(Equation 11.15)

$$PASP = BP_{systolic} - 4\left(V_{PDA}\right)^2$$

where PASP   = pulmonary artery systolic pressure
                     (mm Hg)
     $BP_{systolic}$ = systolic arm blood pressure (mm Hg)
     V_{PDA} = peak systolic PDA velocity gradient (m/s)

4. Estimation of the PASP using Right Ventricular Isovolumic Relaxation Time:

The noninvasive estimation of pulmonary artery systolic pressure was first described by Burstin [34] using the duration of the interval between pulmonary valve closure and tricuspid valve opening (Pc - To) or the right ventricular isovolumic relaxation time (RV_{IVRT}). The principle of this calculation was based on the assumption that this interval increases proportionally with systolic pulmonary artery pressure and is inversely related to heart rate. Based on this premise, Burstin created a nomogram which can be used in the estimation of the PASP from the RV_{IVRT} and the heart rate (Figure 11.16).

In the original article by Burstin, the RV_{IVRT} was measured using phonocardiography and noninvasive pulse tracings. The RV_{IVRT} can also be derived using Doppler echocardiography by three methods: (1) utilising Doppler in association with phonocardiography, (2) utilising the pulmonary artery signal and the tricuspid regurgitant signal, and (3) utilising the RVOT signal and the tricuspid inflow signal. Methods (2) and (3) are illustrated in Figure 11.16. Once the IVRT is determined, the pulmonary artery systolic pressure can be estimated using Burstin's nomogram (Figure 11.17).

34: Burstin, L.: British Heart Journal 29: 393-404, 1967.

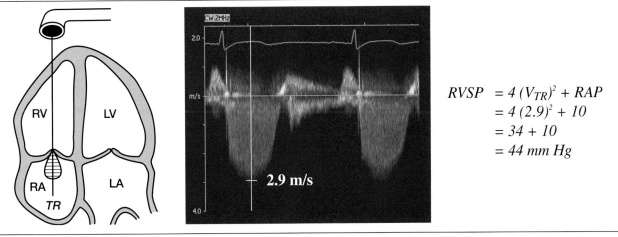

$$RVSP = 4 (V_{TR})^2 + RAP$$
$$= 4 (2.9)^2 + 10$$
$$= 34 + 10$$
$$= 44 \ mm \ Hg$$

Figure 11.13: Estimation of the Right Ventricular Systolic Pressure (RVSP) using the Tricuspid Regurgitant Doppler Signal.
Left, This schematic illustrates how the peak tricuspid regurgitant (TR) velocity is obtained by CW Doppler from the apical four chamber view.
Right, The Doppler signal of the tricuspid regurgitant jet measures approximately 2.9 m/s. Using the simplified Bernoulli equation, the pressure gradient between the right ventricle and right atrium in systole equals 34 mm Hg. Assuming right atrial pressure equals 10 mm Hg, the estimated RVSP is 44 mm Hg.
Abbreviations: LA = left atrium; **LV** = left ventricle; **RA** = right atrium, **RV** = right ventricle; **TR** = tricuspid regurgitation.

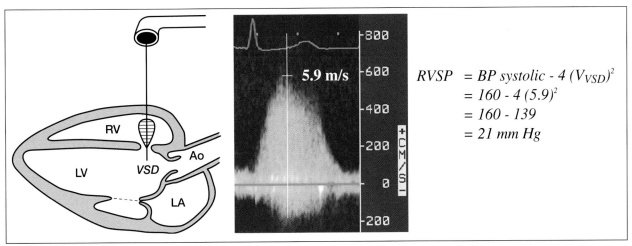

$$RVSP = BP \ systolic - 4 (V_{VSD})^2$$
$$= 160 - 4 (5.9)^2$$
$$= 160 - 139$$
$$= 21 \ mm \ Hg$$

Figure 11.14: Estimation of the Right Ventricular Systolic Pressure (RVSP) using the Doppler Velocity Signal across a Ventricular Septal Defect.
Left, This schematic illustrates how the peak systolic velocity recorded across a ventricular septal defect (VSD) is obtained by CW Doppler from the parasternal long axis view. *Right,* The Doppler signal across the VSD measures approximately 5.9 m/s. Using the simplified Bernoulli equation, the pressure gradient between the left and right ventricle equals 139 mm Hg. If the measured systolic cuff blood pressure is 160 mm Hg, the estimated RVSP is 21 mm Hg.
Abbreviations: Ao = aorta; **LA** = left atrium; **LV** = left ventricle; **RA** = right atrium, **RV** = right ventricle; **VSD** = ventricular septal defect.

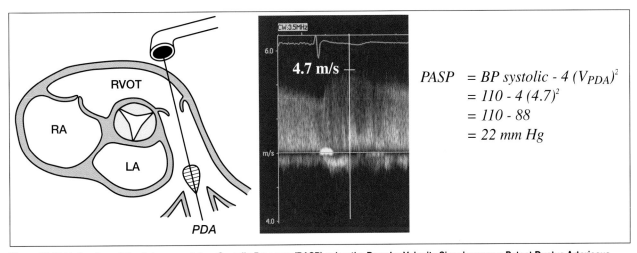

$$PASP = BP \ systolic - 4 (V_{PDA})^2$$
$$= 110 - 4 (4.7)^2$$
$$= 110 - 88$$
$$= 22 \ mm \ Hg$$

Figure 11.15: Estimation of the Pulmonary Artery Systolic Pressure (PASP) using the Doppler Velocity Signal across a Patent Ductus Arteriosus.
Left, This schematic illustrates how the peak systolic velocity recorded across a patent ductus arteriosus (PDA) is obtained by CW Doppler from the parasternal short axis view. *Right,* The systolic Doppler signal across the PDA measures approximately 4.7 m/s. Using the simplified Bernoulli equation, the pressure gradient between the aorta and pulmonary artery equals 88 mm Hg. If the measured systolic cuff blood pressure is 110 mm Hg, the estimated PASP is 22 mm Hg.
Abbreviations: RA = right atrium; **RVOT** = right ventricular outflow tract; **LA** = left atrium.

Estimation of the Diastolic Pulmonary Artery Pressure:

In the presence of pulmonary regurgitation, the pulmonary artery end-diastolic pressure (PAEDP) can be determined.

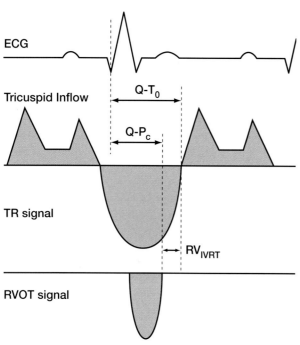

Figure 11.16: Determination of the Right Ventricular Isovolumic Relaxation Time (RV$_{IVRT}$).
The RV$_{IVRT}$ can be determined by measuring (1) the interval from the Q wave of the ECG to tricuspid valve opening (Q-T$_o$) and (2) the interval from the Q wave of the ECG to pulmonary valve closure (Q-P$_c$). The point of tricuspid valve opening can be measured using the tricuspid inflow signal or the tricuspid regurgitant (TR) signal as shown above. Pulmonary valve closure is determined using the RVOT signal. The RV$_{IVRT}$ is then determined by subtracting the Q-T$_o$ from the Q-P$_c$.

Estimation of the PAEDP using the Pulmonary Regurgitant Doppler Signal:

The pulmonary regurgitant velocity reflects the pressure gradient between the pulmonary artery and the right ventricle during diastole. Hence, the end-diastolic velocity represents the end-diastolic pressure gradient between the pulmonary artery and the right ventricle (Figure 11.18). If the right ventricular end-diastolic pressure (RVEDP) is added to this gradient, the PAEDP can be estimated from the following equation:

(Equation 11.16)

$$PAEDP = 4 \left(V_{PR-ED} \right)^2 + RVEDP$$

where PAEDP = pulmonary artery end-diastolic pressure (mm Hg)

V_{PR-ED} = peak end-diastolic velocity of PR signal (m/s)

RVEDP = right ventricular end-diastolic pressure (mm Hg)

In the absence of tricuspid stenosis, the right ventricular end-diastolic pressure is equivalent to the RAP; therefore:

(Equation 11.17)

$$PAEDP = 4 \left(V_{PR-ED} \right)^2 + RAP$$

where PAEDP = pulmonary artery end-diastolic pressure (mm Hg)

V_{PR-ED} = peak end-diastolic velocity of PR signal (m/s)

RAP = mean right atrial pressure (mm Hg)

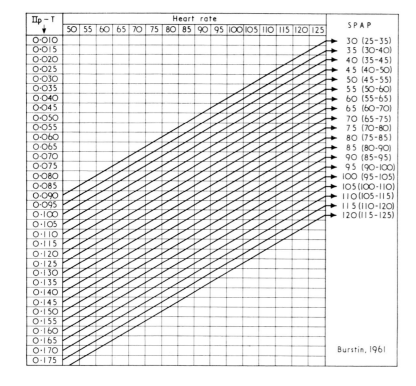

Figure 11.17: Estimation of Pulmonary Artery Systolic Pressure from the Right Ventricular Isovolumic Relaxation Time and Heart Rate (Burstin's Nomogram).
This table may be used in the estimation of the pulmonary artery systolic pressure (SPAP) from the RV$_{IVRT}$ (IIp - T), measured in seconds, and the heart rate. For example, with an IIp-T interval of 0.120 seconds and a heart rate of 95 bpm, the estimated SPAP is 95 mm Hg.
From Burstin, L.: Determination of pressure in the pulmonary artery by external graphic recordings. *British Heart Journal* 29:396, 1967. Reproduced with permission from the BMJ Publishing Group.

Estimation of the Mean Pulmonary Artery Pressure:
The mean pulmonary artery pressure (MPAP) can be estimated by using: (1) the peak pulmonary regurgitant velocity, and (2) from the right ventricular and pulmonary artery acceleration times.

1. Estimation of the MPAP using the Peak Pulmonary Artery Regurgitant Velocity:

As mentioned, the pulmonary regurgitant velocity reflects the pressure gradient between the pulmonary artery and the right ventricle during diastole. It has also been shown that the peak velocity of the pulmonary regurgitant Doppler signal in early diastole also correlates with the MPAP (Figure 11.19) [35]. Thus,

(Equation 11.18)

$$MPAP \approx 4\left(V_{PR\text{-}P}\right)^2$$

where MPAP = mean pulmonary artery measure (mm Hg)

$V_{PR\text{-}P}$ = peak pulmonary regurgitant velocity in early diastole

2. Estimation of the MPAP using the Right Ventricular Acceleration Time:

In the past, right ventricular systolic time intervals such as the pre-ejection period, acceleration time, and right ventricular ejection time have been used in the

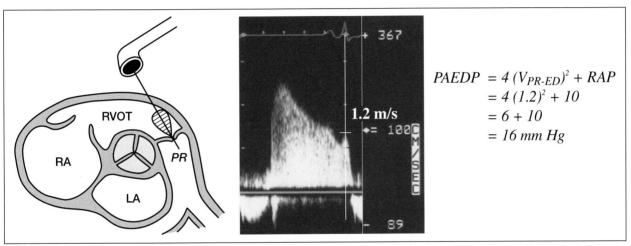

$$PAEDP = 4 (V_{PR\text{-}ED})^2 + RAP$$
$$= 4 (1.2)^2 + 10$$
$$= 6 + 10$$
$$= 16 \ mm \ Hg$$

Figure 11.18: Estimation of the Pulmonary Artery End-Diastolic Pressure (PAEDP) using the Pulmonary Regurgitant Doppler Velocity Signal.
Left, This schematic illustrates how the end-diastolic pulmonary regurgitant (PR) velocity is obtained by CW Doppler from the parasternal short axis view. *Right,* The end-diastolic PR Doppler signal, recorded from the Q wave of the ECG, measures approximately 1.2 m/s. Using the simplified Bernoulli equation, the end-diastolic pressure gradient between the pulmonary artery and the right ventricle equals 6 mm Hg. Assuming that the right ventricular end-diastolic pressure equals the RAP and that the right atrial pressure is 10 mm Hg, the estimated PAEDP is 16 mm Hg.
Abbreviations: LA = left atrium; **PR** = pulmonary regurgitation; **RA** = right atrium, **RVOT** = right ventricular outflow tract.

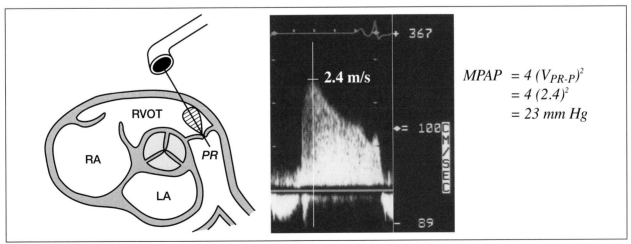

$$MPAP = 4 (V_{PR\text{-}P})^2$$
$$= 4 (2.4)^2$$
$$= 23 \ mm \ Hg$$

Figure 11.19: Estimation of the Mean Pulmonary Artery Pressure (MPAP) using the Pulmonary Regurgitant Doppler Velocity Signal.
Left, This schematic illustrates how the pulmonary regurgitant (PR) velocity is obtained by CW Doppler from the parasternal short axis view. *Right,* The early diastolic PR Doppler signal measures approximately 2.4 m/s. Using the simplified Bernoulli equation, the MPAP is approximately 23 mm Hg.
Abbreviations: LA = left atrium; **PR** = pulmonary regurgitation; **RA** = right atrium, **RVOT** = right ventricular outflow tract.

35: Masuyama, T. et al.: Circulation 74: 484-492, 1986.

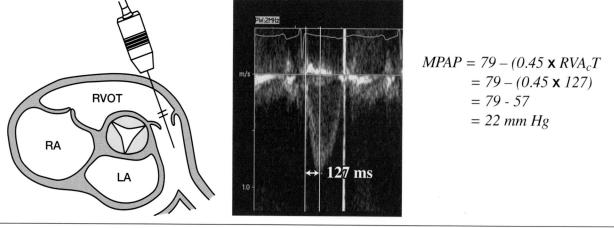

$$MPAP = 79 - (0.45 \times RVA_cT$$
$$= 79 - (0.45 \times 127)$$
$$= 79 - 57$$
$$= 22 \; mm \; Hg$$

Figure 11.20: Estimation of the Mean Pulmonary Artery Pressure (MPAP) using the Right Ventricular Acceleration Time (RVA$_c$T).
Left, This schematic illustrates how the RVA$_c$T is obtained using PW Doppler with the PW sample volume placed within the RVOT. *Right,*
The Doppler signal of the RVA$_c$T measures 127 ms. Using equation 11.19, the estimated MPAP equals 22 mm Hg.
Abbreviations: LA = left atrium; **RA** = right atrium, **RVOT** = right ventricular outflow tract.

estimation of the pulmonary artery pressure. The interval, which correlates most closely with the pulmonary artery pressure, is the right ventricular acceleration time (RVA$_c$T). The RVA$_c$T is the time interval between the onset of flow to the peak systolic flow. As the pulmonary artery pressure increases, there is an increase in the resistance of blood flow from the right ventricle into the pulmonary artery resulting in shortening of the RVA$_c$T. The RVA$_c$T can be measured by PW Doppler echocardiography when the sample volume is placed within the RVOT or proximal main pulmonary artery.Using this technique, three regression equations have been described relating the RVA$_c$T to the MPAP.

(i) Method described by Mahan et al. (1983):
Using this method, the RVA$_c$T is measured utilising PW Doppler with the sample volume placed within the RVOT (Figure 11.20). The RVA$_c$T was found to have a linear relationship with the MPAP such that:

(Equation 11.19)

$$MPAP = 79 \; \left(0.45 \times RVA_cT\right)$$

where MPAP = mean pulmonary artery pressure (mm Hg)
  RVA$_c$T = right ventricular acceleration time (ms)

(ii) Method described by Kitabatake et al. (1983):
Using this method, the RVA$_c$T is measured utilising PW Doppler with the sample volume placed within the RVOT. The RVA$_c$T was found to have a curvilinear relationship with the MPAP such that:

(Equation 11.20)

$$MPAP = 90 \; \left(0.62 \times RVA_cT\right)$$

where MPAP = mean pulmonary artery pressure (mm Hg)
  RVA$_c$T = right ventricular acceleration time (ms)

(iii) Method described by Debastani et al. (1987):
Using this method, the RVA$_c$T is obtained with PW Doppler with the sample volume placed in the proximal main pulmonary artery. The regression equation used to express the MPAP, when the RVA$_c$T was 120 ms or less [36], is as follows:

(Equation 11.21)

$$\log_{10} MPAP = 0.0068 \left(RVA_cT\right) + 2.1$$

where MPAP = mean pulmonary artery pressure (mm Hg)
  RVA$_c$T = right ventricular acceleration time (ms)

Estimation of Right Atrial Pressure using 2-D Echocardiography:
As seen above, many Doppler-derived pressure gradients used to estimate right heart pressures also require estimation of the RAP. There are several methods used in the estimation of the RAP including the use of an empirical value of 10 mm Hg and assessment of the jugular venous pressure (JVP). When the JVP is normal or slightly elevated, a RAP of 14 mm Hg is assumed. When the JVP is significantly elevated, a RAP of 20 mm Hg is assumed. 2-D echocardiography has also been used in the estimation of the RAP by observation of the calibre and reactivity of the inferior vena cava (IVC) with respiration.

Theoretical Considerations:
The RAP can be estimated by the examination of the IVC from the subcostal window. The IVC is a highly compliant vessel that acts as a capacitance reservoir for the right atrium. The calibre and respiratory response of this vessel reflects right-sided haemodynamics.
During inspiration, there is normally an increase in the venous return to the right heart and a decreased pressure within the IVC. This leads to a decrease in both the

---

36: A good correlation between the MPAP and the RVA$_c$T was found when the RVA$_c$T was 120 ms or less. When the acceleration time was greater than 120 ms, the correlation between the MPAP and the acceleration time was not as good.

blood volume and the intraluminal pressure within the IVC resulting in the collapse of the diameter of this vessel. *During expiration*, the reverse occurs.

That is, there is reduced venous return to the right heart resulting in an increase in the intraluminal pressure within the IVC and, hence, expansion of this vessel. Figure 11.21 demonstrates the normal respiratory response of the IVC as seen from the subcostal window.

This normal inspiratory collapse of the IVC is altered (diminished or absent) when flow to the right heart is impeded by increased right-sided filling pressures. Dilatation or distension of the IVC and/or dilatation of the hepatic veins may also ensue. Therefore, it is the maximal size and the degree of collapse of the IVC during respiration that is a useful indicator of the RAP (Table 11.6).

On occasions, there may be minimal change noted in the inspiratory diameter of the IVC due to variations in the force of inspiratory effort and the inability of some patients to inspire deeply (due to severe breathlessness). In these patients a "sniff" manoeuvre may be required to differentiate patients with a normal RAP from those with a genuinely increased RAP. A "sniff" accentuates the normal inspiratory response by generating a sudden decrease in intrathoracic pressure and a reduction in the diameter of the IVC.

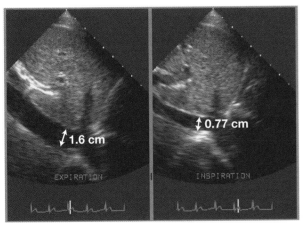

Figure 11.21: The Normal Respiratory Response of the IVC. *Left,* this image demonstrates measurement of the IVC during expiration. *Right,* this image demonstrates measurement of the IVC during inspiration. The size and degree of respiratory collapse allows the non-invasive estimation of the RAP. In this example, the IVC measures 1.6 cm at expiration and 0.77 cm at inspiration. Therefore, using Table 11.6, the estimated RAP is between 5 - 10 mm Hg.

Estimation of Left Heart Pressures:
Estimation of the Left Atrial Pressure:
The mitral regurgitant Doppler signal represents the pressure difference between the left ventricle and left atrium during systole (Figure 11.22). If the left ventricular systolic pressure is known, then it is possible to estimate the left atrial pressure (LAP) using the following equation:

(Equation 11.22)

$$LAP = LVSP - 4\left(V_{MR}\right)^2$$

where LAP   = systolic left atrial pressure (mm Hg)
       LVSP = left ventricular systolic pressure (mm Hg)
       V_{MR} = peak velocity of the MR signal (m/s)

In the absence of LVOT obstruction, the left ventricular systolic pressure is equal to the systolic arm blood pressure measured by cuff sphygmomanometer, therefore:

(Equation 11.23)

$$LAP = BP_{systolic} - 4\left(V_{MR}\right)^2$$

where LAP   = left atrial pressure (mm Hg)
       $BP_{systolic}$ = systolic arm blood pressure (mm Hg)
       V_{MR} = peak velocity of the MR signal (m/s)

Estimation of Left Ventricular End-Diastolic Pressure:
The aortic regurgitant Doppler signal represents the pressure difference between the aorta and left ventricle during diastole (Figure 11.23). By measuring the end-diastolic velocity of the aortic regurgitant signal (measured at the onset of the QRS complex of the ECG), it is possible to estimate the left ventricular end-diastolic pressure (LVEDP). If the aortic diastolic pressure is known, LVEDP can be calculated using the following equation:

(Equation 11.24)

$$LVEDP = AoDP - 4\left(V_{AR-ED}\right)^2$$

where LVEDP = left ventricular end-diastolic pressure (mm Hg)
      AoDP   = aortic diastolic pressure (mm Hg)
      V_{AR-ED} = peak end-diastolic velocity of AR signal (m/s)

Table 11.6: Estimation of the Mean Right Atrial Pressure.

IVC Size (cm)		Changes with respiration or "sniff"	Estimated Mean RAP (mm Hg)
Small	< 1.5	collapse	0 - 5
Normal	1.5 - 2.5	↓ by ≥ 50 %	5 - 10
Normal	1.5 - 2.5	↓ by ≤ 50 %	10 - 15
Dilated	> 2.5	↓ by < 50 %	15 - 20
Dilated + dilated hepatic vein		no change	> 20

From Otto, C.M. and Pearlman, A.S.: <u>Textbook of Clinical Echocardiography.</u> W.B. Saunders Company. pp.110, 1995. Reproduced with permission from W.B. Saunders Company.

The aortic diastolic pressure can be determined by cuff sphygmomanometer, therefore,

(Equation 11.25)

$$LVEDP \quad BP_{diastolic} \quad 4 \left(V_{AR-ED}\right)^2$$

where LVEDP   = left ventricular end-diastolic pressure (mm Hg)

BP$_{diastolic}$ = diastolic arm blood pressure (mm Hg)

V$_{AR-ED}$ = peak end-diastolic velocity of AR signal (m/s)

Elevation in the LAP and the LVEDP can also be identified from the diastolic filling parameters of the left ventricle (see "Assessment of Left Ventricular Diastolic Function" in this Chapter).

Limitations of Intracardiac Pressure Estimation:
Absolute pressure versus estimated pressure:
Pressures derived by Doppler calculations provide an *estimation* only of the actual pressure. Although correlations between the Doppler- and the catheter-derived pressures are excellent (see Appendix 3), Doppler-derived pressures are not exact due to numerous potential errors as described below.

Inaccurate velocity measurements:
As previously mentioned, poor alignment of the Doppler beam with the direction of blood flow will lead to an underestimation of the peak velocity which will, in turn, underestimate or overestimate the actual intracardiac pressure. *Underestimation* occurs when the Doppler-derived pressure is used in isolation or when added to another pressure. *Overestimation* of the actual pressure occurs when the Doppler-derived pressure is subtracted

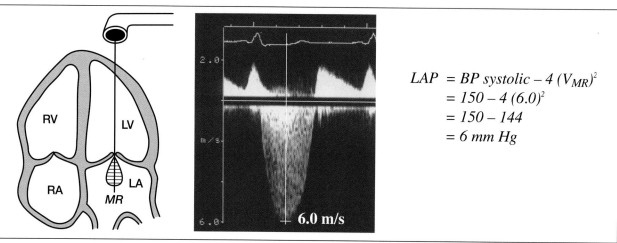

$$LAP = BP \; systolic - 4 \; (V_{MR})^2$$
$$= 150 - 4 \; (6.0)^2$$
$$= 150 - 144$$
$$= 6 \; mm \; Hg$$

Figure 11.22: Estimation of the Left Atrial Pressure (LAP) using the Mitral Regurgitant Doppler Velocity Signal.
Left, This schematic illustrates how the peak mitral regurgitant (MR) velocity is obtained by CW Doppler from the apical four chamber view. *Right,* The peak MR Doppler signal measures approximately 6.0 m/s. Using the simplified Bernoulli equation, the pressure gradient between the left ventricle and left atrium is 144 mm Hg. If the measured systolic cuff blood pressure is 150 mm Hg, the estimated systolic left atrial pressure is 6 mm Hg.
Abbreviations: LA = left atrium; **LV** = left ventricle; **MR** = mitral regurgitation; **RA** = right atrium; **RV** = right ventricle.

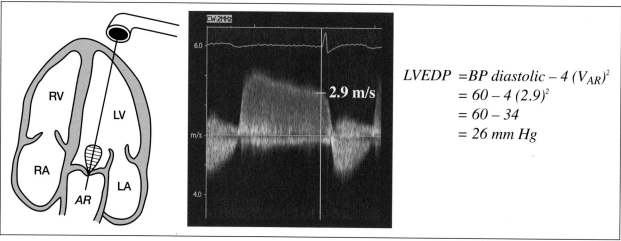

$$LVEDP = BP \; diastolic - 4 \; (V_{AR})^2$$
$$= 60 - 4 \; (2.9)^2$$
$$= 60 - 34$$
$$= 26 \; mm \; Hg$$

Figure 11.23: Estimation of the Left Ventricular End-Diastolic Pressure (LVEDP) using the Aortic Regurgitant Doppler Velocity Signal.
Left, This schematic illustrates how the end-diastolic aortic regurgitant (AR) velocity is obtained by CW Doppler from the apical five chamber view. *Right,* The end-diastolic AR signal measures 2.9 m/s. Using the simplified Bernoulli equation, the pressure gradient between the aorta and left ventricle at end-diastole equals 34 mm Hg. If the measured diastolic cuff blood pressure is 60 mm Hg, the estimated LVEDP is 26 mm Hg.
Abbreviations: AR = aortic regurgitation; **LA** = left atrium; **LV** = left ventricle; **RA** = right atrium; **RV** = right ventricle.

from another pressure; for example, in the measurement of the RVSP using the peak VSD velocity and the systolic cuff blood pressure. Therefore, interrogation for the optimal Doppler signal, from multiple acoustic windows, is mandatory. Colour flow imaging may be useful in the localisation of the jet direction.

Non-simultaneous measurements:

Measurement of the peak velocity across a VSD during systole estimates the maximum instantaneous pressure gradient between the left and right ventricles during systole. However, the right ventricle and left ventricle do not contract simultaneously (the right ventricle begins to contract slightly before the left ventricle). Therefore, the maximum instantaneous pressure gradient may not equal the true systolic pressure difference between these two ventricles.

Blood pressure measurement errors:

Sphygmomanometer errors are typically ± 5 - 10 mm Hg. Furthermore, the cuff blood pressure measurement is erroneous in the presence of left ventricular outflow obstruction (such as aortic stenosis) or significant peripheral vascular disease. Underestimation or overestimation of intracardiac pressures can occur if erroneous blood pressures are measured.

Right ventricular acceleration time:

The right ventricular acceleration time (RVA_cT) is dependent upon the cardiac output and heart rate. Hence, the accuracy of the RVA_cT in the estimation of the MPAP is also dependent on the heart rate and cardiac output. When using the method described by Mahan et al. for the estimation of the MPAP, the heart rate must be between 60 to 100 beats per minute. Furthermore, increased cardiac output or stroke volume through the right heart chambers such as occurs with atrial septal defects, may normalise the acceleration times even when pulmonary artery pressures are elevated resulting in an underestimation of the actual MPAP.

The RVA_cT should be acquired with the PW sample volume located centrally within the RVOT just proximal to the pulmonary valve to avoid contamination of the Doppler signal by systolic flutter of the valve leaflets and eddy currents.

When using the method described by Debastini et al. for determining MPAP, accuracy is increased when the acceleration time is 120 ms or less.

Right Ventricular Isovolumic Relaxation Time (RV_{IVRT}) Errors:

Increased right atrial pressures, which may occur in right heart failure or significant TR, will shorten this interval as tricuspid valve opening occurs earlier. This will result in an underestimation of the pulmonary artery systolic pressure. Furthermore, in patients with heart failure and a low cardiac output, opening of the tricuspid valve may not occur until atrial contraction resulting in prolongation of this interval.

In patients with pulmonary regurgitation, misinterpretation of the pulmonary regurgitant signal with tricuspid inflow may occur. Failure to discriminate between these two signals will result in a shortening of the RV_{IVRT} (the pulmonary regurgitant signal begins before tricupsid valve opening).

Estimation of low pressures:

The left atrial and left ventricular end-diastolic pressures are relatively low pressures which are derived from the subtraction of two significantly higher pressures (refer to equations 11.23 and 11.25). Since Doppler velocities are squared in the calculation of the pressure gradient, an underestimation of velocity will result in overestimation of the actual pressure.

Misinterpretation of Doppler Signals:

Differentiating between tricuspid and mitral regurgitant signals is crucial if they are to be used in the estimation of intracardiac pressures. 2-D guidance and colour flow imaging will help to overcome this problem. Other factors that aid in the differentiation of these two signals include (1) the peak velocity (mitral regurgitant signal is invariably greater than 4 m/s), (2) the duration of the two signals (TR signal is longer than the MR signal), and (3) the inflow velocities (tricuspid diastolic flow velocity is usually lower than the mitral inflow signal).

Arrhythmias:

Multiple Doppler echocardiographic measurements are required to reduce measurement inaccuracies that may occur due to beat-to-beat variation. In sinus rhythm, an average of 3 to 5 beats is recommended. Arrhythmias such as atrial fibrillation require additional averaging (8 to 10 beats) due to increased variation in the R-R interval.

Fluctuation of the R-R interval due to arrhythmias significantly hampers the estimation of the PASP when using the RV_{IVRT}. Accurate recording of this interval is crucial as a difference of 10 ms will result in a 10 mm Hg disparity in the estimated pressure (see Figure 11.17).

Use of an Empirical Constant or the Jugular Venous Pressure for the Mean Right Atrial Pressure:

In some studies, an empirical constant of 10 mm Hg is used for the RAP in the determination of the RVSP and PAEDP. A normal mean RAP is 4 mm Hg, therefore, the addition of this empirical constant may lead to overestimation of normal pressures. Conversely, underestimation of the pulmonary artery diastolic pressure may result if this empirical constant is assumed for the RAP when the right ventricular end-diastolic pressure is elevated.

The clinical assessment of the jugular venous pressure (JVP) can also be used in the estimation of the RAP. In patients with a normal or mildly elevated JVP, the RAP is estimated at 14 mm Hg; for those patients with a significantly elevated JVP, a value of 20 mm Hg is used for the RAP. However, the use of these values tends to result in an overestimation of PASP in patients with normal pressures. Furthermore, accurate measurement of the JVP is particularly difficult in small children, obese patients and patients with markedly elevated right atrial pressures.

For these reasons, it is recommended that the IVC size and reactivity with respiration be used in the estimation of the RAP.

References and Suggested Reading:

General References:

- Feigenbaum, H.: <u>Echocardiography.</u> 5th Ed. Lea & Febiger, 1994.
- Hatle, L. and Angelson, B.: <u>Doppler Ultrasound in Cardiology: Physical Principles and Clinical Application.</u> 2nd Ed. Lea & Febiger, 1985.
- Nishimura, R.: Quantitative hemodynamics by Doppler echocardiography; A noninvasive alternative to cardiac catheterization. *Progress in Cardiovascular Disease. 4:309-342,1994.*
- Oh, J.A., Seward, J.B., Tajik, A.J.: <u>The Echo Manual.</u> Little Brown and Company. 1994.
- Otto, C.M. and Pearlman, A.S.: <u>Textbook of Clinical Echocardiography.</u> W.B. Saunders Company. 1995
- Weyman, A.: <u>Principles and Practice of Echocardiography.</u> 2nd ed. Lea & Febiger,1994.
- Yoganathan, A.P. et al.: Review of hydrodynamic principles for the cardiologist: applications to the study of blood flow and jets by imaging techniques. *Journal of the American College of Cardiology 12: 1344-1353.*

Determination of Pressure Gradients:

- Baumgartner, H. et al.: Discrepancies between Doppler and catheter gradients in aortic prosthetic valves in vitro. A manifestation of localized pressure gradients and pressure recovery. *Circulation 82:1467-1475,1990.*
- Baumgartner, H. et al.: Effect of prosthetic valve design on the Doppler-catheter gradient correlation: An in vitro study of normal St. Jude, Medtronic-Hall, Starr-Edwards and Hancock valves. *Journal of the American College of Cardiology 19:324-332,1992.*
- Burstow, D.J. et al.: Continuous wave Doppler echocardiographic measurement of prosthetic valve gradients: A simultaneous Doppler-catheter correlative study. *Circulation 80:504-514,1989.*
- Connolly, H.M. et al.: Doppler hemodynamic profiles of 86 normal tricuspid valve prostheses. *Journal of the American College of Cardiology 17: 69A, 1991.*
- Currie, P.J. et al.: Continuous-wave Doppler echocardiographic assessment of severity of calcific aortic stenosis: a simultaneous Doppler-catheter correlative study in 100 adult patients. *Circulation 71:1162-1169,1985.*
- Currie, P.J. et al.: Continous wave Doppler determination of right ventricular pressure: A simultaneous Doppler-catheterization study in 127 patients. *Journal of the American College of Cardiology 6:750-756,1985.*
- Currie, P.J. et al.: Instantaneous pressure gradient: A simultaneous Doppler and dual catheter correlative study. *Journal of the American College of Cardiology 7:800-806,1986.*
- Ge, Z. et al.: Simultaneous measurement of left atrial pressure by Doppler echocardiography and catheterization. *International Journal of Cardiology 37:243-251,1992.*
- Ge, Z. et al.: Noninvasive evaluation of interventricular pressure gradients across ventricular septal defect. A simultaneous study of Doppler echocardiography and cardiac catheterization. *American Heart Journal 124:176-182,1992.*

- Ge, Z-M. et al.: Quantification of left-sided intracardiac pressures and gradients using mitral and aortic regurgitant velocities by simultaneous left and right catheterization and continuous-wave Doppler echocardiography. *Clinical Cardiology 16:863-870,1993.*
- Hatle, L. et al.: Noninvasive assessment of atrioventricular pressure half-time by Doppler ultrasound. *Circulation 60:1096-1104,1979.*
- Kosturakis, D. et al.: Noninvasive quantification of stenotic semilunar valve areas by Doppler echocardiography. *Journal of the American College of Cardiology 3:1256-1262,1984.*
- Lei, M-H. et al.: Reappraisal of quantitative evaluation of pulmonary regurgitation and estimation of pulmonary artery pressure by continuous wave Doppler echocardiography. *Cardiology 86: 249-256, 1995.*
- Lengyel, M. et al.: Doppler hemodynamic profiles of 456 clinically and echo-normal mitral valve prostheses. Circulation 82 (suppl III): 43,1990.
- Levine, R.A. et al.: Pressure recovery distal to a stenosis: potential cause of gradient "overestimation" by Doppler echocardiography. *Journal of the American College of Cardiology 13: 706-715, 1989.*
- Lima, C.O. et al.: Noninvasive prediction of transvalvular pressure gradient in patients with pulmonary stenosis by quantitative two-dimensional echocardiographic Doppler studies. *Circulation 67:866-871,1983.*
- Marx, G.R. et al.: Accuracy and pitfalls of Doppler evaluation of the pressure gradient in aortic coarctation. *Journal of the American College of Cardiology 7: 1379-1385, 1986.*
- Masuyama, T. et al.: Continuous-wave Doppler echocardiographic detection of pulmonary regurgitation and its application to noninvasive estimation of pulmonary artery pressure. *Circulation 74:484-492,1986.*
- Miller, F.A. et al.: Normal aortic valve prosthesis Hemodynamics: 609 prospective Doppler examinations. *Circulation 80 (suppl II): 169,1989.*
- Murphy, .D.J. et al.: Continuous-wave Doppler in children with ventricular septal defect: Noninvasive estimation of interventricular pressure gradient. *American Journal of Cardiology 57:428-432,1986.*
- Nishimura, R.A., Tajik, A.J.: Determination of left-sided pressure gradients by ultilizing Doppler aortic and mitral regurgitant signals: Validation by simultaneous dual catheter and Doppler studies. *Journal of the American College of Cardiology 11:317-321,1988.*
- Nishimura, R.A. et al: Accurate measurement of the transmitral gradient in patients with mitral stenosis: A simultaneous catheterization and Doppler echocardiography study. *Journal of the American College of Cardiology 24:152-158,1994.*
- Otto, C.M. and Pearlman, A.S.: Doppler echocardiography in adults with symptomatic aortic stenosis. *Archives of Internal Medicine 148: 2553-2560, 1988.*
- Otto, C.M. et al.: Doppler echocardiographic findings in adults with severe symptomatic valvular aortic stenosis. *American Journal of Cardiology 68: 1477-1484, 1991.*
- Sagar, K.B. et al.: Doppler echocardiographic evaluation of Hancock and Bjork-Shiley prosthetic valves. *Journal of the American College of Cardiology 7:681-687,1986.*

- Simpson, I.A. et al.: Clinical value of Doppler echocardiography in the assessment of adults with aortic stenosis. *British Heart Journal 53:636-639,1985.*
- Smith, M.D. et al.: Systematic correlation of continuous-wave Doppler and hemodynamic measurements in patients with aortic stenosis. *American Heart Journal 111:245-252,1986.*
- Stamm, R.B., Martin, R.P.: Quantification of pressure gradients across stenotic valves by Doppler ultrasound. *Journal of the American College of Cardiology 2:707,718,1983.*
- Stewart, S.F.C. et al.: Errors in pressure gradient measurement by continuous wave Doppler ultrasound: Type, size and age effects in bioprosthetic aortic valves. *Journal of the American College of Cardiology 18:769-779,1991.*
- Teien, D. et al.: Noninvasive estimation of the mean pressure difference in aortic stenosis by Doppler ultrasound. *British Heart Journal 56: 450-455, 1986.*
- Teirstein, P.S. et al.: The accuracy of Doppler ultrasound measurement of pressure gradients across irregular, dual, and tunnel-like obstructions to blood flow. *Circulation 72: 577-584, 1985.*
- Vandervoort, P.M. et al.: Pressure recovery in bileaflet heart valve prostheses. *Circulation 92: 3464-3472, 1995.*
- Wilkins, G.T. et al.: Validation of continuous-wave Doppler echocardiographic measurements of mitral and tricuspid prosthetic valve gradients: A simultaneous Doppler-catheter study. *Circulation 74:786-795,1986.*

Intracardiac Pressure Estimation:
- Burstin, L.: Determination of pressure in the pulmonary artery by external graphic recordings. *British Heart Journal 29:393-404,1967.*
- Chan, K-L., et al.: Comparison of three Doppler ultrasound methods in the prediction of pulmonary artery pressure. *Journal of the American College of Cardiology 9:549-554,1987.*
- Currie, P.J. et al.: Continuous-wave Doppler determination of right ventricular pressure: A simultaneous Doppler-catheterization study in 127 patients. *Journal of the American College of Cardiology 6: 750-756, 1985.*
- Debastini, A. et al.: Evaluation of pulmonary artery pressure and resistance by pulsed Doppler echocardiography. *American Journal of Cardiology 59: 662-668, 1987.*
- Ge, Z., et al.: Simultaneous measurement of pulmonary artery diastolic pressure by Doppler echocardiography and catheterization with patent ductus arteriosus. *American Heart Journal 125:263-266,1993.*
- Ge, Z., et al.: Noninvasive evaluation of interventricular pressure gradient across ventricular septal defect: a simultaneous study of Doppler echocardiography and cardiac catheterization. *American Heart Journal 124:176-182, 1992.*
- Ge, Z., et al.: Noninvasive evaluation of right ventricular and pulmonary artery systolic pressures in patients with ventricular septal defects: Simultaneous study of Doppler and catheterization data. *American Heart Journal 125:1073-1081,1993.*
- Ge, Z. et al.: Simultaneous measurement of left atrial pressure gradients by Doppler echocardiography and catheterization. *International Journal of Cardiology 37:243-251, 1992.*
- Ge, Z. et al.: Quantification of left-sided intracardiac pressures and gradients using mitral and aortic regurgitant velocities by simultaneous left and right catheterization and continuous-wave Doppler echocardiography. *Clinical Cardiology. 16:863-870, 1993.*
- Gorscan, J. et al.: Noninvasive estimation of left atrial pressure in patients with congestive heart failure and mitral regurgitation by Doppler echocardiography. *American Heart Journal 121: 858-863,1991.*
- Grayburn, P.A. et al.: Quantitative assessment of the haemodynamic consequences of aortic regurgitation by means of continuous wave Doppler recordings. *Journal of the American College of Cardiology 10:135-141,1987.*
- Hatle, L., et al.: Non-invasive estimation of pulmonary artery systolic pressure with Doppler ultrasound. *British Heart Journal 45:157-165,1981.*
- Kitabatake, A., et al.: Noninvasive evaluation of pulmonary hypertension by pulsed Doppler technique. *Circulation 68:302-309,1983.*
- Lee, R.T., et al.: Prospective Doppler echocardiographic evaluation of pulmonary artery diastolic pressure in the Medical Intensive Care Unit. *American Journal of Cardiology 64:1366-1370,1989.*
- Lei, M-H., et al.: Reappraisal of quantitative evaluation of pulmonary regurgitation and estimation of pulmonary artery pressure by continuous wave Doppler. *Cardiology 86:249-256,1995.*
- Mahan, G. et al.: Estimation of pulmonary artery pressure by pulsed Doppler echocardiography (Abstract). *Circulation 68 (suppl III): 367, 1983.*
- Marx, G.R., et al.: Doppler echocardiographic estimation of systolic pulmonary artery pressure in pediatric patients with interventricular communications. *Journal of the American College of Cardiology 6:1132-1137,1985.*
- Marx, G.R. et al.: Doppler echocardiographic estimation of systolic pulmonary artery pressure in patients with aortic-pulmonary shunts. *Journal of the American College of Cardiology 7: 880-885, 1986.*
- Masauyama, T., et al.: Continuous-wave Doppler echocardiographic detection of pulmonary regurgitation and its application in noninvasive estimation of pulmonary artery pressure. *Circulation 74: 484-492, 1986.*
- Murphy, D.J. et al.: Continuous-wave Doppler in children with ventricular septal defect: noninvasive estimation of interventricular pressure gradient. *American Journal of Cardiology 57: 428-432, 1986.*
- Musewe, N.N. et al.: Doppler echocardiographic measurement of pulmonary artery pressure from ductal Doppler velocities in the Newborn. *Journal of the American College of Cardiology 15: 446-456, 1990.*
- Stevenson, J.G.: Comparison of several noninvasive methods for estimation of pulmonary artery pressure. *Journal of the American Society of Echocardiography 2:157-171,1989.*
- Yock, P.G., Popp, R.L.: Noninvasive estimation of right ventricular systolic pressure by Doppler ultrasound in patients with tricuspid regurgitation. *Circulation 70: 657-662, 1984.*

Intracardiac Shunt Calculations (QP:QS):

- Cloez, J-L. et al.: Determination of pulmonary to systemic blood flow ratio in children by a simplified Doppler echocardiographic method. *Journal of the American College of Cardiology 11: 825-830, 1988.*

- Dittman, H. et al.: Accuracy of Doppler echocardiography in quantification of left to right shunts in adult patients with atrial septal defect. *Journal of the American College of Cardiology 11: 338-342, 1988.*

- Kitatabake, A. et al.: Noninvasive evaluation of the ratio of pulmonary to systemic flow in atrial septal defect by duplex Doppler echocardiography. *Circulation 69: 73-79, 1984.*

- Kurokawa, S. et al.: Noninvasive evaluation of the ratio of pulmonary to systemic flow in ventricular septal defect by means of Doppler two-dimensional echocardiography. *American Heart Journal 116: 1033-1044, 1988.*

- Meijboom, E.J. et al.: A two-dimensional Doppler echocardiographic method for calculation of pulmonary and systemic blood flow in a canine model with variable-sized left-to-right extracardiac shunt. *Circulation 68: 437-445, 1983.*

- Sabry, A.F. et al.: Comparison of four Doppler echocardiographic methods for calculating pulmonary-to-systemic shunt flow ratios in patients with ventricular septal defect. *American Journal of Cardiology 75: 611-614, 1995.*

- Sanders, S.P. et al.: Measurement of systemic and pulmonary blood flow and QP;QS ratio using Doppler and two-dimensional echocardiography. *American Journal of Cardiology 51: 953-956, 1983.*

- Valdes-Cruz, L.M. et al.: A pulsed Doppler echocardiographic method for calculating pulmonary and systemic blood flow in atrial level shunts: validation studies in animals and initial human experience. *Circulation 69: 80-86, 1984.*

- Vargas Barron, J. et al.: Clinical utility of two-dimensional Doppler echocardiographic techniques for estimating pulmonary to systemic blood flow ratios in children with left to right shunting atrial septal defect, ventricular septal defect or patent ductus arteriosus. *Journal of the American College of Cardiology 3: 169-178, 1984.*

Chapter 12
Valve Area Calculations

Valve areas can be estimated by Doppler echocardiography by application of the continuity principle. Using this principle, it is theoretically possible to determine any valve area, native or prosthetic. Two other methods which can be employed in the estimation of stenotic mitral valve areas include the pressure half-time (PHT) method and the proximal isovelocity surface area (PISA) technique. The clinical significance of valve areas with the severity of valvular stenosis are listed in Table 12.1.

Table 12.1: Clinical Significance of Valve Areas in Valvular Stenosis.

AORTIC STENOSIS [1]	
Aortic Valve Area	
Normal	> 2.0 cm^2
Mild	> 1.0 cm^2
Moderate	$0.76 - 1.0$ cm^2
Severe	≤ 0.75 cm^2
MITRAL STENOSIS [2]	
Mitral Valve Area	
Normal	$4 - 6$ cm^2
Mild	> 1.5 cm^2
Moderate	$1.0 - 1.5$ cm^2
Severe	< 1.0 cm^2
TRICUSPID STENOSIS [3]	
Tricuspid Valve Area	
Normal	> 7.0 cm^2
Severe	< 1.0 cm^2

Sources: (1) Oh et al., *Journal of the American College of Cardiology* 11:1227-1234,1988; (2) Nishimura, R.A. and Tajik, A.J., *Progress in Cardiovascular Disease* 34:309-342,1994; (3) Alexander, R.W., Schlant, R.C., Fuster, V. Hurst's. The Heart. 9th Edition. McGraw-Hill, pp. 1837 & 18431998.

Continuity Equation for the Calculation of Valve Areas

Typically, the severity of valvular stenosis is determined by the maximum and/or mean pressure gradient across that valve. However, pressure gradients are flow dependent and are affected, therefore, by the stroke volume and cardiac output. Thus, in situations where the stroke volume is increased (high cardiac output states), pressure gradients may be increased in the absence of a significant stenosis. Conversely, low pressure gradients may be found in the presence of severe stenosis when the stroke volume is reduced (low cardiac output states). Therefore, overestimation or underestimation of the severity of valvular stenosis may occur if the Doppler-derived pressure gradients are used in isolation.

Flow rates also affect prosthetic valve pressure gradients; for example, high pressure gradients may occur across a normally functioning prosthetic valve when examined under high flow rates. Henceforth, calculation of the *effective* valve area by the continuity equation provides a better indication of prosthetic valve function.

Studies validating the accuracy and reliability of the continuity equation in the determination of native and prosthetic valve areas are tabulated in Appendix 6.

Theoretical Considerations:
As previously discussed, the continuity principle is based on the principle of the conservation of mass which simply states "what goes in, must come out". Providing that there is no loss of fluid from the system, flow through a stenotic valve (Q_{sten}) must equal the flow proximal to it (Q_{prox}) so that $Q_{sten} = Q_{prox}$. Since flow (Q) is equal to the product of the mean velocity (V) and the cross-sectional area (CSA), this relationship can be written:

(Equation 12.1)

$$CSA_{prox} \times V_{prox} = CSA_{sten} \times V_{sten}$$

Therefore, to calculate the stenotic valve area, equation 12.1 is simply rearranged to:

(Equation 12.2)

$$CSA_{sten} = \frac{CSA_{prox} \times V_{prox}}{V_{sten}}$$

where CSA_{prox} = cross-sectional area proximal to a stenosis (cm^2)
CSA_{sten} = cross-sectional area of stenotic valve (cm^2)
V_{prox} = mean velocity proximal to stenosis (m/s)
V_{sten} = mean velocity through stenosis (m/s)

Because flow within the heart is pulsatile, the velocity time integral (VTI) rather than the mean velocity is used, thus:

(Equation 12.3)

$$CSA_{sten} = \frac{CSA_{prox} \times VTI_{prox}}{VTI_{sten}}$$

where CSA_{prox} = cross-sectional area proximal to a stenosis (cm^2)
CSA_{sten} = cross-sectional area of stenotic valve (cm^2)
VTI_{prox} = velocity time integral proximal to stenosis (cm)
VTI_{sten} = velocity time integral through stenosis (cm)

Doppler Echocardiographic Determination of the Aortic Valve Area:
The continuity principle is most commonly used in the calculation of the area of the stenotic aortic valve which is illustrated in Figure 12.1. The prosthetic aortic valve area (AVA) can also be calculated in the same manner.

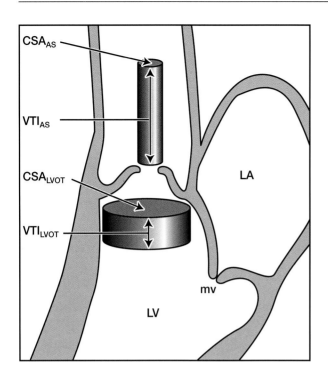

Figure 12.1: Calculation of the Aortic Valve Area by the Continuity Equation.
The continuity principle states that flow through the stenotic aortic valve (Q_{AS}) must be equal to the flow proximal to; that is, the flow within the LVOT (Q_{LVOT}). Thus, $Q_{AS} = Q_{LVOT}$. Since flow is pulsatile within the heart, the volumetric flow is a product of the integrated velocity over time (VTI) and the cross-sectional area (CSA); hence,

$$Q_{LVOT} = CSA_{LVOT} \times VTI_{LVOT} \text{ and } Q_{AS} = CSA_{AS} \times VTI_{AS}$$

Therefore, since $Q_{LVOT} = Q_{AS}$

$$CSA_{LVOT} \times VTI_{LVOT} = CSA_{AS} \times VTI_{AS}$$

By rearranging this equation, the stenotic aortic valve area (CSA_{AS}) can be determined:

$$CSA_{AS} = \frac{CSA_{LVOT} \times VTI_{LVOT}}{VTI_{AS}}$$

Doppler Echocardiographic Determination of the Mitral, Tricuspid, and Pulmonary Valve Areas:
The mitral, tricuspid, and pulmonary valve areas (native or prosthetic) can also be derived by application of the continuity principle. However, it is not always easy to measure the flow proximal to these stenotic valves (especially in the atrioventricular valves). Fortunately, measurement of flow through the LVOT is relatively easy and, providing that flow through both the stenotic valve and the LVOT are equal, flow through the LVOT can be substituted for the flow proximal to the stenotic valve. Hence, the unknown valve area can be calculated by:

(Equation 12.4)

$$CSA_{sten} = \frac{CSA_{LVOT} \times VTI_{LVOT}}{VTI_{sten}}$$

where CSA_{LVOT} = cross-sectional area of left ventricular outflow tract (cm²)
CSA_{sten} = cross-sectional area of stenotic/prosthetic valve (cm²)
VTI_{LVOT} = velocity time integral through left ventricular outflow tract (cm)
VTI_{sten} = velocity time integral through stenotic/prosthetic valve (cm)

Limitations of the Continuity Equation:
Assumptions of Volumetric Flow Calculations:
Calculation of the valve area by the continuity equation is based on the determination of the volumetric flow rate or stroke volume. Stroke volume calculations are, in turn, based on a simple hydraulic formula which determines the volumetric flow rate through a cylindrical tube under steady flow conditions. In order to apply this concept to the heart, certain assumptions regarding flow properties and conditions are made. These assumptions include that:

(1) flow is occurring in a rigid, circular tube, (2) there is a uniform velocity across the vessel, (3) the derived CSA is circular, (4) the CSA remains constant throughout the period of flow, and (5) the sample volume remains in a constant position throughout the period of flow.
However, blood vessels are elastic and, therefore, change throughout the duration of flow within the cardiac cycle. In addition, annular diameters may change throughout the period of flow and, while the left and right ventricular outflow tracts assume a circular configuration, the same may not be said for the atrioventricular valves that assume a more elliptical shape.

Determination of the CSA of the LVOT:
Determination of the CSA of the LVOT is derived by measuring the diameter of the LVOT during systole. The CSA is then calculated by squaring the diameter and multiplying this by 0.785. Therefore, any error in the measurement of the diameter is magnified. Suboptimal imaging and excessive calcification of the LVOT annulus further prejudices the accuracy of this measurement.
When calculating the effective orifice area of the prosthetic aortic valve, measurement of the LVOT diameter may prove difficult due to reverberations arising from the dense sewing ring of the prosthesis. Therefore, it is sometimes necessary to substitute the prosthetic valve size for the LVOT diameter. However, one should be aware of the fact that the LVOT diameter and the prosthetic valve size are not always equal. For example, the prosthetic valve size may be larger than the LVOT diameter when the prosthetic aortic valve is implanted superior to the valve annulus or when there is progressive narrowing of the LVOT due to fibrosis, scarring or calcification which may occur with "aging" of prosthetic valves. Therefore, the direct substitution of the prosthetic ring size for the LVOT is not recommended. Substitution

Method of Calculation of Valve Areas using the Continuity Principle:
Below, is a "step-by-step" method for calculation of a stenotic or prosthetic valve area using the continuity principle.

Method for calculation of valve area by the continuity equation
Step 1: measure the CSA of the LVOT (CSA_{LVOT}): from the parasternal long axis view, measure the LVOT diameter (D): - measure during systole - measure from inner edge to inner edge determine CSA of LVOT annulus (cm^2): - $CSA = 0.785 \times D^2$ **Step 2: measure the VTI of the LVOT (VTI_{LVOT}):** from the apical 5 chamber view, measure the VTI of the LVOT: - using PW Doppler, place the sample volume just proximal to the aortic valve - measure during the same phase of the cardiac cycle (systole) - trace the leading edge velocity to obtain the VTI (cm) **Step 3: measure the VTI of the stenotic/prosthetic valve (VTI_{sten}):** using CW Doppler, measure the VTI across the stenotic valve: - interrogate from multiple windows to ensure highest velocity signal is obtained - trace the leading edge velocity to obtain the VTI (cm) **Step 4: calculate the unknown stenotic/prosthetic valve area (CSA_{sten}):** $$CSA_{sten}\ (cm^2) = \frac{CSA_{LVOT} \times VTI_{LVOT}}{VTI_{sten}}$$

Technical Consideration for determination of mitral, tricuspid and/or pulmonary valve areas: Flow through the LVOT can only be substituted for flow proximal to a stenotic/prosthetic valve when flow through both the stenotic/prosthetic valve and the LVOT are equal. In the presence of significant aortic regurgitation, the flow through the LVOT will be greater than flow through the stenotic/prosthetic valve and, therefore, valve area will be overestimated. In this instance, the RVOT VTI and CSA can be substituted for the LVOT parameters provided that there is no intracardiac shunt or significant pulmonary regurgitation.

of the prosthetic valve size for the LVOT diameter should only be done when the LVOT cannot be accurately measured.

Failure to Obtain the Peak Velocity:
As previously mentioned, when there is a large angle (θ) between ultrasound beam and the direction of blood flow, a significant underestimation of the true velocity occurs. Therefore, failure to align the ultrasound beam parallel to the direction of blood flow will result in the underestimation of the actual peak velocity. This *underestimation* of the peak velocity will ultimately result in the *overestimation* of the valve area by the application of the continuity equation. Consequently, meticulous Doppler interrogation, utilising multiple transducer positions to obtain the peak velocity, is mandatory.

Erroneous Velocity Time Integral Measurements:
Calculation of the valve area assumes that flow within the LVOT is laminar. Therefore, for accurate results, it is necessary to position the sample volume where the flow profile is uniform. Correct positioning of the sample volume in the LVOT is particularly important in the

assessment of the AVA in aortic stenosis. In this instance, the sample volume should be positioned 0.5 to 1.5 cm proximal to aortic valve to avoid flow acceleration which may occur immediately proximal to this stenotic valve.

Inappropriate Application of the "Simplified" Continuity Equation:
Since the peak velocities through the outflow tract and the aortic valve occur during the same ejection period, calculation of the AVA can be simplified by substituting the peak velocities for the VTI. However, application of this simplified version of the continuity equation becomes less accurate in situations when the peak velocities through the LVOT and aortic valve do not occur simultaneously. This situation typically occurs when there are alterations in the shape of the LVOT and variable aortic flow profiles.

Differential flow through CSA_{prox} and CSA_{sten}:
Assessment of the valve area by the continuity equation requires that flow through the CSA proximal to the stenosis and the CSA of the stenosis are equal. Therefore, differential flow such as valvular regurgitation or intracardiac shunt flow may invalidate the calculation of

the valve area by the continuity equation. For example, when calculating the MVA when there is coexistent aortic regurgitation, the flow through the LVOT and the mitral valve is not equal (there is greater flow through the LVOT). Hence, calculation of the MVA by this method will be overestimated. Furthermore, calculation of the MVA in the presence of mitral regurgitation will also invalidate the MVA calculation. In this instance, the stroke volume through the mitral valve will be greater than that through the LVOT. When calculating the AVA in the presence of a coexistent membraneous ventricular septal defect, flow through the LVOT will be greater than flow through the aortic valve (some flow through the LVOT will be shunted across the ventricular septal defect into the right ventricle). Hence, the AVA will be overestimated.

Low Cardiac Output States:
Underestimation of the AVA determined by the continuity equation may occur in patients with a low cardiac output. For example, in situations where there is poor myocardial contractility and/or reduced flow through the aortic valve, calculation of the "resting" AVA may significantly underestimate the true anatomical valve area. Small valve areas due to a low cardiac output can be differentiated from small valve areas due to significant stenosis by "normalising" or increasing the cardiac output through the valve. "Normalisation" of the cardiac output can be achieved by exercise or dobutamine infusion. Increasing the cardiac output results in an increase in both the LVOT velocity as well as the velocity across the aortic valve. In patients with mild aortic stenosis, the increase in the LVOT velocity is greater than the increase in the transaortic velocity and, hence, the "effective" AVA will increase. In patients with true severe aortic stenosis, increasing the cardiac output will not significantly alter the relationship between the LVOT gradient and the transaortic gradient, and, therefore, the AVA will remain unchanged.

Estimation of Prosthetic Effective Orifice Areas:
The accuracy of the Doppler-derived effective orifice area (EOA) in prosthetic valves is dependent upon the valve type. Significant underestimation of the EOA may occur in the St. Jude prosthetic valve in the aortic position due to localised high velocities and pressure recovery distal to the valve. In this situation, the peak velocities are not representative of the mean velocity distribution across the prosthetic orifice. Determination of the EOA using the VTI rather than the peak velocity was shown to improve the correlation between the EOA calculated by the continuity and Gorlin equations.

Technical Consideration:
The normal EOA value for prosthetic valves is dependent on the valve type, size and position of the valve. Therefore, when evaluating possible obstruction of a prosthetic valve, the ranges that are used in the assessment of the severity of native valve stenoses do not apply.

Pressure Half-Time and Deceleration Time Methods for Calculation of Mitral Valve Areas

The pressure half-time (PHT) and deceleration time (DT) can be used in the estimation of the mitral valve area (MVA) in patients with mitral stenosis. The principal advantage of the PHT in the estimation of the MVA is that it is independent of the cardiac output or coexistent mitral regurgitation. Therefore, this method is useful in the assessment of the severity of mitral stenosis in situations where the mean transmitral pressure gradients may be misleading. For instance, overestimation of the severity of mitral stenosis using the transmitral pressure gradient may occur when there is coexistent mitral regurgitation. In this instance, increased transmitral gradients occur because of increased flow across the regurgitant valve. Conversely, underestimation in the severity of mitral stenosis may occur when there is a low mean transmitral pressure gradient in the setting of a low cardiac output. Calculation of the MVA by the PHT can readily overcome these potential misinterpretations. For example, patients with mitral regurgitation but only mild mitral stenosis will have a short PHT despite increased transmitral pressure gradients. Conversely, in patients with a low cardiac output, prolongation of the PHT will be evident with significant stenosis even when there is a low transmitral pressure gradient. Studies validating the accuracy and reliability of the PHT in the calculation of the MVA are tabulated in Appendix 7.

Theoretical Considerations:
In the presence of mitral stenosis, the pressure gradient between the left atrium and left ventricle is increased throughout diastolic period and the rate of decline of the early peak velocity is prolonged. Prolongation of this diastolic deceleration time occurs because a longer time is required for the left atrium to empty into the left ventricle through the stenotic mitral valve. The rate of decline of the pressure difference between the left atrium and left ventricle can be measured by the pressure half-time (PHT). The PHT is defined as the time required for the pressure to decay to half its original value.

In Doppler echocardiography, velocity rather than pressure is displayed on the Doppler spectrum. Since velocity and pressure are related, the PHT can also be measured from the velocity spectrum (Figure 12.2). It is important to note, however, that the PHT is not equal to the velocity half-time. In fact, the pressure corresponding to one-half of the peak pressure ($P_{1/2}$) is derived from the following equation:

(Equation 12.5)

$$P_{1/2} = \frac{V_{peak}}{\sqrt{2}}$$

$$or$$

$$= \frac{V_{peak}}{1.414}$$

Technical Consideration:
Due to the relationship between pressure and velocity, the PHT can be derived from the velocity spectrum. Recall that the relationship between pressure (P) and velocity (V) is expressed by the following equation:

(Equation 5.12)

$$\Delta P = 4V^2$$

Therefore, using the velocity Doppler curve the pressure point (P) which corresponds to one-half of the peak pressure (P_{peak}) can be derived as follows:

$$P = \tfrac{1}{2} P_{peak}$$

$$4(V)^2 = \tfrac{1}{2} 4(V_{peak})^2$$

$$V^2 = \frac{4(V_{peak})^2}{4 \times 2}$$

$$V^2 = \frac{(V_{peak})^2}{2}$$

$$V = \frac{\sqrt{(V_{peak})^2}}{\sqrt{2}}$$

$$V = \frac{V_{peak}}{\sqrt{2}}$$

$$V = \frac{V_{peak}}{1.414}$$

Another method for determining the velocity corresponding to the one-half of the pressure is derived by *multiplying* the peak velocity by 0.707.

Hatle and Angelsen [37], observed that a PHT greater than 220 ms usually equated to a MVA of 1.0 cm². Based on this observation, a formula for the calculation of the MVA using the PHT and an empirical constant of 220 was derived:

(Equation 12.6)

$$MVA = \frac{220}{PHT}$$

The PHT is also related to the deceleration time (DT) which is the time taken for the peak early diastolic velocity to fall to zero. However, the early diastolic velocity does not always fall to zero. But since the deceleration slope of the mitral velocity curve is usually linear, this slope can be easily extrapolated to the zero baseline enabling the measurement of the DT (Figure 12.3).

The relationship between the PHT and the DT is such that the PHT is equal to 29% of the DT and, therefore, can be expressed by:

(Equation 12.7)

$$PHT = 0.29 \times DT$$

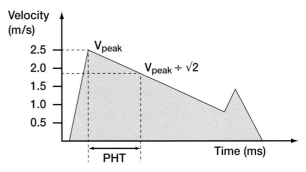

Figure 12.2: Method of Measuring the Pressure Half-Time from the Doppler Velocity Spectrum.
This schematic illustrates how the pressure half-time (PHT) is measured from the mitral velocity spectrum. The PHT is the time required for the pressure to decay to half its original value. Using the velocity spectrum, the PHT is equal to the time taken for the peak velocity (V_{peak}) to fall to $V_{peak} \div \sqrt{2}$. In this example, the V_{peak} is 2.5 m/s; therefore, the $V_{peak} \div \sqrt{2}$ is 1.8 m/s. Hence, the PHT is equal to the time taken for the velocity to fall from 2.5 m/s to 1.8 m/s.

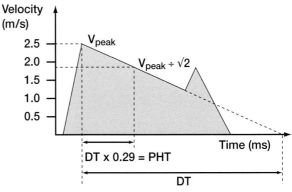

Figure 12.3: Method of Measuring the Deceleration Time from the Doppler Velocity Spectrum.
This schematic illustrates how the deceleration time (DT) is measured from the mitral velocity spectrum. The DT is the time required for the velocity slope to fall from the peak velocity (V_{peak}) to zero. Normally, the mitral velocity does not fall all the way to the zero baseline and, hence, the deceleration slope must be extrapolated to the zero baseline. Observe that the PHT is equal to 29% of the DT; hence, the PHT can be derived by multiplying the DT by 0.29.

37: Hatle, L. and Angelsen, B.: Doppler Ultrasound in Cardiology. Physical Principles and Clinical Applications. U.S.A.: Lea and Febiger, 1985. pp: 118-122.

By combining equations 12.6 and 12.7, it is also possible to calculate the MVA from the DT:

(Equation 12.8)

$$MVA = \frac{220}{0.29 \times DT}$$
$$= \frac{759}{DT}$$

Limitations of the PHT in the Calculation of the MVA
Non-linear (Curvilinear) Early Diastolic Slope:
In the majority of cases, the diastolic pressure decay between the left atrium and left ventricle follows a straight line, thus, enabling accurate measurements of the PHT and the MVA. A non-linear or curvilinear decay of the diastolic pressure gradient can lead to erroneous calculations of the MVA if the PHT is measured incorrectly. The portion of the curvilinear slope measured is dependent on: (1) the end-diastolic pressure gradient and (2) the part of the slope considered to be most representative. Figure 12.4 illustrates the various methods that may be used in the determination of the PHT when there is a curvilinear slope and a high end-diastolic gradient. Of these methods, method C appears to provide the most accurate estimation of the MVA by the PHT.

Post Balloon Mitral Valvuloplasty:
Immediately following balloon mitral valvuloplasty, the accuracy of the calculated MVA by the PHT declines. This has been attributed to the fact that the PHT is not only inversely related to the MVA, but is also directly proportional to other factors such as the peak transmitral gradient and chamber compliance. In the normal clinical situation, left atrial and ventricular compliance counteract one another. However, immediately

following balloon mitral valvuloplasty abrupt changes in left atrial pressure and compliance occur altering the relationship between the PHT and the MVA. This adverse effect on the PHT appears to be short-term as studies performed 24 to 48 hours after balloon mitral valvuloplasty correlate equally as well with the haemodynamic valve areas determined prior to the procedure.

Significant Aortic Regurgitation:
Misinterpretation between the mitral stenotic signal and the aortic regurgitant signal is possible. Differentiation between these two signals can be easily recognised by observation of the timing of each signal. Aortic regurgitation commences at the closure of the aortic valve while mitral inflow begins following the isovolumic relaxation period (time interval between aortic valve closure and mitral valve opening).
Severe aortic regurgitation may also lead to overestimation of the MVA by shortening the PHT. In this instance, the PHT is shortened due to a marked and rapid increase in the left ventricular end-diastolic pressure which effectively reduces the diastolic pressure gradient between the left atrium and the left ventricle.

Cardiac Rhythm Disturbances:
In the presence of sinus tachycardia or first degree atrioventricular heart block, the deceleration slope prior to atrial contraction may be so short that accurate measurement of the PHT is not possible. In addition, atrial flutter with frequent atrial contractions may produce a falsely short PHT and, therefore, will overestimate the MVA.

Prosthetic Mitral Valve Areas:
The PHT method for determining MVA in prosthetic valves has not been validated. In fact, it has been suggested that the PHT in prosthetic valves is reflective of non-prosthetic factors such as the left ventricular diastolic function rather than the effective valve area. Application of the continuity equation in the estimation of the effective valve area provides a more accurate indication of prosthetic mitral valve function.

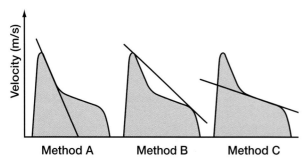

Figure 12.4: Methods used in the Determination of the Pressure Half-Time (PHT) in Curvilinear Doppler Spectrums.
Method A measures the pressure half-time in early diastole by following the early diastolic slope.
Method B measures the pressure half-time by the "mean" slope method which measures the slope from the peak early diastolic velocity to the peak end-diastolic velocity.
Method C measures the pressure half-time by measuring the slope from mid-diastole to end-diastolic velocity.

Method of Calculation of the Mitral Valve Area using the Pressure Half-time and Deceleration Time:
The MVA can be derived from both the PHT and the DT. Below, are "step-by-step" methods for calculation of the MVA using these two techniques.

Method for calculation of the mitral valve area by the PHT and DT

Step 1:   optimise the CW Doppler signal through the mitral valve:
   a)   usually best from apical window
   b)   colour flow imaging may facilitate alignment with stenotic jet

Step 2:   measure the peak E velocity (V_{peak})

Step 3:   calculate the pressure half-time (ms):
   a)   determine point marking $1/2$ of the pressure ($P^{1/2}$)
   $$P^{1/2} = V_{peak} \div \sqrt{2}$$
   $$= V_{peak} \div 1.4$$
   b)   draw vertical lines to the baseline from V_{peak} and $P^{1/2}$
   c)   measure the time interval between these two points (PHT)

Step 4:   calculate the mitral valve area (MVA):

$$MVA \ (cm^2) = \frac{220}{PHT}$$

where 220 = empirically derived constant

Method for calculation of the mitral valve area by the deceleration time

Step 1:   optimise the CW Doppler signal through the mitral valve:
   a) usually best from apical window
   b) colour flow imaging may facilitate alignment with stenotic jet

Step 2:   measure the peak E velocity (Vpeak)

Step 3:   calculate the deceleration time (ms):
   a) from Vpeak extrapolate a line to the zero baseline
   b) measure the time interval between these two points (DT)

Step 4:   calculate the mitral valve area (MVA):

$$MVA \ (cm^2) = \frac{759}{DT}$$

where 759 = 220 ÷ 0.29 (remember: PHT = 0.29 x DT)

Proximal Isovelocity Surface Area Method for Calculation of the Mitral Valve Areas

The proximal isovelocity surface area (PISA) principle can be applied in the calculation of the area of a narrowed orifice (regurgitant or stenotic). This technique has been used in the calculation of the MVA in patients with mitral stenosis.

The principal advantage of the PISA technique in the estimation of the MVA lies in the fact that this method is unaffected by many factors which are known to significantly hamper the calculation of the MVA by other echocardiographic techniques such as 2-D planimetry, the continuity equation and the PHT methods. For example, the PISA method can be used when there is mitral leaflet calcification, thickening or distortion, and/or associated mitral or aortic regurgitation.

Studies validating the accuracy and reliability of the PISA method in the calculation of the MVA are tabulated in Appendix 8.

Theoretical Considerations:
Calculation of the area of a narrowed orifice by the PISA method is essentially based upon the continuity principle which states that flow proximal to a narrowed orifice must equal flow through the narrowed orifice providing that there is no fluid lost from the system.

Calculation of flow proximal to a narrowed orifice can be determined by assuming that as flow converges toward this narrowed orifice, it accelerates in a laminar manner forming a series of concentric hemispheric shells of uniform velocity (isovelocity). As flow advances closer to the narrowed orifice, the area of each hemispheric shell decreases and the velocity of each shell increases (Figure 12.5). The flow rate at any given hemispheric shell proximal to the narrowed orifice is a product of the area and the velocity of that shell and is expressed by the following equation:

(Equation 12.9)

$$Q = 2\pi r^2 V_r$$

where Q = flow rate (cc/s)
$2\pi r^2$ = area of a hemispheric shell derived from the radius [r] (cm²)
Vr = velocity at the radial distance (cm/s)

Based on the conservation of mass (the continuity principle), blood passing through a given hemisphere must ultimately pass through the narrowed orifice.
In other words, the flow rate through any given hemisphere must equal the flow rate through the narrowed orifice so that:

(Equation 12.10)

$$2\pi r^2 V_r = A_o \times V_o$$

where A_o = area of the narrowed orifice (cm²)
V_o = peak velocity through the narrowed orifice (cm/s)
$2\pi r^2$ = area of a hemispheric shell derived from the radius [r] (cm²)
Vr = velocity at the radial distance (cm/s)

Therefore, by rearranging the above equation, the area through the narrowed orifice (A_o) can be calculated:

(Equation 12.11)

$$A_o = \frac{2\pi r^2 V_r}{V_o}$$

Application of the PISA Principle in Echocardiography:
The radial distance (r) and the velocity at the radial distance (V_r) can be identified by CFI. The radial distance is measured as the proximal distance from the first aliased velocity (blue-red interface) to the narrowed orifice. The velocity at the radial distance is equivalent to the Nyquist limit as depicted on the colour velocity bar; hence, V_r becomes V_N:

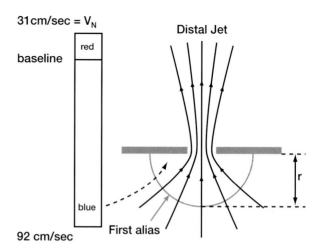

Figure 12.5: The Proximal Isovelocity Surface Area (PISA) Principle applied in the Calculation of a Stenotic or Regurgitant Orifice Area.
Flow proximal to a narrowed orifice, whether it be stenotic or regurgitant, streamlines towards the orifice. Points in which flow has the same velocity form concentric hemispheric isovelocity contours. These hemispheres are easily identified by colour flow imaging as aliasing which occurs as velocities exceed the Nyquist limit. The isovelocity surface area is equal to $2\pi r^2$, where r is the radial distance from the orifice to the first aliased velocity. The velocity at the radial distance is equal to the Nyquist limit of the colour bar (V_N).

(Equation 12.12)

$$A_o = \frac{2\pi r^2 V_N}{V_o}$$

where A_o = area of the narrowed orifice (cm²)
V_o = peak velocity through the narrowed orifice (cm/s)
$2\pi r^2$ = area of a hemispheric shell derived from the radius [r] (cm²)
V_N = aliased velocity identified as the Nyquist limit (cm/s)

Application of the PISA Principle in Mitral Valve Stenosis:
This principle can be applied to the assessment of the MVA in mitral stenosis where: (1) the stenotic MVA is the narrowed orifice and (2) the peak velocity through the narrowed orifice is the peak early diastolic velocity (peak E wave velocity) through the stenotic mitral valve:

(Equation 12.13)

$$MVA = \frac{2\pi r^2 V_N}{V_{MS}}$$

where MVA = mitral valve area (cm²)
$2\pi r^2$ = area of a hemispheric shell derived from the radius [r] (cm²)
V_N = aliased velocity identified as the Nyquist limit (cm/s)
V_{MS} = peak early diastolic mitral velocity (cm/s)

However calculation of the MVA is not this simple. The PISA principle is actually based on flow approaching a narrowed orifice that conforms to a flat planar surface. In mitral stenosis, the mitral leaflets form a funnel so that the flow convergence region proximal to the stenotic orifice is, in fact, more wedge-shaped with an angle of α (see Figure 12.6). To account for the altered shape of the flow profile, an angle correction factor of α/180 has been derived. This angle correction factor is based upon the following facts: (1) if the mitral valve leaflets were laid out flat, flow would converge toward the orifice over an arc of 180° from any direction, and (2) in mitral stenosis, flow can only converge to the narrowed orifice over an arc of α degrees. Therefore, accounting for the angle correction factor, the MVA can be derived from the following equation:

(Equation 12.14)

$$MVA = \frac{2\pi r^2\, V_N}{V_{MS}} \times \left(\frac{\alpha}{180}\right)$$

where　MVA = mitral valve area (cm²)

　　　$2\pi r^2$ = area of a hemispheric shell derived from the radius [r] (cm²)

　　　V_N = aliased velocity identified as the Nyquist limit (cm/s)

　　　V_{MS} = peak mitral E velocity (cm/s)

　　　α/180 = angle correction factor

Limitations of the PISA Method for Calculating the MVA.
Assumptions of PISA Calculations:

The PISA model is based on the hemispherical flow convergence area. However, the mitral stenotic orifice may be elliptical. Furthermore, the geometry of the isovelocity shell changes with: (1) the flow rate, (2) the pressure gradient, and (3) the orifice size and shape.

Effective Valve Area versus Anatomical Valve Area:

Calculation of the MVA by the PISA technique is determined by the peak velocity of the stenotic mitral signal (the early diastolic E wave) rather than the integration of flow over the entire diastolic filling period. Hence, the maximum flow rate and the MVA are measured at the *vena contracta* in early diastole providing an estimation of the "effective" orifice area. The "effective" orifice area is generally smaller than the anatomical valve area. Despite this, the mitral valve area calculated by the PISA technique has correlated well with other independent measures of the MVA (see Appendix 8).

Radius Measurements:

Accurate calculations of the MVA by the PISA technique are dependent upon the precise measurement of the radial distance between the stenotic orifice and the first aliased velocity. Since the valve area is derived by squaring the radius (equation 12.14), failure to measure the correct radius may result in a significant underestimation or overestimation of the MVA. Furthermore, the relatively small size of the proximal

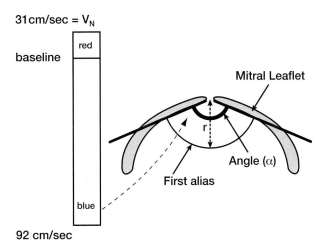

Figure 12.6: Funnel-shaped Flow Convergence Region Proximal to the Mitral Valve Orifice.
Angle a is the angle of the mitral valve leaflets proximal to the orifice in the region containing the flow convergence region.

convergence region to the field of view may limit the accuracy of this measurement. Methods that may be employed to overcome problems in the radial measurement include magnification of the proximal flow convergence region and reduction of the aliasing velocity. Reduction of the aliased velocity effectively increases the radial distance and can be achieved by shifting the colour baseline toward the direction of flow. However, reducing the aliased velocity also has potential limitations. At very low aliasing velocities, overestimation of the mean velocity displayed by the colour Doppler may result due to suppression of low velocities by colour wall filters. Therefore, resulting in an overestimation of the proximal flow convergence region.

Measurement of Angle α:

Measurement of angle α must be done off-line using a protractor. The angle formed by the stenotic mitral valve leaflets is three dimensional. Therefore, the correction for angle α which is performed in one imaging plane (usually the apical four chamber view) may not be representative of the true leaflet geometry and may not account for variations within the geometry of the leaflets.

Atrial Fibrillation:

As mentioned, precise measurement of the radial distance between the stenotic orifice to the first aliased velocity is crucial to the accuracy of the calculated MVA since the valve area is derived by squaring the radius. Failure to measure the correct radius may result in a significant underestimation or overestimation of the MVA. Beat-to-beat variations that occur with atrial fibrillation may magnify errors in the radius measurement. Minimisation of this potential error can be achieved by averaging multiple measurements of the radius.

References and Suggested Reading:
Continuity Equation:
- Baumgartner, H. et al.: Doppler assessment of prosthetic valve orifice area: An in vitro study. *Circulation 85:2273-2283,1992.*
- Bednarz, J.E. et al.: An echocardiographic approach to the assessment of aortic stenosis. *Journal of the American Society of Echocardiography 9: 286-294, 1996.*
- Bitar, J.N. et al.: Doppler echocardiographic assessment with the continuity equation of St. Jude mechanical prostheses in the mitral valve position. *American Journal of Cardiology 76:287-293,1995.*
- Chafizadeh, E.R., Zoghbi, W.A.: Doppler echocardiographic assessment of the St. Jude medical prosthetic valve in the aortic position using the continuity equation. *Circulation 83:213-223,1991.*
- Come, P.C. et al.: Echocardiographic assessment of aortic valve area in elderly patients with aortic stenosis and of changes in valve area after percutaneous balloon valvuloplasty. *Journal of the American College of Cardiology 10:115-124,1987.*
- Danielson, R. et al.: Factors affecting Doppler echocardiographic mitral valve area assessment in aortic stenosis. *American Journal of Cardiology 63:1107-1111,1989.*
- Dumesnil, J.G. et al.: Validation and applications of indexed aortic prosthetic valve areas calculated by Doppler echocardiography. *Journal of the American College of Cardiology 16: 637-643, 1990.*
- Karp, K. et al.: Accurate estimation of the valve area in mitral stenosis by application of the continuity equation. *Journal of Cardiovascular Ultrasonography 7:293,1988.*
- Mohan, J.C. et al.: Improved Doppler assessment of the Bjork-Shiley mitral prothesis using the continuity equation. *International Journal of Cardiology 43:321-326,1994.*
- Nakatani, S. et al.: Value and limitations of Doppler echocardiography in the quantification of stenotic mitral valve area: Comparison of the pressure half-time and continuity equation methods. *Circulation 77:78,1988.*
- Nakatani, S. et al.: Time related changes in mitral valve area after balloon mitral valvuloplasty assessed by Doppler continuity equation method. *Circulation 78:II-487,1988.*
- Nishimura, R.A. et al.: Doppler evaluation of results of percutaneous aortic balloon valvuloplasty in calcific aortic stenosis. *Circulation 78:791-799,1988.*
- Oh, J.K. et al.: Prediction of the severity of aortic stenosis by Doppler aortic valve area determination: Prospective Doppler-catheter correlation in 100 patients. *Journal of the American College of Cardiology 11:1227-1234,1988.*
- Otto, C.M. et al.: Determination of the stenotic aortic valve area in adults using Doppler echocardiography. *Journal of the American College of Cardiology 7:509-517,1986.*
- Otto, C.M. and Pearlman, A.S.: Doppler echocardiography in adults with symptomatic aortic stenosis. *Archives of Internal Medicine 148: 2553-2560, 1988.*

- Pibarot, P. et al.: Substitution of left ventricular outflow tract diameter with prosthesis size is inadequate for calculation of the aortic prosthetic valve area by the continuity equation. *Journal of the American Society of Echocardiography 8: 511-517, 1995.*
- Rask, L.P. et al.: Flow dependence of the aortic valve area in patients with aortic stenosis: assessment by application of the continuity equation. *Journal of the American Society of Echocardiography 9: 295-299, 1996.*
- Richards, K.L. et al.: Calculation of aortic valve area by Doppler echocardiography: a direct application of the continuity equation. *Circulation 73: 964-969, 1986.*
- Robson, D.J., Flaxman, J.C.: Measurement of the end-diastolic pressure gradient and mitral valve area in mitral stenosis by Doppler ultrasound. *Eur Heart J 5:660-,1984.*
- Rothbart, R.M. et al.: Determination of aortic valve area by two-dimensional and Doppler echocardiography in patients with normal and stenotic bioprosthetic valves. *Journal of the American College of Cardiology 15:817-824,1990.*
- Skjaerpe, T. et al.: Noninvasive estimation of valve area in patients with aortic stenosis by Doppler ultrasound and two-dimensional echocardiography. *Circulation 72:810-818,1985.*
- Stoddard, M.F. et al.: Immediate and short-term effects of aortic balloon valvuloplasty on left ventricular diastolic function and filling in humans. *Journal of the American College of Cardiology 14:1218-1228,1989.*
- Teirstein, P. et al.: Doppler echocardiographic measurement of aortic valve area in aortic stenosis: a noninvasive application of the Gorlin formula. *Journal of the American College of Cardiology 8:1059-1065,1986.*
- Wranne, B. et al.: Stenotic lesions. *Heart (supplement 2): 75: 36-42, 1996.*
- Zoghbi, W.A. et al.: Accurate noninvasive quantification of stenotic aortic valve area by Doppler echocardiography. *Circulation 73:452-459,1986.*

Pressure Half-time Method for Calculation of Mitral Valve Areas:
- Abascal, V. et al.: Echocardiographic evaluation of mitral valve structure and function in patients followed for at least 6 months after percutaneous balloon mitral valvuloplasty. *Journal of the American College of Cardiology 12:606-615,1988.*
- Chambers, J.B.: Mitral pressure half-time: is it a valid measure of orifice area in artificial heart valves? *Journal of Heart Valve Disease 2: 571-577, 1993.*
- Chen, C. et al.: Reliability of the Doppler pressure half-time method for assessing effects of percutaneous mitral balloon valvuloplasty. *Journal of the American College of Cardiology 13:1309-1313,1989.*
- Come, P.C. et al.: Noninvasive assessment of mitral stenosis before and after percutaneous balloon mitral valvuloplasty. *American Journal of Cardiology 61:817-825,1988.*

- Gonzalez, M.A. et al.: Comparison of two-dimensional and Doppler echocardiography and intracardiac hemodynamics for quantification of mitral stenosis. *American Journal of Cardiology 60:327-332,1987.*
- Hatle, L. et al.: Noninvasive assessment of atrioventricular pressure half-time by Doppler ultrasound. *Circulation 60: 1096-1104, 1979.*
- Oh, J.K. et al.: Characteristic Doppler echocardiographic pattern of mitral inflow velocity in severe aortic regurgitation. *Journal of the American College of Cardiology. 14: 1712-1717, 1989.*
- Nakatani, S. et al. : Value and limitations of Doppler echocardiography in the quantification of stenotic mitral valve area: Comparison of the pressure half-time and continuity equation methods. *Circulation 11: 78-85, 1988.*
- Reid ,C. et al.: Mechanism of increase in mitral valve area and influence of anatomic features in double-balloon catheter balloon valvuloplasty in adults with mitral stenosis: A Doppler and two-dimensional echocardiographic study. *Circulation 76:628-636,1987.*
- Sagar, K.B. et al.: Doppler echocardiographic evaluation of Hancock and Bjork-Shiley prosthetic valves. Journal of the American College of Cardiology 7: 681-687, 1986.
- Smith, M.D. et al.: Comparative accuracy of two-dimensional echocardiography and Doppler pressure half-time methods in assessing the severity of mitral stenosis in patients with and without prior commissurotomy. *Circulation 73: 100-107, 1986.*
- Smith, M.D. et al.: Measurement of mitral pressure half-time in patients with curvilinear spectral patterns. (Abstract) *Circulation 78: II - 78, 1998.*
- Smith, M.D. et al.: Value and limitations of Doppler pressure half-time in quantifying mitral stenosis: A comparison with micromanometer catheter recordings. *Am Heart J 121:480-488,1991.*
- Stamm, R.B., Martin, R.P.: Quantification of pressure gradients across stenotic valves by Doppler ultrasound. *Journal of the American College of Cardiology 2: 707-718, 1983.*

- Tabbalat, R.A., Haft, J.I.: Effect of severe pulmonary hypertension on the calculation of mitral valve area in patients with mitral stenosis. *Am Heart J 121:488-493,1991.*
- Thomas, J.D. et al.: Inaccuracy of mitral pressure half-time immediately after percutaneous mitral valvotomy. *Circulation 78: 980-993, 1988.*
- Thomas, J.D. et al.: Doppler pressure half-time: a clinical tool in search of theoretical justification. *Journal of the American College of Cardiology 10: 923-929, 1987.*
- Wilkins, G.T. et al.: Validation of continuous-wave Doppler echocardiographic measurement of mitral and tricuspid prosthetic valve gradients: A simultaneous Doppler-catheter study. *Circulation 74: 786-795, 1986.*

Proximal Isovelocity Surface Area for Calculation of the Mitral Valve Area:

- Aguilar, J.A. et al.: Calculation of the mitral valve area with the proximal convergent flow method with Doppler-color in patients with mitral stenosis. (English abstract only) *Arch Inst Cardiol Mex 64:257-263,1994.*
- Centamore, G. et al.: Validity of the proximal isovelocity surface area color Doppler method for calculating the valve area in patients with mitral stenosis: Comparison with the two-dimensional echocardiographic method. (English Abstract only) *G Ital Cardiol 22:1201-1210,1992.*
- Deng, Y-B. et al.: Estimation of mitral valve area in patients with mitral stenosis by the flow convergence region method: Selection of aliasing velocity. *Journal of the American College of Cardiology 24:683-689,1994.*
- Rifkin, R.D. et al.: Comparison of proximal isovelocity surface area method with pressure half-time and planimetry in the evaluation of mitral stenosis. *Journal of the American College of Cardiology 26:458-465,1995.*
- Rodriguez, L. et al.: Validation of the proximal flow convergence method: Calculation of orifice area in patients with mitral stenosis. *Circulation 88:1157-1165,1993.*

Chapter 13
Doppler Quantification of Regurgitant Lesions

Valvular regurgitation can be assessed indirectly, semiquantitatively, and quantitatively by Doppler echocardiography. Indirect indicators of significant valvular regurgitation include increased forward flow velocities, increased intensity of the regurgitant Doppler signal, and flow reversals. Valvular regurgitation can be assessed semiquantitatively by jet area ratios. Quantitative measurements of valvular regurgitation include calculation of regurgitant volumes, regurgitant fractions, and the effective regurgitant orifice area. Various Doppler echocardiographic parameters and values used as indicators of the severity of valvular regurgitation are summarised in Appendix 9.

Indirect Indicators of Significant Regurgitation

Indirect clues to the presence of significant regurgitation are summarised in the Table 13.1. In particular, the shapes of the spectral signal and flow reversal are especially helpful in the indirect assessment of valvular regurgitation.

Increased Forward Flow Velocities:
Theoretical Considerations:
In the presence of significant valvular regurgitation, the stroke volume through that valve will be increased. This increase in the stroke volume results from an increase in the antegrade (forward) flow through the incompetent valve (remember that the stroke volume is a product of the CSA and the mean velocity or VTI). Thus, the greater the severity of regurgitation, the higher the velocity of the antegrade or forward flow through that valve.

Limitations of Increased Forward Velocities as an Indicator of Significant Regurgitation:
In the presence of valvular stenosis, both the forward velocity and the mean gradient are usually increased. Therefore, an increase in these parameters may not be helpful in semiquantitating the severity of valvular regurgitation. However, a *disproportionate* increase in velocities (particularly in the mean mitral valve gradient) may still be of value. For example, an increase

in both the peak and mean mitral inflow velocities with a normal pressure half-time suggests that the increase in these velocities is not a result of mitral stenosis but may be due to significant valvular regurgitation.

Increased Intensity of Regurgitant Signal:
Theoretical Considerations:
The continuous-wave Doppler signal intensity (CWSI) can be used in the indirect assessment of the severity of valvular regurgitation, particularly when compared with the intensity of antegrade flow. Semiquantification of the severity of regurgitation by the CWSI assumes that the intensity or amplitude of the returning Doppler signal is proportional to the number of blood cells moving within the Doppler beam at that instant in time. Therefore, the intensity of this signal should increase with increasing regurgitant volumes. For example, a weak Doppler signal is indicative of relatively mild valvular regurgitation; whereas a strong signal of equal intensity to the antegrade signal is suggestive of significant regurgitation.

Limitations of Increased Intensity of the Regurgitant Signal as an Indicator of Significant Regurgitation:
The absolute CWSI can be affected by machine factors, anatomic factors, physiological factors and technical factors. Machine factors that may affect the CWSI include gain and wall filter settings. Anatomic factors which may affect the CWSI include chest wall thickness and chamber size, both of which can lead to significant attenuation of the ultrasound beam and, therefore, an underestimation of the CWSI. In this situation, comparison of the CWSI of the regurgitant jet with antegrade CWSI may be especially helpful. Physiological factors that may affect the CWSI include jet volume, shape, and direction as well as atrial and ventricular function. Poor ultrasound beam alignment with the regurgitant jet is a technical factor which may result in an underestimation of the CWSI.

Shape of Regurgitant Spectral Doppler Signal:
The shape of the spectral CW Doppler signal is determined by the variation in the pressure gradient

Table 13.1: Indirect Indicators of Significant Regurgitation.

Doppler Parameter	Significant Regurgitation
● Forward flow velocities	● Increased (indicative of increased stroke volumes)
● Intensity of regurgitant signal	● Strong compared to forward flow signal
● Shape of regurgitant signal	● Rapid "drop-off" of signal (see below)
● Duration of regurgitant signal	● Shortened (finishes prior to end of diastole - PR)
● Flow reversals	● Systolic flow reversal into veins entering atrium (MR/TR) ● Diastolic flow reversal in descending & abdominal aorta (AR)

across the regurgitant valve over the flow period. Using the modified Bernoulli equation, the velocity at any point on the Doppler trace can be translated to the instantaneous pressure gradient across the valve at that instant in time. Two distinct Doppler signs have been recognised as reliable indicators of significant regurgitation: (1) the "V" cut-off sign (for atrioventricular valves), and (2) a shortened pressure half-time or deceleration slope (for semilunar valves).

(i) The "V" Cut-Off Sign for Atrioventricular Valve Regurgitation:

The "V" cut-off sign is an indicator of significant atrioventricular (AV) valve regurgitation. This cut-off sign occurs in middle-to-late systole and is caused by a high "V-wave" in the atrial pressure trace.

Theoretical Considerations:

In the presence of AV valve regurgitation, the Doppler velocity spectrum reflects the pressure gradient between the ventricle and atrium during systole. When there is mild valvular regurgitation, the atrial pressure is usually normal; thus, the pressure gradient between ventricle and the atrium is relatively high and remains constantly high throughout the entire systolic period. In the presence of significant AV valve regurgitation, the atrial pressure may be increased toward the end of systole. Hence, the pressure gradient between these two chambers in mid-to-late systole is lessened. This reduction in the pressure difference between the atrium and the ventricle is reflected in the Doppler spectral trace producing a "V-shaped" Doppler signal (Figure 13.1).

(ii) Shortened Pressure Half-Time (Deceleration Slope) for Semilunar Valve Regurgitation:

As stated, the Doppler velocity spectrum reflects the pressure gradient between two chambers or vessels. In aortic regurgitation, the Doppler velocity spectrum represents the pressure gradient between the aorta and left ventricle during diastole. In the case of pulmonary regurgitation, the Doppler velocity spectrum represents the pressure gradient between the pulmonary artery and right ventricle during diastole. The rapidity in which the pressures between the aorta or pulmonary artery and their respective ventricles equalise is a function of the severity of the regurgitation.

Although the majority of research into the shortening of the deceleration slope or pressure half-time has been performed on aortic regurgitant jets (discussed in detail below), the same concept can also be applied to the shape of the pulmonary regurgitant Doppler signal.

Theoretical Considerations:

Alterations in the shape of the aortic regurgitant Doppler signal are based on the assumption that the aortic valve acts as a restrictive orifice that controls the rate of regurgitant flow from the aorta to the left ventricle during diastole. Therefore, the regurgitant flow rate between these two sites as well as the rate of decline of the diastolic pressure gradient will vary depending on the regurgitant orifice size. For example, the larger the

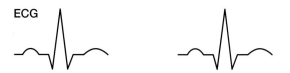

ECG

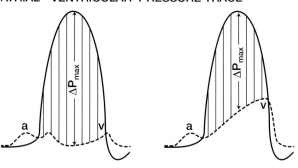

ATRIAL - VENTRICULAR PRESSURE TRACE

DOPPLER VELOCITY CURVES

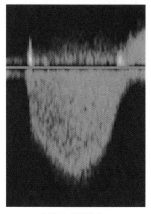
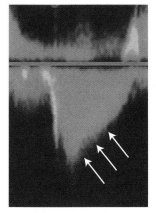

Mild AV Valve Regurgitation   Severe AV Valve Regurgitation

Figure 13.1: The Shape of the Doppler Signal as an Indicator of Significant Atrioventricular Valve Regurgitation.
In AV valve regurgitation, the regurgitant Doppler velocity signal is a function of the pressure gradient between the atrium and the ventricle during systole. This schematic illustrates pressure tracings of the atrium and the ventricle, and the Doppler velocity spectrum during systole. The atrial pressure trace consists of an *a* wave which represents an increase in atrial pressure with atrial contraction, and a *v* wave which represents an increase in atrial pressure during ventricular systole due to venous return into the atria.
Left, In mild AV valve regurgitation, the pressure gradient between the atrium and the ventricle is high and this gradient remains relatively constant throughout the entire systolic period. This results in a symmetrical, U-shaped Doppler velocity curve.
Right, In severe AV valve regurgitation, the pressure gradient between the ventricle and atrium is high initially as for mild AV valve regurgitation. However, with a corresponding increase in the *v* wave of the atrial pressure trace, the gradient between the ventricle and atrium decreases toward the latter half of systole. This results in a rapid and asymmetric, V-shaped Doppler velocity curve *(triple arrows).*

regurgitant orifice, the greater the rate of decline of the diastolic pressure gradient between the aorta and the left ventricle. Conversely, the smaller the regurgitant orifice, the slower the rate of decline. Since the Doppler velocity spectrum of the aortic regurgitant jet reflects the pressure difference between the aorta and left ventricle during diastole, this Doppler spectrum can be used to determine the rate of decline of the pressure gradient and, hence, indirectly, the size of the regurgitant orifice.

The maximum Doppler velocity of the regurgitant signal occurs following aortic valve closure when the pressure difference between the aorta and left ventricle is greatest. The magnitude of the Doppler regurgitant jet then decreases throughout diastole as the pressure difference between the aorta and left ventricle lessens due to: (1) the fall in the aortic diastolic pressure (due to a combination of forward run-off to the periphery as well as regurgitation back into the left ventricle), and (2) the rise in the left ventricular diastolic pressure (due to a combination of normal mitral inflow and the aortic regurgitant volume).

In mild aortic regurgitation, the early diastolic pressure gradient is high. This gradient then gradually declines throughout diastole due to a gradual decline in the aortic diastolic pressure and only a small increase in the left ventricular end-diastolic pressure (LVEDP). In the presence of severe aortic regurgitation, two important pressure changes occur (1) the aortic diastolic pressure falls rapidly, and (2) the LVEDP increases. This results in rapid decline or decay of the pressure gradient over the diastolic period (Figure 13.2).

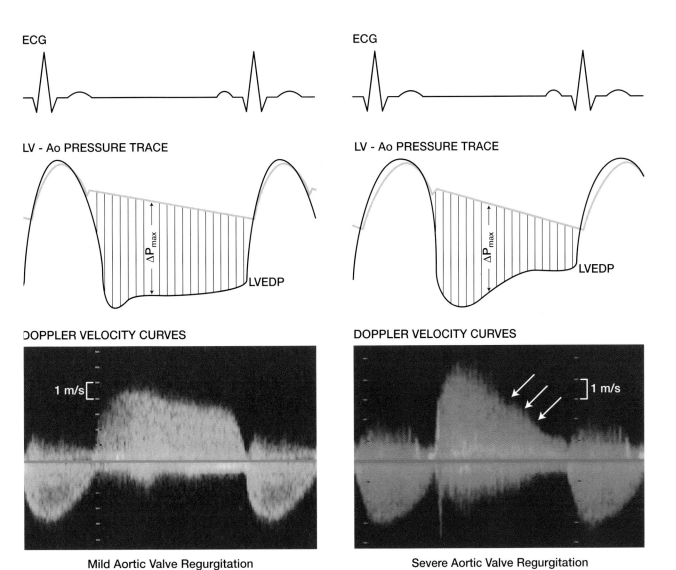

Mild Aortic Valve Regurgitation   Severe Aortic Valve Regurgitation

Figure 13.2: The Shape of the Doppler Velocity Signal as an Indicator of Aortic Regurgitation.
The regurgitant Doppler signal is a function of the pressure gradient between the aorta and left ventricle during diastole. This schematic illustrates aortic and left ventricular pressure tracings, and the Doppler velocity spectrum during diastole.
Left, In mild aortic regurgitation, the pressure difference between the aorta and left ventricle in early diastole is high. This gradient then *gradually* decreases throughout diastole due to a gradual decline in the aortic diastolic pressure and only a small increase in the left ventricular end-diastolic pressure (LVEDP). The resultant Doppler spectrum depicts a *flat* deceleration slope.
Right, In severe aortic regurgitation, the aortic pressure drops rapidly during diastole and the LVEDP rises rapidly. This results in a rapid decline of the diastolic slope of the regurgitant Doppler velocity curve *(triple arrows)*.

The rate of decline of the aortic regurgitant velocity spectrum has been quantitated using both the deceleration rate or, more commonly, the pressure half-time (Figure 13.3). The deceleration slope or rate is derived from the peak velocity and the deceleration time and can be expressed by:

(Equation 13.1)

$$DS = \frac{V_{peak}}{DT}$$

where DS   = deceleration slope (m/s²)
       V_{peak} = peak velocity (m/s)
       DT   = deceleration time (s)

Measurement of the pressure half-time (PHT) is analogous to that used in the Doppler assessment of mitral stenosis. Recall that the PHT is defined as the time required for the pressure to decay to half its original value. In Doppler echocardiography, velocity rather than pressure is displayed on the Doppler spectrum. Since velocity (V) and pressure are related, the PHT can be measured from the velocity spectrum:

(Equation 12.5)

$$P_{1/2} = \frac{V_{peak}}{\sqrt{2}}$$

$$or$$

$$= \frac{V_{peak}}{1.414}$$

The PHT is also related to the deceleration time (DT) such that the PHT is equal to 29% of the DT:

(Equation 12.7)

$$PHT = 0.29 \times DT$$

where PHT = pressure half-time (ms)
       DT   = deceleration time (ms)

Clinical Significance of the Deceleration Slope and Pressure Half-time in Aortic Regurgitation:

Although investigators have reported reasonable correlations between the DS, the PHT and the severity of aortic regurgitation, significant overlap between grades exists. In general, a DS of > 3.5 m/s² and a PHT of < 200 ms is indicative of severe aortic regurgitation (refer to Table 13.2 and Figure 13.4).

Limitations of the Shape of the Regurgitant Doppler Signal as an Indicator of Significant Regurgitation:
Others factors affecting the shape of the regurgitant signal:
The PHT method for the estimation of orifice size relies on the passage of flow from one chamber with a single outlet into another chamber with a single inlet. Such a situation exists with mitral stenosis where the PHT method is successfully applied to the estimation of the MVA.
However, with aortic regurgitation, the aorta has a "double outlet" (to the periphery and to the left ventricle) and the

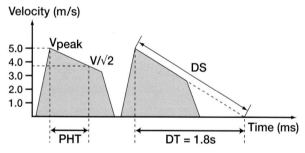

Figure 13.3: Method of Measuring the Pressure Half-Time and Deceleration Slope from the Continuous-Wave Doppler Velocity Spectrum of Aortic Regurgitation.
This schematic illustrates how the pressure half-time (PHT) and deceleration slope (DS) are measured from the Doppler velocity spectrum of aortic regurgitation.
Left, The PHT is the time required for the pressure to decay to half its original value. Using the velocity spectrum, the PHT is equal to the time taken for the peak velocity (V_{peak}) to fall to $V_{peak} \div \sqrt{2}$. In this example, the V_{peak} is 5.0 m/s and the V/√2 is 3.5 m/s. Hence, the PHT is equal to the time taken for the velocity to fall from 5.0 m/s to 3.5 m/s.
Right, The DS is measured by dividing the peak velocity (V_{peak}) by the deceleration time (DT). In this example, the V_{peak} is 5.0 m/s and the DT is 1.8 s. Thus, the DS is equal to 5.0 m/s ÷ 1.8 m/s which equates to 2.8 m/s².
The PHT can also be derived from the DT (equation 11.31). In this example, the DT is 1.8 s or 1800 ms. Using equation 11.31, the PHT is equal to 1800 x 0.29 (522 ms).

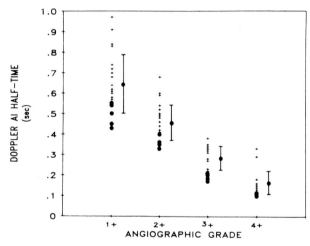

Figure 13.4: Relationship between the Doppler Pressure Half-time and the Severity of Aortic Regurgitation.
The Doppler pressure half-time (PHT) is plotted as a function of the angiographic grade of aortic regurgitation (AR) in 86 patients (25 patients = mild [1⁺] AR; 27 patients = moderate [2⁺] AR; 18 patients = moderately severe [3⁺] AR; 16 patients = severe [4⁺] AR). Patients with identical PHTs are plotted as a **single cross** or **circle**. Patients with a LVEDP greater than 26 mm Hg are represented as **solid circles**. Means and standard deviations for Doppler PHT are plotted for each angiographic range.
Observe the high sensitivity and specificity for a PHT of < 200 ms as an indicator of severe [4+] AR.
From Teague, S. M. et al.: Quantification of aortic regurgitation utilising continuous wave Doppler ultrasound. *Journal of the American College of Cardiology. 8:596, 1986.* Reproduced with permission from the American College of Cardiology.

Table 13.2: Sensitivity and Specificity of a Deceleration Slope of > 3.5 m/s² as an Indicator of Severe Aortic Regurgitation.

First Author (Year)	Pt. Pop.	Sensitivity	Specificity
Labovitz (1986) [1]	25	26%	100%
Masuyama (1986) [2]	30	60%	100%
Grayburn (1987) [3]	31	26%	100%
Beyer (1987) [4]	15	67%	89%
Wilkenshiff (1994) [5]	73	91%	76%
Dolan (1995) [6]	156	64%	99%

Sources: **(1)** Labovitz, A. J. et al, *Journal of the American College of Cardiology 8: 1341-1347, 1986*: patient population: mild AR = 9; moderate AR = 9; severe AR = 7; **(2)** Masuyama, T. et al., *Circulation 73: 460-466, 1986*: patient population: mild AR = 7; moderate AR = 13; severe AR = 10; **(3)** Grayburn, P. A. et al., *Journal of the American College of Cardiology 10: 135-141, 1987*: patient population: mild AR = 5; moderate AR = 7; severe AR = 19; **(4)** Beyer, R. W. et al., *American Journal of Cardiology 60: 852-856, 1987*: patient population: mild AR = 5; moderate AR = 4; severe AR = 6; **(5)** Wilkenshiff, U. M. et al.:, *European Heart Journal 15: 1227-1234, 1994*: patient population: mild AR = 22; moderate AR = 26; severe AR = 32; **(6)** Dolan, M. S. et al., *American Heart Journal 129: 10141020, 1995*: patient population: mild AR = 64; moderate AR = 44; severe AR = 48.

left ventricle has a "double inlet" (from the mitral valveand from the regurgitant aortic valve). Thus, the aortic diastolic pressure decay is not only related to the severity of aortic regurgitation but also to the systemic vascular resistance (afterload) as well as aortic and left ventricular compliance. Therefore, an increase in the systemic vascular resistance or a reduction in left ventricular compliance, results in an increase in the rate of decline of the PHT without any change in regurgitant orifice size. For example, shortening of the PHT in the absence of significant regurgitation may be seen in patients who have a "stiff", noncompliant ventricle with increased LVEDP.

Suboptimal Doppler Recordings:
High quality Doppler recordings of the regurgitant signals may not be feasible in all patients. In these instances, the shape of the spectral Doppler recording will be of little use in the semiquantitation of the severity of regurgitation. Furthermore, poor or inadequately aligned Doppler signals prohibit the indirect assessment of the shape of the Doppler curve. For example, poor alignment of the ultrasound beam with the direction of the regurgitant jet may underestimate or overestimate the PHT of the regurgitant jet.

Heart Rate:
Increasing heart rate can lead to an overestimation of the severity of regurgitation when using the PHT. For instance, when the heart rate is increased, there is a concomitant increase in the end-diastolic gradient between the aorta and left ventricle due to a decrease in the LVEDP. Furthermore, an increased heart rate may

result in a very short slope and, thus, reduce the accuracy of this measurement. For these reasons, the influence of heart rate should be considered in the serial evaluation of patients with aortic regurgitation when using the PHT.

Flow Reversal Velocities:
Reversal of blood flow into the pulmonary veins with mitral regurgitation, the hepatic veins with tricuspid regurgitation, and in the descending and abdominal aorta with aortic regurgitation also provide indirect evidence of the severity of valvular regurgitation.

(i) Flow Reversal in Atrioventricular Valve Regurgitation:
In the presence of significant (at least moderate) AV valve regurgitation, the regurgitant jet "displaces" a significant volume of blood, already in the atrium, backward. This results in systolic flow reversal into the veins draining into the atrium. In the case of significant tricuspid valve regurgitation, systolic flow reversal into the hepatic veins can be detected from the subcostal window when the PW Doppler sample is placed within the hepatic vein (Figure 13.5).

Likewise, when there is significant mitral regurgitation, systolic flow reversal into the pulmonary veins may be detected when the PW Doppler sample is placed within the right upper pulmonary vein from the apical four chamber view.

More recently, the pulmonary venous Doppler spectrum has been quantitated using the systolic to diastolic pulmonary venous flow velocity ratio. Using this method, the systolic to diastolic pulmonary venous flow velocity ratio was obtained by integrating the systolic and diastolic components of the pulmonary venous Doppler spectrum (see Figure 13.6). This ratio provides a reasonably sensitive and specific parameter for assessing the severity of mitral regurgitation. The clinical significance of this ratio in the assessment of the various grades of mitral regurgitation is listed in Table 13.3.

(ii) Flow Reversal in Semilunar Valve Regurgitation:
Regurgitation of the semilunar valves results in reversal of flow downstream from the valve. Hence, when these valves become significantly incompetent, diastolic flow reversal within the great vessels occurs. The velocity and the duration of flow reversal during diastole provides an index of the severity of regurgitation.

Pan-diastolic flow reversal within the descending thoracic aorta is typically seen with at least moderate aortic regurgitation (Figure 13.7). In particular, an end-diastolic flow velocity of > 18 cm/s has been reported to predict moderate to severe aortic regurgitation with a sensitivity of 88% and a specificity of 92% [38].

Pan-diastolic flow reversal within abdominal aorta (Figure 13.8) has also been reported as an extremely sensitive and specific sign of severe aortic regurgitation (sensitivity of 100% and specificity of 97%) [39].

38: Tribouilloy, C. et al.: British Heart Journal 65: 37-40, 1991. (Patient population: mild AR = 8; moderate AR = 18; moderately severe AR = 22; severe AR = 13). 39: Takenaka, K. et al.: American Journal of Cardiology 57: 1340-1343, 1986. (Patient population: no AR = 10; mild AR = 13; moderate AR = 9; severe AR = 11).

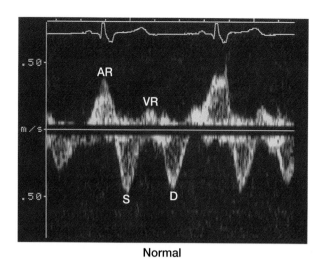

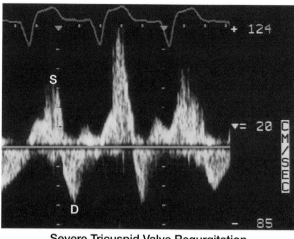

| Normal | Severe Tricuspid Valve Regurgitation |

Figure 13.5: Hepatic Venous Systolic Flow Reversal: Normal and with Significant Tricuspid Regurgitation.
Left, This is an example of the normal hepatic venous Doppler flow profile recorded from the subcostal window. There are normally four components to the normal flow profile: systolic forward flow (S); diastolic forward flow (D); atrial flow reversal (AR); and ventricular flow reversal (VR). Observe that forward flow signals are depicted below the zero baseline and reversed flow signals are depicted above the zero baseline.
Right, This is an example of the hepatic venous flow profile in a patient with significant tricuspid regurgitation. Observe that the systolic (S) component of this signal appears above the zero baseline indicating that flow is directed toward the transducer as blood is displaced *backward* into the hepatic vein.

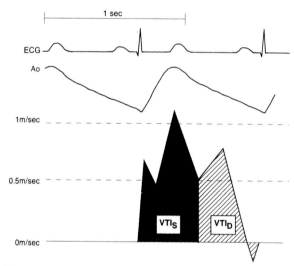

Figure 13.6: Calculation of the Systolic to Diastolic Velocity Time Integral Ratio (VTIs/VTId).
This schematic illustrates how the systolic VTI to diastolic VTI ratio (VTI_s/VTI_d) is obtained from the pulmonary venous Doppler trace. The VTI_s is determined by planimetry of the systolic component of the pulmonary venous Doppler trace (dark hatched signal). The VTI_d is determined by planimetry of the diastolic component of the pulmonary venous Doppler trace (light hatched signal). The VTI_s/VTI_d ratio is then simply derived by dividing the VTI_s by the VTI_d. Observe that the VTI_d also includes the atrial reversal component of the pulmonary venous flow profile.
Abbreviations: Ao = aortic pressure signal; **ECG** = electrocardiogram.
From Seiler, C. et al.: Quantitation of mitral regurgitation using the systolic/diastolic pulmonary venous flow velocity ratio. *Journal of the American College of Cardiology 31: 1385, 1998.* Reproduced with permission from the American College of Cardiology.

Table 13.3: Clinical Significance of the VTIs/VTId Ratio in Mitral Regurgitation.

Severity of MR	VTI_s/VTI_d Ratio	Sensitivity	Specificity
Mild	> 1.0	84 %	84 %
Moderate	0.5 - 1.0	57 %	81 %
Moderately severe	0.0 - 0.5	33 %	85 %
Severe	< 0.0	52 %	96 %

Source: Seiler, C. et al., *Journal of the American College of Cardiology 31: 1383-1390, 1998:* patient population: mild MR = 31; moderate MR = 28; moderately severe MR = 18; severe MR = 23.

Limitations of Flow Reversal as an Indicator of Significant Regurgitation:

Coexistent left-to-right shunts or other anomalies of the aorta:

Retrograde pan-diastolic flow reversal within the abdominal aorta in the absence of significant aortic regurgitation can also be demonstrated in patients with the following conditions: (1) a significant left-to-right shunt through either a patent ductus arteriosus or other aorto-pulmonary shunts, (2) aortic coarctation, (3) aortic dissection, or (4) aortic aneurysm. False positive results may occur because of continuous flow in these conditions.

Arrhythmias:

In the presence of atrial fibrillation, flow reversals within the pulmonary and hepatic veins are less useful as indicators of significant mitral or tricuspid valve regurgitation. This is because of blunting of the systolic component of the venous signal which is commonly seen with this arrhythmia.

Premature ventricular contractions or cardiac pacemaker contractions may cause systolic flow reversal in the absence of significant AV valve regurgitation. False positive results occur under these circumstances because of an increase in the atrial pressure during ventricular systole at the time when the AV valve is closed.

Poor setting of wall filters:
Wall filters are necessary to avoid artefacts produced by wall motion. However, poor setting of these filters may also produce misleading results. Flow reversal velocities are typically low; therefore, flow reversals may not be detected if the wall filters are set too high. Therefore, it is important that the wall filters are set as low as possible when assessing the pulmonary and hepatic veins, and the descending and abdominal aorta.

Effect of respiration:
Flow velocities within the right side of the heart vary with normal respiration. In particular, there is an increase in the systolic, diastolic and atrial reversal flow velocities of the hepatic vein with inspiration. Hence, it is important to be aware of this normal variation to avoid misleading results.

Left atrial compliance and pressures:
When the left atrium is severely dilated and compliant, systolic flow reversal into the pulmonary veins may be absent even when there is severe mitral regurgitation. In this situation, all of the excess regurgitant volume is accommodated within the atrium without displacement into the pulmonary veins.

Furthermore, systolic flow reversal may also occur with increased left atrial pressure independent of the severity of mitral regurgitation. In this instance, increased left atrial pressure reverses the atrial-to-pulmonary venous pressure gradient leading to systolic flow reversal.

Eccentric jets:
Systolic flow reversal into the pulmonary veins may occur even in the absence of significant mitral regurgitation. This false positive result may occur when the regurgitant jet is eccentric and is aimed directly into the vein producing systolic flow reversal.

Duration of Regurgitant Signal:
The duration of the regurgitant signal is particularly helpful in the assessment of pulmonary regurgitation. In patients with severe pulmonary regurgitation, the regurgitant signal may be seen to terminate well before the end of diastole (Figure 13.9). Early termination of the Doppler signal with severe pulmonary regurgitation occurs when there is a rapid rise in the right ventricular diastolic pressure and equalisation of the pulmonary and right ventricular diastolic pressures.

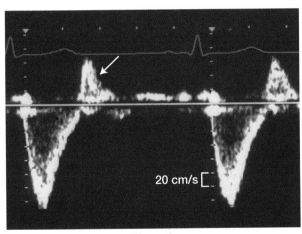

Normal

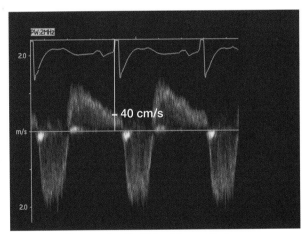

Severe Aortic Valve Regurgitation

Figure 13.7: Descending Aorta Diastolic Flow Reversal: Normal and with Significant Aortic Regurgitation.
Left, This is an example of a normal descending aortic Doppler flow profile recorded from the suprasternal window. Observe that during early diastole, there is a short period of low velocity flow reversal (less than one-third of diastole and less than 60 cm/s). This flow is directed toward the transducer and is, therefore, displayed above the zero baseline. This flow represents retrograde movement of blood flow back toward the aortic valve.
Right, This is an example of the pan-diastolic flow reversal within the descending thoracic aorta in a patient with severe aortic regurgitation. Observe that flow reversal occupies the entire diastolic period (pan-diastolic) and that the end-diastolic velocity exceeds 20 cm/s.

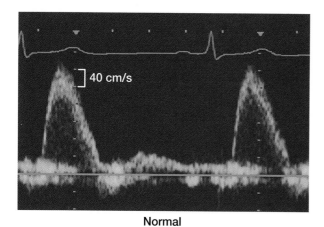 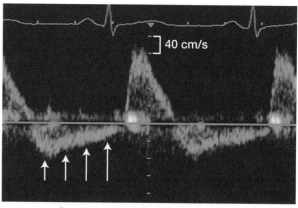

Normal   Severe Aortic Valve Regurgitation

Figure 13.8: Abdominal Aorta Diastolic Flow Reversal: Normal and with Significant Aortic Regurgitation.
Left, This is an example of a normal abdominal aortic Doppler flow profile recorded from the subcostal window. Observe that normal systolic flow is directed toward the transducer and that there is minimal forward flow during diastole.
Right, This is an example of the pan-diastolic flow reversal within the abdominal aorta in a patient with severe aortic regurgitation. Observe that flow reversal (seen below the zero baseline) occupies the entire diastolic period (*arrows*).

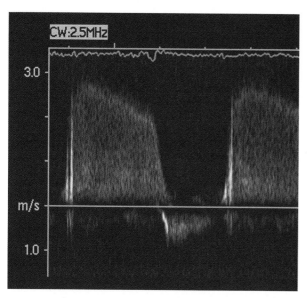 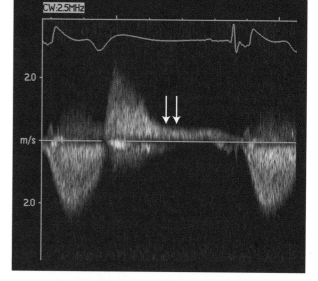

Mild Pulmonary Valve Regurgitation   Severe Pulmonary Valve Regurgitation

Figure 13.9: Duration of the regurgitant signal as an indicator of the severity of regurgitation.
Left, This is an example of a continuous-wave Doppler signal obtained in a patient with mild pulmonary regurgitation. Observe that the deceleration slope of this signal is quite long. Also note that the duration of this signal continues throughout the entire diastolic period.
Right, This is an example of a continuous-wave Doppler signal obtained in a patient with severe pulmonary regurgitation. Observe that the deceleration slope of this signal is extremely steep. Also note that the duration of this signal is very short and terminates well before the end of diastole (*arrows*).

Colour Flow Doppler Imaging of Regurgitant Jets

Colour flow Doppler imaging (CFI) allows the semiquantification of regurgitant valve lesions by providing real-time, colour-encoded visualisation of regurgitant blood flow. Hence, CFI provides a rapid and accurate means of mapping the area of regurgitant jets in multiple orthogonal planes. Because of the ease in which CFI identifies regurgitant jets, attempts have been made to quantify the severity of regurgitation by measurement of various parameters. These parameters include: (1) the aortic regurgitant jet height and the aortic regurgitant jet height to LVOT diameter ratio, and (2) the regurgitant jet area and regurgitant jet area to receiving chamber area ratio.

Regurgitant Jet Height and Regurgitant Jet Height / Left Ventricular Outflow Tract Diameter Ratio:

Measurement of the maximum length of the aortic regurgitant jet into the cavity of the left ventricle has been used as an indicator of the severity of regurgitation. However, the maximal height of the regurgitant jet at its origin (JH) or the ratio of the regurgitant jet height to the diameter of the left ventricular outflow tract (JH/LVOH) provides a better estimation of the severity of regurgitation. Figure 13.10 illustrates the measurement technique for determining the JH and the JH/LVOH ratio.

Clinical Significance of the Regurgitant JH and the Regurgitant JH/LVOH Ratio in Aortic Regurgitation:

Although investigators have reported reasonable correlations between the JH and the JH/LVOH as indicators of the various grades of severity of aortic regurgitation (AR), significant overlap between grades exists. In general, a JH of 8 mm provides a good discriminator between grades 1-2/4 AR and grades 3-4/4 AR. A JH/LVOH of > 40% provides a good discriminator between grades 1-2/4 AR and grades 3-4/4 AR while a JH/LVOH of < 25% identifies those patients with mild AR (refer to Figure 13.11) [40]. Furthermore, the JH/LVOH has been found to be the best indicator for predicting the severity of aortic regurgitation (Figure 13.12).

Regurgitant Jet Area and Regurgitant Jet Area / Receiving Chamber Area Ratio:

Comparison of the regurgitant jet area (RJA) and the area of the chamber into which the valve leaks has also been shown to provide semiquantitative evaluation of the severity of valvular regurgitation. Figures 13.13 and 13.14 illustrate the measurement technique for determining the regurgitant jet area and the regurgitant jet area-to-receiving chamber area ratio in the evaluation of aortic and mitral regurgitation.

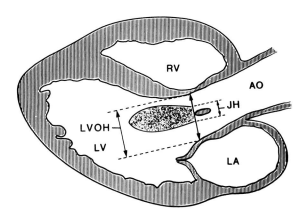

Figure 13.10: Measurement of the Regurgitant Jet Height and the Regurgitant Jet Height-to-Left Ventricular Outflow Tract Diameter Ratio.

The *regurgitant jet height* (JH) is measured as the maximal anteroposterior diameter (height) of the regurgitant jet, just below the aortic valve, as seen from the parasternal long axis view of the left ventricle. The *LVOT diameter* is measured at end-diastole, at the same location as the regurgitant jet. The *regurgitant jet height-to-LVOT* diameter ratio (JH/LVOH) is simply calculated by dividing the maximal regurgitant jet height by the diameter of the LVOT.

Abbreviations: AO = aorta; **JH** = maximal regurgitant jet height; **LA** = left atrium; **LV** = left ventricle; **LVOH** = left ventricular outflow tract diameter or height; **RV** = right ventricle. From Perry, G. J. et al.: Evaluation of aortic insufficiency by Doppler color flow mapping. Journal of the *American College of Cardiology 9: 953, 1987.* Reproduced with permission from the American College of Cardiology.

Clinical Significance of the RJA and the RJA-to-Receiving Chamber Area in Valvular Regurgitation:

Good correlations between the absolute regurgitant jet area (RJA) and angiographic grades of mitral regurgitation (MR) and tricuspid regurgitation (TR) have been reported. In patients with MR, a RJA of ≥ 8 cm² indicates severe regurgitation (sensitivity of 82%, specificity of 94%) and a RJA of ≤ 4 cm² indicates mild MR (sensitivity of 85%, specificity of 75%) [41].

In patients with TR, a RJA of ≥ 8 cm² is also indicative of severe regurgitation (sensitivity of 71%, specificity of 91%) [42].

In patients with aortic regurgitation (AR), a RJA/LVOA of 25 % discriminates between those patients with mild to moderate AR from those patients with moderately severe to severe AR (sensitivity of 92%, specificity of 93%) [43].

Good correlations between the regurgitant jet area-to-receiving chamber area and angiographic grades of both mitral and aortic regurgitation have also been reported (refer to Tables 13.4 and 13.5). Note that the values reported for differentiating between the various grades of mitral regurgitation have also been translated to the evaluation of tricuspid regurgitation [44].

40: Dolan, M. S. et al.: American Heart Journal 129: 1014 - 1020, 1995. 41: Spain, M.G. et al.: Journal of the American College of Cardiology 13: 585-590, 1989. 42: Grossman, G. et al.: European Heart Journal 19: 652-659, 1998. 43: Quantification of aortic regurgitation by Doppler echocardiography: A practical approach. American Heart Journal 129: 10141020, 1995. 44: Yamachika, S. et al.: Journal of the American Society of Echocardiography. 10: 159-168, 1997.

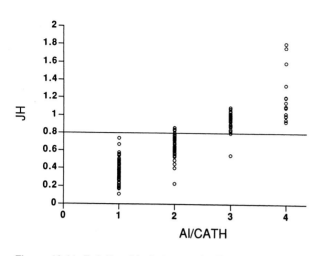 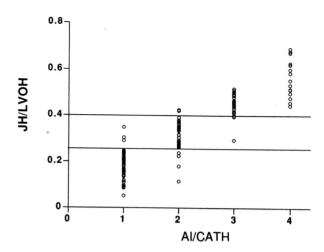

Figure 13.11: Relationship between the Regurgitant Jet Height and the Regurgitant Jet Height-to-Left Ventricular Outflow Tract Diameter Ratio and the Severity of Aortic Regurgitation.

The maximum regurgitant jet height (JH) and the regurgitant jet height-to-left ventricular outflow tract diameter ratio (JH/LVOH) are plotted as a function of the angiographic grade of aortic regurgitation (AR) in 156 patients (64 patients = mild [1] AR; 44 patients = moderate [2] AR; 48 patients = moderately severe [3] to severe [4] AR).

Left, This graph indicates the individual values for JH and their correlation with angiographic severity of aortic regurgitation (AI/CATH). Observe that the cut-off point of 0.8 cm (8 mm) provides a good discriminator between grades 1-2/4 AR and grades 3-4/4 AR (sensitivity of 97% and specificity of 98%).

Right, This graph indicates the individual values JH/LVOH and their correlation with angiographic severity of aortic regurgitation (AI/CATH). Observe that the cut-off point of 0.4 (40%) provides a good discriminator between grades 1-2/4 AR and grades 3-4/4 AR (sensitivity of 94% and specificity of 97%) while a cut-off point of 0.25 (25%) separates those patients with mild (1/4) AR from those patients with greater degrees of AR (sensitivity of 95% and specificity of 96%).

From Dolan, M. S. et al.: Quantification of aortic regurgitation by Doppler echocardiography: A practical approach. *American Heart Journal 129: 1018, 1995.* Reproduced with permission from Mosby, Inc., St. Louis, MO. USA.

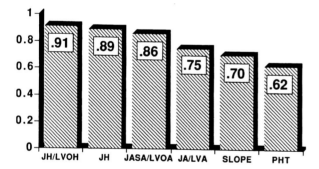

Figure 13.12: Comparison of Various Colour Flow Doppler and Continuous-wave Doppler Parameters versus Angiographic Grading of Aortic Regurgitation.

All correlations are expressed as the correlation coefficient. Observe that the colour flow Doppler parameters have higher correlations with the angiographic grading of aortic regurgitation compared with CW Doppler parameters such as the slope and PHT. (JH and JH/LVOH measurements obtained in 156 patients; JASA/LVOA measurements obtained in 152 patients; JA/LVA obtained in 140 patients; CW Doppler parameters obtained in 161 patients).

Abbreviations: JA/LVA = regurgitant jet area-to-left ventricular area; **JASA/LVOA** = parasternal short axis regurgitant jet area-to-left ventricular outflow tract area ratio; **JH** = regurgitant jet height; **JH/LVOH** = regurgitant jet height-to-left ventricular outflow tract height; **PHT** = pressure half-time of regurgitant jet. From Dolan, M. S. et al.: Quantification of aortic regurgitation by Doppler echocardiography: A practical approach. *American Heart Journal 129: 1017, 1995.* Reproduced with permission from Mosby, Inc., St. Louis, MO. USA.

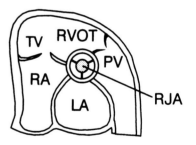

Figure 13.13: Measurement of the Regurgitant Jet Area and the Regurgitant Jet Area-to-Left Ventricular Outflow Area Ratio.

The *regurgitant jet area (RJA)* is measured from the parasternal short axis view at the level of the LVOT. The *left ventricular outflow tract area (LVOA)* is measured at end-diastole, at the same location as the regurgitant jet. The *regurgitant jet area-to-left ventricular outflow tract area ratio (RJA/LVOA)* is simply calculated by dividing the maximal regurgitant jet area by the area of the LVOT. This value is typically expressed as a percentage.

Abbreviations: LA = left atrium; **PV** = pulmonary valve; **RA** = right atrium; **RJA** = regurgitant jet area; **RVOT** = right ventricular outflow tract ; **TV** = tricuspid valve.

From Perry, G.J. et al.: Evaluation of aortic insufficiency by Doppler color flow mapping. *Journal of the American College of Cardiology 9: 952-959, 1987.* Reproduced with permission from the American College of Cardiology.

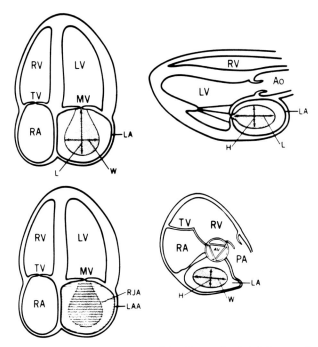

Figure 13.14: Measurement of the Regurgitant Jet Area and the Regurgitant Jet Area-to-Left Atrial Area Ratio from Multiple Orthogonal Planes.

The regurgitant jet area (RJA) and left atrial area (LAA) are measured from multiple orthogonal planes including: (1) the apical four chamber view *(top left)*; (2) the parasternal long axis view *(top right)*; (3) the apical four chamber view *(bottom left)*; and (4) the parasternal short axis view *(bottom right)*. The *regurgitant jet area-to-left atrial area ratio (RJA/LAA)* is simply calculated by dividing the maximal regurgitant jet area (RJA) by the area of the left atrium (LAA). This value is typically expressed as a percentage.

Abbreviations: Ao = aorta; **AV** = aortic valve; **H** = maximum height of the regurgitant jet; **L** = maximum length of the regurgitant jet; **LA** = left atrium; **LAA** = left atrial area; **LV** = left ventricle; **MV** = mitral valve; **RA** = right atrium; **RJA** = regurgitant jet area; **RV** = right ventricle; **TV** = tricuspid valve; **W** = maximum width of the regurgitant jet.

From Helmcke, F. et al.: Color Doppler assessment of mitral regurgitation with orthogonal planes. *Circulation* 75: 176, 1987. Reproduced with permission from Lippincott, Williams & Wilkins.

Table 13.4: Clinical Significance of the Regurgitant Jet Area/Left Atrial Area Ratio (RJA/LAA) in Mitral Regurgitation.

Severity of MR	RJA/LAA (%)	Sensitivity	Specificity
Mild	< 20	73 - 94 %	92 - 100%
Moderate	20 - 40	94 %	95 %
Severe	> 40	65 - 94 %	95 - 96%

Sources: Combined sources from Helmcke, F. et al., *Circulation 75: 175-183, 1987* and Spain, M.G. et al., *Journal of the American College of Cardiology 13: 585-590, 1989*. Helmcke study: patient population: no MR = 65; mild [1] MR = 36; moderate [2] MR = 18; severe [3] MR = 28; Spain study: patient population: mild [1] MR = 20; moderate [2] MR = 16; severe [3] MR = 11.

Table 13.5: Clinical Significance of the Regurgitant Jet Area/Left Ventricular Outflow Tract Area Ratio (RJA/LVOA) in Aortic Regurgitation.

Severity of AR	RJA/LVOA (%)	Sensitivity	Specificity
Mild	< 4	80 %	100%
Moderate	4 - 24	100 %	95 %
Moderately severe	25 - 59	100 %	100 %
Severe	≥ 60	100 %	100 %

Source: Perry, G.J et al.: *Journal of the American College of Cardiology. 9: 952-959, 1987*: patient population: mild [1] AR = 6; moderate [2] AR = 6; moderately severe [3] AR = 6; severe [4] AR = 11.

Limitations of Colour Flow Doppler Imaging in the Assessment of Valvular Regurgitation:

The principal limitation of CFI in the evaluation of valvular regurgitation lies in the large number of factors which affect the regurgitant jet size and shape. These factors can be divided into two groups: (1) technical factors and (2) physiological factors (see Table 13.6).

Wall Jets:

The regurgitant jet size is influenced by the location or direction of the jet with respect to adjacent walls of the receiving chamber. This factor is particularly important with eccentric jets. Eccentric regurgitant jets tend to adhere to adjacent structures such as chamber walls (hence, known as "wall jets" or "impinging jets"). This affects both the shape and area of regurgitant jets (Figure 13.15). Wall jets can appear significantly smaller than free jets due to jet distortion and loss of jet momentum. Therefore, underestimation of the severity of the regurgitant lesion may occur with eccentric regurgitant jets.

Influence of Co-Existent Jets:

A potential problem exists in the evaluation of aortic regurgitation by CFI when there is coexistent mitral stenosis or a prosthetic mitral valve in-situ. In these situations, the transmitral flow stream may be abnormally directed such that aortic regurgitant jets merge with the mitral inflow jet. This merger between these two jets can obscure or falsely magnify the aortic regurgitant jet area.

Instrument Settings:

The displayed area of the regurgitant jet by CFI is affected by numerous instrument settings such as gain settings, pulse repetition frequency, and transducer frequency. These factors can alter "perceived" regurgitant jet size independent of any actual change in the regurgitant volume. In particular, improper gain settings may lead to erroneous quantification of the severity of regurgitation. For example, excessively low gain settings will underestimate the severity while excessively high gain settings will clutter the image with noise making it difficult to identify the true outline of the regurgitant jet area.

The regurgitant jet area is also inversely related to the

Table 13.6: Physiological and Technical Factors affecting Colour Flow Doppler Imaging in the Assessment of Valvular Regurgitation.

Physiological Factors	Technical Factors
• Driving pressure	• Gain settings
• Receiving chamber size & compliance	• Transducer frequency
• Wall jets	• Incident angle
• Regurgitant volume	• Filter settings
• Size and shape of regurgitant orifice	• Pulse repetition frequency
• Influence of coexistent jets	• Frame rate
• Mitral regurgitation of ischaemic origin	• Attenuation of ultrasound energy
	• Suboptimal imaging of regurgitant jet

pulse repetition frequency which is directly related to the transducer frequency. Therefore, low frequency transducers (2.5 MHz) should be used to optimise the regurgitant jet signal.

Incident Angle:
Nonparallel alignment of the ultrasound beam with the regurgitant jet produces lower Doppler frequency shifts. Thus, regurgitant jets may be misinterpreted as laminar or nondisturbed flow.

Furthermore, accuracy of the JH/LVOH is dependent upon the angle of the transducer with respect to the JH and the LVOH. Typically, interrogation of the

regurgitant jet is performed by careful manipulation and angulation of the ultrasound beam in order to obtain the maximum JH. However, the maximal jet JH and the maximal LVOH may not occur in the same imaging plane (see Figure 13.16). The LVOT is circular, therefore, if the LVOT is not transected through its exact centre, underestimation of the true diameter (height) will occur. This will result in an overestimation of the JH/LVOH and the severity of aortic regurgitation.

Regurgitant Volumes and Regurgitant Fractions

Utilisation of spectral Doppler in conjunction with 2-D imaging can be used in the quantification of valvular regurgitation by measurement of regurgitant fractions and regurgitant volumes. These calculations are primarily based on the measurement of stroke volumes and the continuity principle. Calculation of the regurgitant volume can also be calculated using the PISA technique (see "Effective Regurgitant Orifice

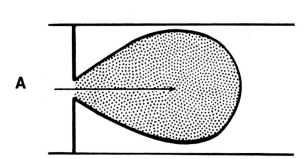

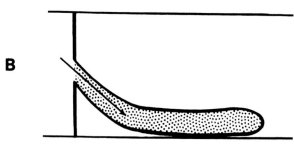

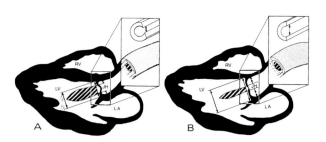

Figure 13.16: The Effect of the Transducer Angle and the Regurgitant Jet Height and Left Ventricular Outflow Tract Diameter.
This schematics illustrate the effect of the transducer angle on the measurement of the regurgitant jet height (JH) and the left ventricular outflow tract height (LVOH).
A, In this image, the aortic regurgitant JH is maximised. However, because of the eccentricity of the regurgitant jet, the LVOH is decreased. This would result in an overestimation of the JH/LVOH ratio.
B, In this image of the same patient, the LVOH is maximised but the aortic regurgitant JH is decreased, underestimating the JH/LVOH ratio.
In order to obtain an accurate measure of the JH/LVOH ratio, the JH from image *A* and the LVOH from image *B* should be used.
From Reynolds, T. et al.: The JH/LVOH method in the quantification of aortic regurgitation: How the cardiac sonographer may avoid an important potential pitfall. *Journal of the American Society of Echocardiography. 4: 107, 1991.* Reproduced with permission from Mosby Inc., St. Louis, MO, USA.

Figure 13.15: Wall Jets versus Free Jets.
In this schematic, both the wall jet and the free jet have the same regurgitant orifice size and volume.
A, Observe that the free jet flows into the centre of the chamber, essentially filling the chamber.
B, Observe that the wall jet is directed into the wall of the receiving chamber. As a result, the jet clings to the wall and transfers all its momentum to the wall, thus, truncating the jet. Therefore, the area of the regurgitant jet appears smaller despite the fact that the regurgitant orifice and regurgitant volume is the same as for the free jet (*A*).
From Feigenbaum, H.: Echocardiography. 5th Edition. Lea and Febiger. pp: 42, 1994. Reproduced with permission from Lippincott, Williams & Wilkins and from the author.

Areas" - Proximal Isovelocity Surface Area Method). The clinical significance of regurgitant volumes and regurgitant fractions are listed in Table 13.9 (page 177). Studies validating the accuracy of Doppler echocardiography in determination of the regurgitant fraction are tabulated in Appendix 10.

Theoretical Considerations:

Calculation of the regurgitant volume and regurgitant fraction are based upon the calculation of the stroke volume through the regurgitant valve and the stroke volume through a competent valve.

In the absence of valvular regurgitation or an intracardiac shunt, the stroke volume through all valves will be equal. When a valve becomes incompetent, the stroke volume through this valve will be higher as the total forward stroke volume across the regurgitant valve is a product of the normal forward stroke volume plus the regurgitant volume (see Figures 13.17 and 13.18). Thus, the regurgitant volume, defined as the volume of blood that regurgitates (leaks) through an incompetent valve, can be calculated when the stroke volume through a competent valve and the stroke volume through the regurgitant valve are known; hence,

(Equation 13.2)

$$RVol\ (cc) = SV_{RV} - SV_{CV}$$

where RVol = regurgitant volume (cc)
  SV_{RV} = total stroke volume across the regurgitant valve (cc)
  SV_{CV} = forward stroke volume through a competent valve (cc)

Technical consideration:

From Figures 13.17 and 13.18, it can also be appreciated that the left ventricular stroke volume is increased with both aortic and mitral regurgitation. Thus, the stroke volume of the left ventricle can also be used to determine the total forward stroke volume through the mitral valve in mitral regurgitation and the total forward stroke volume through the left ventricular outflow tract with aortic regurgitation.

The **regurgitant fraction** is defined as the fraction or percentage of the total stroke volume that regurgitates (leaks) through an incompetent valve and is equal to:

(Equation 13.3)

$$RF(\%) = \frac{RVol}{SV_{forward}} \times 100$$

where RF = regurgitant fraction (%)
  RVol = regurgitant volume (cc)
  $SV_{forward}$ = total forward stroke volume across regurgitant valve (cc)

Regurgitant volumes and regurgitant fractions can be calculated across any cardiac valve. More commonly, however, these calculations are implemented in the quantitative assessment of the left-sided regurgitant valves; that is, in the assessment of mitral and aortic regurgitation. Table 13.7 lists the variables required for the calculation of the regurgitant volume and regurgitant fraction in each of these valves.

Method of Calculation of the Regurgitant Volume and Regurgitant Fraction:

The various methods that can be used for the calculation of the regurgitant volume and regurgitant fraction include:
(1) calculation of the total stroke volume through the regurgitant valve and the normal stroke volume through a competent valve;
(2) calculation of the total stroke volume of the left ventricle and the normal stroke volume;
(3) calculation of the forward stroke volume and flow reversal in the aortic arch (aortic regurgitation).

"Step-by-step" methods for calculation of the regurgitant fraction and regurgitant volume in aortic and mitral regurgitation are outlined on the following pages.

Table 13.7: Variables required in the Measurement of the Regurgitant Volume and Regurgitant Fraction in Aortic and Mitral Regurgitation.

Valvular Regurgitation	Total Stroke Volume (cc)	Forward Stroke Volume (cc)
MR without AR	$CSA_{MV} \times VTI_{MV}$	$CSA_{LVOT} \times VTI_{LVOT}$
MR with AR (no intracardiac shunt)	$CSA_{MV} \times VTI_{MV}$	$CSA_{RVOT} \times VTI_{RVOT}$
AR without MR	$CSA_{LVOT} \times VTI_{LVOT}$	$CSA_{MV} \times VTI_{MV}$
AR with MR (no intracardiac shunt)	$CSA_{LVOT} \times VTI_{LVOT}$	$CSA_{RVOT} \times VTI_{RVOT}$
AR (using the forward and reverse flows from the aortic arch)	$CSA_{Ao\text{-}diast} \times VTI_{Ao\text{-}diast}$	$CSA_{Ao\text{-}sys} \times VTI_{Ao\text{-}sys}$

Abbreviations: AR = aortic regurgitation; **CSA$_{Ao\text{-}dias}$** = cross-sectional area of the aortic arch in diastole; **CSA$_{Ao\text{-}sys}$** = cross-sectional area of the aortic arch in systole; **CSA$_{LVOT}$** = cross-sectional area of the left ventricular outflow tract; **CSA$_{MV}$** = cross-sectional area of mitral valve annulus; **CSA$_{RVOT}$** = cross-sectional area of the right ventricular outflow tract; **MR** = mitral regurgitation; **VTI$_{Ao\text{-}dias}$** = velocity time integral of diastolic envelope of flow reversal from the descending thoracic aorta; **VTI$_{Ao\text{-}sys}$** = velocity time integral of systolic envelope of forward flow from the descending thoracic aorta; **VTI$_{LVOT}$** = velocity time integral of left ventricular outflow tract; **VTI$_{MV}$** = velocity time integral of mitral valve annulus; **VTI$_{RVOT}$** = velocity time integral of right ventricular outflow tract.

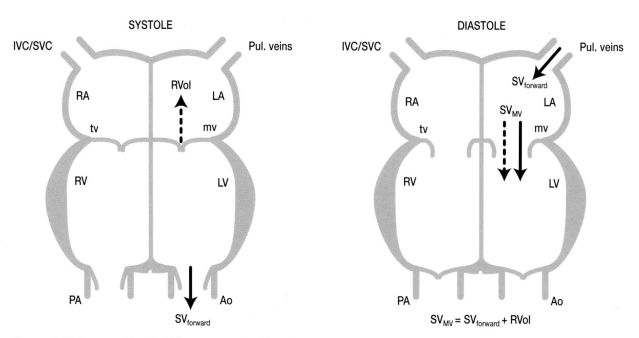

Figure 13.17: Increased Stroke Volume across the Mitral Valve in Mitral Regurgitation.
This schematic illustrates why the stroke volume across the mitral valve is increased with mitral regurgitation.
Left, During systole, the left ventricle contracts and ejects blood in two directions: (1) forward into the aorta and around the body to the systemic circulation (normal forward stroke volume = $SV_{forward}$) and (2) backward across the incompetent mitral valve into the left atrium (regurgitant volume = RVol).
Right, During diastole, the total stroke volume across the mitral valve (SV_{MV}) into the left ventricle is increased as the stroke volume through the mitral valve includes the stroke volume returning to the heart via the pulmonary veins ($SV_{forward}$) plus the regurgitant volume (RVol).
Therefore, if $SV_{forward}$ and SV_{MV} are determined, it is possible to calculate the regurgitant volume.

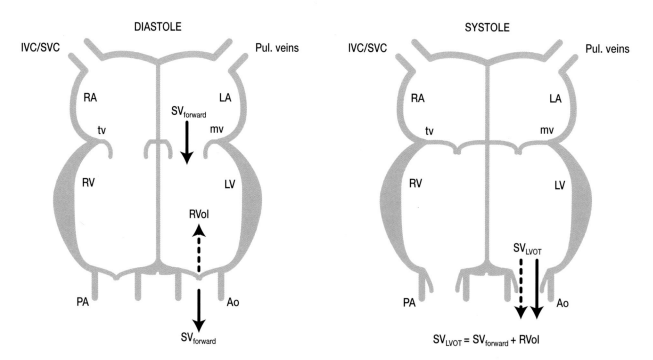

Figure 13.18: Increased Stroke Volume across the Left Ventricular Outflow Tract in Aortic Regurgitation.
This schematic illustrates why the stroke volume across the left ventricular outflow tract is increased with aortic regurgitation.
Left, During diastole, following aortic valve closure, blood travels in two directions: (1) forward to the systemic circulation ($SV_{forward}$) and (2) backward into the left ventricle through the incompetent aortic valve (regurgitant volume = RVol). *At the same time,* the returning forward stroke volume enters the left ventricle via the mitral valve ($SV_{forward}$). Therefore, the volume of the left ventricle is increased.
Right, During systole, the total stroke volume through the left ventricular outflow tract (SV_{LVOT}) is increased as it includes the returning forward stroke volume through the mitral valve ($SV_{forward}$) plus the regurgitant volume (RVol).
Therefore, if $SV_{forward}$ and SV_{LVOT} are determined, it is possible to calculate the regurgitant volume.

Method (1) for calculation of regurgitant volume and regurgitant fraction

Step 1: **Calculate the stroke volume through the left ventricular outflow tract (LVOT):**
  a) measure the diameter of the LVOT:
   - from the parasternal long axis view of the LV during systole
   - measured at the level of the aortic annulus
   - measured from the inner edge to the inner edge of aortic cuspal insertion

  b) assuming a circular shape of the LVOT, calculate the area of the LVOT (cm²):

   - $CSA = 0.785 \times D^2$

  c) measure the VTI of the LVOT (cm):
   - from the apical five chamber view
   - P-W Doppler sample volume positioned in centre of LVOT proximal to aortic valve
   - VTI is traced along the leading edge velocity

  d) calculate the LVOT stroke volume (SV):

   - $SV\ (cc) = CSA\ (cm^2) \times VTI\ (cm)$

Step 2: **Calculate the stroke volume through the mitral valve (MV):**
  a) measure the mitral valve annulus diameter:
   - from the apical four chamber view at mid-diastole
   - measured from the inner edge to the inner edge

  b) assuming a circular shape of the mitral valve, calculate the mitral valve area (cm²):

   - $CSA = 0.785 \times D^2$

  c) measure the VTI from the mitral annulus (cm):
   - from the apical four chamber view
   - P-W Doppler sample volume positioned **at the level** of mitral valve annulus
   - VTI is traced along the modal velocity

  d) calculate the stroke volume (SV) across the mitral valve:

   - $SV\ (cc) = CSA\ (cm^2) \times VTI\ (cm)$

Step 3: **Calculate the Regurgitant Volume (cc) and Regurgitant Fraction (%):**
  a) for mitral valve regurgitation:

$$RVol\ (cc) = SV_{MV} - SV_{LVOT}$$

$$RF(\%) = \frac{SV_{MV} - SV_{LVOT}}{SV_{MV}} = \frac{RVol}{SV_{MV}}$$

  b) for aortic valve regurgitation:

$$RVol\ (cc) = SV_{LVOT} - SV_{MV}$$

$$RF(\%) = \frac{SV_{LVOT} - SV_{MV}}{SV_{LVOT}} = \frac{RVol}{SV_{LVOT}}$$

Technical Consideration:
Calculation of the regurgitant fraction for pulmonary and tricuspid regurgitation can also be performed using the method described above by simply substituting the calculation of the mitral stroke volume with either the tricuspid or pulmonary stroke volume (step 2).

Method (2) for calculation of regurgitant volume and regurgitant fraction

Step 1: **calculate the stroke volume of the left ventricle by 2-D echo (SV_{2D}):**
   a) using Simpson's Biplane method:
   - calculate the left ventricular end-diastolic volume (LVEDV)
   - calculate left ventricular end-systolic volume (LVESV)
   - calculate the stroke volume (cc):

$$SV_{2D} = LVEDV - LVESV$$

For Mitral Regurgitation:

Step 2: **calculate the stroke volume through the left ventricular outflow tract (LVOT):**
   a) measure the diameter of the LVOT:
   - from the parasternal long axis view of the LV during systole
   - measured at the level of the aortic annulus
   - measured from the inner edge to the inner edge of aortic cuspal insertion

   b) assuming a circular shape of the LVOT, calculate the area of the LVOT (cm²):

   - $CSA = 0.785 \times D^2$

   c) measure the VTI of the LVOT (cm):
   - from the apical five chamber view
   - P-W Doppler sample volume positioned in centre of LVOT proximal to aortic valve
   - VTI is traced along the leading edge velocity

   d) calculate the LVOT stroke volume (SV):

   - $SV\ (cc) = CSA\ (cm^2) \times VTI\ (cm)$

Step 3: **calculate the regurgitant volume (cc) and regurgitant fraction (%):**

$$RVol\ (mls) = SV_{2D} - SV_{LVOT}$$

$$RF(\%) = \frac{SV_{2D} - SV_{LVOT}}{SV_{2D}} = \frac{RVol}{SV_{2D}}$$

For Aortic Regurgitation:

Step 2: **calculate the stroke volume through the mitral valve (MV):**
   a) measure the mitral valve annulus diameter:
   - from the apical four chamber view at mid-diastole
   - measured from the inner edge to the inner edge

   b) assuming a circular shape of the mitral valve, calculate the mitral valve area (cm²):

   - $CSA = 0.785 \times D^2$

   c) measure the VTI from the mitral annulus (cm):
   - from the apical four chamber view
   - P-W Doppler sample volume positioned **at the level** of mitral valve annulus
   - VTI is traced along the modal velocity

   d) calculate the stroke volume (SV) across the mitral valve:

   - $SV\ (cc) = CSA\ (cm^2) \times VTI\ (cm)$

Step 3: **calculate the regurgitant volume (cc) and regurgitant fraction (%):**

$$RVol\ (mls) = SV_{2D} - SV_{MV}$$

$$RF(\%) = \frac{SV_{2D} - SV_{MV}}{SV_{2D}} = \frac{RVol}{SV_{2D}}$$

Method (3) for calculation of the regurgitant fraction in aortic regurgitation

Step 1:   **calculate the systolic stroke volume (SV$_{systolic}$):**
   a) measure the systolic diameter of the aortic arch:
   - from the suprasternal long axis view of the aorta during systole
   - measured at the top of the aortic arch
   - measured from the inner edge to the inner edge of aortic lumen

   b) assuming a circular shape of the aortic lumen, calculate the aortic lumen area (cm²):

   - $CSA = 0.785 \times D^2$

   c) measure the systolic VTI (cm):
   - from the suprasternal long axis view of the aorta
   - P-W Doppler sample volume positioned proximal to the head and neck vessels
   - VTI of the systolic envelope is traced along the leading edge velocity

   d) calculate the systolic forward stroke volume (SV$_{systolic}$):

   - $SV (cc) = CSA (cm^2) \times VTI (cm)$

Step 2:   **calculate the diastolic stroke volume (SV$_{diastolic}$):**
   a) measure the diastolic diameter of the aortic arch:
   - from the suprasternal long axis view of the aorta during systole
   - measured at the top of the aortic arch
   - measured from the inner edge to the inner edge of aortic lumen

   b) assuming a circular shape of the aortic lumen, calculate the aortic lumen area (cm²):

   - $CSA = 0.785 \times D^2$

   c) measure the *diastolic* VTI (cm):
   - from the suprasternal long axis view of the aorta
   - P-W Doppler sample volume positioned just distal to the left subclavian artery within the descending aorta
   - the VTI of the *diastolic* envelope is traced along the leading edge velocity

   d) calculate the diastolic reversed stroke volume (SV$_{diastolic}$):

   - $SV (cc) = CSA (cm^2) \times VTI (cm)$

Step 3:   **Calculation of Regurgitant Fraction (%):**

$$RF(\%) = \frac{SV_{diastolic}}{SV_{systolic}}$$

Technical Considerations:

Method (1) is considered to be the most accurate method for calculating the regurgitant volume and regurgitant fraction. Method (2) is less accurate as it uses Doppler-derived data and a 2-D geometrical calculation.

Method (2) can be used instead of method (1) when it is difficult to measure the mitral annulus or the LVOT diameter.

Method (3) is rarely used in clinical practice as imaging of the aorta from the suprasternal notch is often challenging.

Limitations of the Regurgitant Volume and Regurgitant Fraction Calculations:

Assumptions of Stroke Volume Calculations.
As previously mentioned, stroke volume calculations are based on a simple hydraulic formula which determines the volumetric flow rate through a cylindrical tube under steady flow conditions. Therefore, to apply this concept to the heart, the following assumptions are made: (1) the derived CSA is circular, (2) blood flow is uniform, (3) the CSA remains constant throughout the period of measured flow (systole or diastole), and (4) the sample volume remains in a constant position throughout the period of flow. However, the flow profiles and the diameters from which the CSA is derived may change throughout the period of flow. In addition, while the left and right ventricular outflow tracts assume a circular configuration, the same may not be said for the mitral valve annulus which is more elliptical in its shape.

Errors in Diameter Measurements.
One variable that is used in the calculation of the total and forward stroke volumes is the CSA. Calculation of this measurement involves squaring the diameter. Therefore, any error in the diameter measurement is magnified. Failure to measure the diameter during the correct phase of the cardiac cycle may also lead to significant errors in stroke volume calculations. Diameters and, therefore, the CSA should be measured at the same phase in the cardiac cycle as the VTI; that is, the CSA should be determined at the time when blood flow is passing through that region.

Due to the difficulty of obtaining accurate diameter measurements, an alternative and more simplified technique has been proposed for the calculation of the regurgitant fraction in patients with aortic regurgitation. This technique, proposed by Xie et al [45], assumes that there is a fixed relationship between the ratio of the CSA of the LVOT and the CSA of the mitral annulus (CSA_{LVOT}/CSA_{MV}). From a population of 50 normal subjects, a constant of 0.77 was derived representing this ratio. Therefore, by substituting the derived constant of 0.77 for the CSA measurements, calculation of the regurgitant fraction can be simplified to:

(Equation 13.4)

$$RF(\%) = 1 - \left[\frac{1}{0.77} \times \frac{VTI_{MV}}{VTI_{LVOT}}\right] \times 100$$

where RF = regurgitant fraction (%)
1 = total forward stroke volume
1/0.77 = inverted ratio of the constant for CSA_{LVOT}/CSA_{MV}
VTI_{MV} = velocity time integral across the mitral annulus (cm)
VTI_{LVOT} = velocity time integral across the LVOT (cm)

An important potential problem of the application of this simplified technique includes distortion and dilatation of the aortic annulus which may occur in patients with aortic stenosis or Marfan's syndrome. In these circumstances, alterations to the CSA_{LVOT}/CSA_{MV} relationship may occur.

Errors in Measurement of Velocity Time Integrals.
The following factors all contribute to errors in VTI measurements: (1) poor beam alignment with the direction of blood flow, (2) incorrect placement of the PW Doppler sample volume, (3) improper tracing of Doppler trace, and (4) failing to average a sufficient number of beats. Errors in VTI measurements will result in errors in the calculation of the stroke volumes, regurgitant volumes and regurgitant fractions.

Of particular importance, is the overestimation of the mitral VTI which may occur due to: (1) incorrect placement of the PW Doppler sample volume too far into the left ventricle rather than *at* the mitral valve annulus, and (2) failure to trace the modal velocity (brightest line).

"Normal" Regurgitant Fractions.
Multiple measurements of stroke volume variables at two different sites leads to small errors in the calculation of the regurgitant fraction. This leads to a so-called "normal" regurgitant fraction even in patients with no regurgitation. Various values for a "normal" regurgitant fraction have been reported (see Table 13.8). In spite of this, there remains a clear separation between the "normal" regurgitant fraction and regurgitant fractions derived in the cases with significant valvular regurgitation (see Table 13.9).

Presence of Multivalvular Lesions or Intracardiac Shunts.
Calculation of the regurgitant fraction in patients with combined mitral stenosis and mitral regurgitation may not be reliable due to distortion of the mitral valve orifice.

Table 13.8: "Normal" Regurgitant Fractions by Doppler Echocardiography.

First Author (Year)	Pt. Pop.	RF (%)
Kitabatake (1985) [1]	10	2.4 ± 5 *
Rokey (1986) [2]	11	15.7 ± 7.6 *
Tribouilloy (1991) [3]	20	4.2
Enriquez-Sarano (1993) [4]	30	4.8 ± 3.9 *
	20	5.3 ± 4.5 *

* mean ± one standard deviation

Sources: **(1)** Kitabatake, A., et al., *Circulation* 72:523-529,1985; **(2)** Rokey, R., et al., Journal of the *American College of Cardiology* 7:1273-1278,1986; **(3)** Tribouilloy, C., et al., *British Heart Journal* 66:290-294,1991; **(4)** Enriquez-Sarano, M. et al., *Circulation* 87: 841-848, 1993.

45: Xie, G-Y., et al.: Journal of the American College of Cardiology 24:1041-1045,1994.

Table 13.9: Clinical Significance of Regurgitant Volumes and Regurgitant Fractions in Valvular Regurgitation.

Valve / Severity	Regurgitant Volume (cc)	Regurgitant Fraction (%)
Mitral Regurgitation: [1]		
Mild	< 30	< 30
Moderate	30 - 44	30 - 39
Moderately severe	45 - 59	40 - 60
Severe	≥ 60	> 60
Tricuspid Regurgitation: (**)		
Mild	< 30	< 30
Moderate	30 - 44	30 - 39
Moderately severe	45 - 59	40 - 60
Severe	≥ 60	> 60
Aortic Regurgitation: [2]		
Mild	-	< 20
Moderate	-	20 - 40
Moderately severe	-	40 - 60
Severe	-	> 60
Pulmonary Regurgitation: [3]		
Mild	-	< 40
Moderate	-	40 - 60
Severe	-	> 60

(**) values delineated for assessing the various degrees of mitral regurgitation have also been translated to the assessment of tricuspid regurgitation [46].
Sources: (1) Dujardin, K.S. et al., *Circulation 96: 3409-3415, 1997*; **(2)** Nishimura, R.A. et al., *American Heart Journal 124: 995-1001, 1992*; **(3)** Marx, G.R. et al., *American Journal of Cardiology 61: 595-601, 1988.*

Similarly, calculation of the regurgitant fraction is invalid when there is regurgitation through the valve used to calculate the forward stroke volume. Obviously in this situation, the regurgitant fraction will be *underestimated* as the forward stroke volume is *overestimated*.

Calculations of the regurgitant fraction and the regurgitant volume in aortic or mitral regurgitation using the pulmonary (RVOT) flow are also compromised when there is a coexistent intracardiac shunt. In this instance, intracardiac shunt flow will effectively produce unequal flow through the right and left sides of the heart.

Significant Learning Curve of the Operator.
Calculation of the regurgitant fraction is tedious and time consuming. Furthermore, the multiple steps involved in the calculation of this parameter increases the potential for error. Therefore, it is not surprising that a significant learning curve exists in the calculation of this index. Improved accuracy occurs with increasing expertise in measurement technique.

Effective Regurgitant Orifice Areas

Recall that the effective orifice area of stenotic valves can be calculated by application of the continuity principle. Application of this same principle can also be applied to the calculation of the effective regurgitant orifice area (EROA). Fundamentally, this principle is based on the theory of the conservation of mass which simply states "what goes in, must come out". Calculation of the EROA can be performed using: (1) the spectral Doppler technique or (2) by application of the PISA method.

1. Spectral Doppler Technique for Calculation of the Effective Regurgitant Orifice Area.
Theoretical Considerations:
As mentioned above, calculation of the EROA is based on the principle of the conservation of mass which states "what flows in, must flow out". Based on this principle, the EROA is calculated from the premise that the regurgitant volume through an incompetent valve is equal to the flow *at* the regurgitant orifice.

Recall that stroke volume can be calculated from the CSA and the VTI; hence, the regurgitant volume at the regurgitant orifice can be expressed as:

(Equation 13.5)

$$RVol = EROA \times VTI_{RJ}$$

where RVol = regurgitant volume (cc)
EROA = effective regurgitant orifice area (cm²)
VTI_{RJ} = velocity time integral of the regurgitant jet (cm)

Therefore, by rearranging the above equation, the EROA can be derived by:

(Equation 13.6)

$$EROA = \frac{RVol}{VTI_{RJ}}$$

where RVol = regurgitant volume (cc)
EROA = effective regurgitant orifice area (cm²)
VTI_{RJ} = velocity time integral of the regurgitant signal (cm)

46: Yamachika, S. et al.: Journal of the American Society of Echocardiography. 10: 159-168, 1997.

Method of Calculation of the Effective Regurgitant Orifice Area:
Below, is a "step-by-step" method for calculation of the EROA based on the continuity principle.

Method for calculation of the Effective Regurgitant Orifice Area

Step 1: **calculate the stroke volume through the left ventricular outflow tract (LVOT):**
a) measure the LVOT diameter:
- from the parasternal long axis view of the LV during systole at the level of the aortic annulus
- measured from the inner edge to the inner edge of aortic cuspal insertion

b) assuming a circular shape of the LVOT, the LVOT area is calculated (cm²):
- $CSA = 0.785 \times D^2$

c) measure the LVOT VTI (cm):
- from the apical five chamber view, P-W Doppler sample volume positioned in centre of LVOT proximal to aortic valve
- the VTI is traced along the leading edge velocity

d) calculate the LVOT stroke volume (SV):
- $SV\ (cc) = CSA\ (cm^2) \times VTI\ (cm)$

Step 2: **calculate the stroke volume through the mitral valve (MV):**
a) measure the mitral valve annulus diameter:
- from the apical four chamber view at mid-diastole
- measured from the inner edge to the inner edge

b) assuming a circular shape of the mitral valve, the annular area is calculated (cm²):
- $CSA = 0.785 \times D^2$

c) measure the mitral annulus VTI (cm):
- from the apical four chamber view, P-W Doppler sample volume positioned **at the level** of mitral valve annulus
- the VTI is traced along the modal velocity

d) calculate the stroke volume (SV) across the mitral valve:
- $SV\ (cc) = CSA\ (cm^2) \times VTI\ (cm)$

Step 3: **calculate the regurgitant volume (cc):**

For mitral valve regurgitation (MR):
$$RVol_{(MR)} = SV_{(MV)} - SV_{(LVOT)}$$

For aortic valve regurgitation (AR):
$$RVol_{(AR)} = SV_{(LVOT)} - SV_{(MV)}$$

Step 4: **measurement of VTI of regurgitant signal:**
a) optimise CW Doppler spectrum of regurgitant signal
b) trace the VTI of regurgitant signal

Step 5: **calculate the effective regurgitant orifice area (cm²):**

For mitral valve regurgitation (MR):
$$EROA_{(MR)} = RVol_{(MR)} \div VTI_{(MR)}$$

For aortic valve regurgitation (AR):
$$EROA_{(AR)} = RVol_{(AR)} \div VTI_{(AR)}$$

Limitations of Calculation of the Effective Regurgitant Orifice Area:
Calculation of the EROA revolves around the calculation of the regurgitant volume. Therefore, limitations in the calculation of the EROA technique are essentially the same as those outlined for the calculation of the regurgitant volume. In addition, another potential source of error in the calculation of the EROA lies in the measurement of the VTI of the regurgitant signal. In particular, the inability to obtain a complete CW Doppler envelope may occur due to eccentric jets or a large incident angle between the ultrasound beam and regurgitant jet direction.

2. Proximal Isovelocity Surface Area Method for Calculation of the Effective Regurgitant Orifice Area.

Calculation of the effective regurgitant orifice area (EROA) by the proximal isovelocity surface area (PISA) method is simply a variation in the application of the continuity equation. Studies validating the quantitative evaluation of valvular regurgitation by the PISA technique with other techniques are tabulated in Appendix 11.

Theoretical Considerations:
The principles of the PISA method in the calculation of a narrowed orifice area have been previously discussed (see "Proximal Isovelocity Surface Area in the Calculation of the Mitral Valve Area"). This principle can also be applied in the evaluation of valvular regurgitation by calculation of the EROA.
Recall that the flow rate proximal to a narrowed orifice is the product of the hemispheric flow convergent area and the velocity of that isovelocity shell and is expressed by the following equation:

(Equation 12.9)

$$Q = 2\pi r^2 V_r$$

where Q   = flow rate (cc/s)
  $2\pi r^2$ = area of a hemispheric shell (cm²)
  V_r = velocity at the radial distance - r (cm/s)

Based on the continuity principle, blood flow passing through a given hemisphere *must* ultimately pass through the narrowed orifice. Therefore, the flow rate through any given hemisphere must equal the flow rate through the narrowed orifice:

(Equation 12.10)

$$2\pi r^2 V_r = A_o \times V_o$$

where A_o = area of the narrowed orifice (cm²)
  V_o = peak velocity through the narrowed orifice (cm/s)

Therefore, by rearranging the equation (12.9), the area through the narrowed orifice (Ao) can be calculated:

(Equation 12.11)

$$A_o = \frac{2\pi r^2 V_r}{V_o}$$

Application of this PISA Principle in the Calculation of the Effective Regurgitant Orifice Area:
When this principle is applied to the assessment of the effective regurgitant orifice area (EROA), the regurgitant valve acts as the narrowed orifice and the peak velocity through the narrowed orifice is equivalent to the peak velocity of the regurgitant jet. Furthermore, using colour flow Doppler imaging, both the radial distance (r) and the velocity at the radial distance (V_r) can be identified (Figure 13.19). The radial distance (r) is measured as the proximal distance from the first aliased velocity (blue-red interface) to the regurgitant orifice or valve while the velocity at the radial distance (V_r) is equivalent to the Nyquist limit which is depicted on the colour velocity bar; hence, V_r becomes V_N. Therefore, calculation of the EROA can be expressed by the following equation:

(Equation 13.7)

$$EROA = \frac{2\pi r^2 V_N}{V_R}$$

where EROA = effective regurgitant orifice area (cm²)
  $2\pi r^2$ = area of a hemispheric shell derived from the radius [r] (cm²)
  V_N = aliased velocity identified as the Nyquist limit (cm/s)
  V_R = peak regurgitant velocity (cm/s)

Calculation of the Regurgitant Volume from the EROA:
As mentioned previously, the regurgitant volume through an incompetent valve is equal to the flow at the regurgitant orifice. Therefore, assuming that the regurgitant orifice does not change throughout the period of regurgitant flow, the regurgitant volume can also be calculated from the EROA and the VTI of the regurgitant signal (see Figure 13.19):

(Equation 13.5)

$$RVol = EROA \times VTI_{RJ}$$

where RVol = regurgitant volume (cc)
  EROA = effective regurgitant orifice (cm²)
  VTI_{RJ} = velocity time integral of regurgitant jet signal (cm)

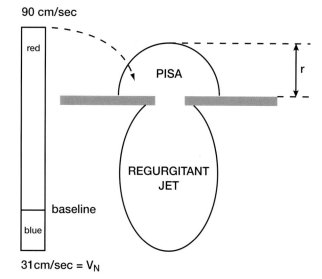

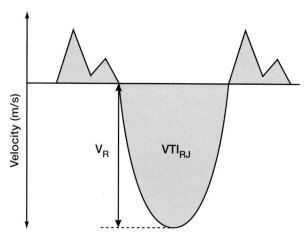

Figure 13.19: Measurement of the Effective Regurgitant Orifice and Regurgitant Volume using the Proximal Isovelocity Surface Area (PISA) Method.
Top, This image represents a colour flow image of the PISA and regurgitant jet. The radial distance (r) is measured between the regurgitant orifice and the aliased velocity (V_N). The radial distance may be optimised by moving the colour Doppler baseline downward to maximise the radius to the first aliased velocity. The aliased velocity (V_N) is recognised as the Nyquist limit on the colour Doppler bar.
Bottom, This image represents the CW Doppler signal of the regurgitant jet measuring the peak regurgitant velocity (V_R) and the velocity time integral (VTI_{RJ}) of the regurgitant jet (shaded area under the Doppler curve).

Simplified Method for Calculation of the Mitral Regurgitant Volume:

Recently, a simplified method for the calculation of the mitral regurgitant volume has been described [47].

This method can be employed when appropriate CW Doppler signals of the mitral regurgitant jet cannot be obtained; in particular, when the regurgitant jet is eccentric. The simplified technique is based on the premise that the ratio between the maximal mitral regurgitant velocity and the VTI of the regurgitant signal

is equal to a constant of 3.25. Hence, the estimated regurgitant volume can be calculated from the regurgitant flow rate and this constant:

(Equation 13.8)

$$RVol = \frac{2 \pi r^2 V_N}{3.25}$$

where RVol = estimated regurgitant volume (cc)
$2\pi r^2$ = area of a hemispheric shell derived from the radius [r] (cm²)
V_N = aliased velocity identified as the Nyquist limit (cm/s)
3.25 = constant

Calculation of the Tricuspid Regurgitant Orifice Area:

Most commonly, the PISA technique is used in the calculation of the mitral EROA; however, this technique can also be used to calculate the aortic EROA and the tricuspid EROA. When using this principle in the calculation of the tricuspid EROA, two important corrections to equation (13.7) are required.

Firstly, it has been found that flattening of the PISA close to the regurgitant tricuspid valve leads to an underestimation of the PISA radius because the aliased velocities (V_N) are a significant proportion of flow velocity at the regurgitant orifice [48]. This error can be corrected by multiplying the flow rate by (V_R / V_R - V_N), where V_R is the peak velocity of the regurgitant signal and V_N is the aliased velocity (Nyquist limit). Secondly, as for mitral stenosis, the global geometry of the regurgitant orifice distorts the PISA such that the isovelocity contours are actually smaller than a hemisphere. This alteration in the shape of the isovelocity contours can be corrected for by multiplying 2π by (α/180), where α is the angle subtended by the valve leaflets. Hence, the equation for the calculation of the tricuspid regurgitant flow rate (Q) in cc/s is expressed:

(Equation 13.9)

$$Q = 2 \pi r^2 V_N \left(\frac{V_R}{V_R - V_N} \right) \left(\frac{\alpha}{180} \right)$$

The tricuspid EROA is, thus, calculated using the following equation:

(Equation 13.10)

$$EROA = \frac{2 \pi r^2 V_N}{V_R - V_N} \left(\frac{\alpha}{180} \right)$$

where EROA = effective regurgitant orifice area (cm²)
$2\pi r^2$ = area of a hemispheric shell derived from the radius [r] (cm²)
V_N = aliased velocity identified as the Nyquist limit (cm/s)
V_R = peak regurgitant velocity (cm/s)
α/180 = angle correction factor

47: Rossi, A. et al.: Journal of the American Society of Echocardiography 11: 138-148, 1998.   48: Rivera, J.M. et al.: American Heart Journal 127: 1354-1362, 1994.

Method of Calculation of the Effective Regurgitant Orifice Area:

As mentioned previously, the EROA calculated by the PISA method can be performed in mitral, aortic or tricuspid regurgitation. However, calculation of the EROA is most commonly performed in patients with mitral regurgitation. Below, is a "step-by-step" method for calculation of the EROA in mitral regurgitation (MR) based on the PISA method. Calculation of the mitral EROA by this technique is also illustrated in Figure 13.20.

Method for the calculation of the EROA in MR by the PISA technique

Step 1: **Optimise the 2-D image of the regurgitant mitral valve orifice:**
   a) from the apical four chamber view
   b) expand on the region of the mitral valve orifice
   c) position the focal zone to level of the valve

Step 2: **Optimise the colour flow Doppler signal of the regurgitant orifice:**
   a) position colour box proximal to mitral valve
   b) decrease aliasing velocity by shifting colour baseline to ~ 30 cm/s

Step 3: **Note the colour aliased velocity (V_N);**
   a) depicted on the colour bar (cm/s)

Step 4: **Measure the radius (r):**
   a) from the first aliased region to mitral valve orifice (cm)

Step 5: **Measure the maximum mitral regurgitant velocity (V_{MR}):**
   a) using CW Doppler
   b) obtain complete Doppler spectrum of regurgitant signal
   c) measure the maximum MR velocity (V_{MR})
   d) convert the velocity measurement to cm/s

Step 6: **Calculate regurgitant flow rate ($Flow_{MR}$):**

$$Flow_{MR} \ (mls/s) = 6.28 \ r^2 \ V_N$$

where $6.28 = 2\pi$

Step 7: **Calculate the effective regurgitant orifice area ($EROA_{MR}$):**

$$EROA_{MR} \ (cm^2) = \frac{Flow_{MR}}{V_{MR}}$$

Step 8: **Convert units of $EROA_{MR}$ from cm² to mm²:**
   a) multiply by 100

Clinical Significance of the Effective Regurgitant Orifice Area and Valvular Regurgitation.

Table 13.10 lists the values which differentiate between the various grades of severity of mitral and aortic regurgitation.

Simplified Method for Evaluating Valvular Regurgitation:

A simplified method for evaluating mitral and tricuspid regurgitation can also be achieved using the flow convergence region proximal to the regurgitant orifice. This method, which simply involves the measurement of the radius of the PISA dome, has been found to separate various angiographic grades of mitral and tricuspid regurgitation (see Table 13.11).

Advantages of the PISA Technique in the Quantification of Valvular Regurgitation.

As mentioned, semi-quantitative echocardiographic techniques such as colour flow imaging are based on the extent of colour flow distribution within the receiving chamber. Eccentric regurgitant jets and other machine factors such as the pulse repetition frequency, colour gain, and the driving pressure of the regurgitant jet may significantly effect the spatial distribution of the regurgitant jet depicted on the colour flow Doppler image. Quantification of the severity of mitral regurgitation by the PISA technique, however, is unaffected by the majority of these factors. Furthermore, calculations based on the PISA method are easier to perform and less time-consuming than the calculation of regurgitant fractions

Table 13.10: Clinical Significance of the EROA and Valvular Regurgitation.

Valve / Severity	EROA (mm²)	Sensitivity	Specificity
Mitral regurgitation: [1]			
Mild	< 20	63%	70%
Moderate	20 - 29	-	-
Moderately severe	30 - 39	-	-
Severe	≥ 40	85%	63%
Aortic regurgitation: [2]			
Severe	≥ 30	90%	90%

Sources: (1) Dujardin, K.S. et al., *Circulation 96: 3409-3415, 1997*: patient population: mild [1] MR = 47; moderate [2] MR = 37; moderately severe [3] MR = 21; severe [4] MR = 75; **(2)** Tribouilloy, C.M. et al., *Journal of the American College of Cardiology 32: 1032-1039, 1998*.

Table 13.11: Clinical Significance of the PISA Radius and Valvular Regurgitation.

Valve / Severity	Aliased Velocity (cm/s)	PISA radius (mm)	Sensitivity	Specificity
Mitral regurgitation: [1]				
Mild	38 cm/s	< 3.5	63%	70%
Moderate		3.5 - 7.5	-	-
Moderately severe		7.5 - 14.5	-	-
Severe		> 14.5	85%	63%
Tricuspid regurgitation: [2]	28 cm/s			
Severe		> 8.5	76 %	91%

Sources: (1) Bargiggia, G.S. et al., *Circulation 8: 148-1489, 1991*: patient population: mild MR = 11; moderate MR = 14; moderately severe MR = 11; severe MR = 9; **(2)** Grossman, G. et al., *European Heart Journal 19: 652-659, 1998*: patient population: mild [1] TR = 22; moderate [2] TR = 24; severe [3] TR = 21.

and regurgitant volumes. Regurgitant volume and regurgitant fraction calculations require multiple measurements from two different flow sites whereas the PISA method only requires the measurement of the radius and the peak regurgitant jet.

The value of the PISA technique in the quantification of prosthetic valve regurgitation has also been recognised [49]. Difficulty in the detection and assessment of mitral prosthetic valve regurgitation is a well known and frequently encountered limitation of transthoracic echocardiography. This important limitation occurs due to masking of the colour flow Doppler signal behind the prostheses. However, detection of mitral prosthetic valve regurgitation can often be identified by the recognition of the flow convergence region proximal to the regurgitant orifice.

Limitations of the PISA Technique in the Quantification of Valvular Regurgitation.
Effective Regurgitant Orifice Area Versus Anatomical Regurgitant Orifice Area.
Calculation of the regurgitant orifice by the PISA technique is determined by measuring the aliased velocity, the radius and the peak regurgitant velocity obtained at one point of the cardiac cycle; thus, providing an estimation of the "effective" regurgitant orifice during that flow period. This concept is particularly important in the evaluation of aortic regurgitation where the regurgitant flow rate by the PISA method and regurgitant velocity are measured in early diastole so that the calculated EROA is actually the *early diastolic* EROA.

In addition, the EROA is smaller than the anatomical regurgitant orifice area.

Radius Measurements.
As mentioned, accurate calculations of a narrowed orifice area by the PISA technique is dependent upon the precise measurement of the radial distance between the narrowed orifice to the first aliased velocity. As the regurgitant orifice is derived by squaring the radius (equation 11.47), failure to measure the correct radius may result in a significant underestimation or overestimation of the EROA. Optimisation of the radial distance can be achieved by shifting the colour Doppler baseline toward the direction of blood flow. This baseline shift results in the magnification of the proximal flow convergence region, a reduction of the aliasing velocity, and an increase in the radial distance. The degree of baseline shift will vary depending upon the regurgitant orifice diameter and the transducer frequency. Aliased velocities that have been used in clinical trials using the PISA technique for the evaluation of valvular regurgitation are listed in Table 13.12.

Atrial Fibrillation.
As mentioned, precise measurement of the radius between the regurgitant orifice to the first aliased velocity is crucial to the accurate calculation of the effective regurgitant orifice area. Therefore, the beat-to-beat variations that occur with atrial fibrillation can be a potential source of error in the measurement of the radius.

49: Yoshida, K., et al.: Journal of the American College of Cardiology 19:333-338,1992.

proximal to the mitral regurgitant orifice. Furthermore, the close proximity of the LVOT to the regurgitant mitral orifice may also alter the overall shape of the flow convergence region.

Mitral Valve Prolapse.

Overestimation of the EROA is problematic in patients with mitral valve prolapse. In these patients, phasic variations of the EROA and regurgitant volume may occur during systole resulting in an overestimation of the EROA by the PISA technique (Figure 13.21). Therefore, measurement of the EROA should be performed in mid to late systole in these patients.

References and Suggested Reading:

Intensity of Regurgitant Signal:
- Bolger, A.F. et al.: Understanding continuous-wave Doppler signal intensity as a measure of regurgitant severity. *Journal of the American Society of Echocardiography 10: 613-622, 1997.*
- Utsunomiya, T. et al.: Can signal intensity of the continuous wave Doppler regurgitant jet estimate severity of mitral regurgitation? *American Heart Journal 123: 166-171, 1992.*

Flow Reversals:
- Diebold, E. et al.: Quantitative assessment of tricuspid regurgitation using pulsed Doppler echocardiography. *British Heart Journal 50: 443-449, 1983.*
- Enriquez-Sarano, M. et al.: Determinants of pulmonary venous flow reversal in mitral regurgitation and its usefulness in determining the severity of regurgitation. *American Journal of Cardiology. 83: 535-541, 1999.*
- Seiler, C. et al.: Quantitation of mitral regurgitation using the systolic/diastolic pulmonary venous flow velocity ratio. *Journal of the American College of Cardiology 31: 1383-1390, 1998.*
- Takenaka, K. et al.: A simple Doppler echocardiographic method for estimating severity of aortic regurgitation. *American Journal of Cardiology 57: 1340-1343, 1986.*
- Tribouilloy, C. et al.: End diastolic flow velocity just beneath the aortic isthmus assessed by pulsed Doppler echocardiography: a new predictor of the aortic regurgitant fraction. *British Heart Journal 65: 37-40, 1991.*

Pressure Half-time in Aortic Regurgitation:
- Beyer, R. W. et al.: Correlation of continuous-wave Doppler assessment of chronic aortic regurgitation with hemodynamics and angiography. *American Journal of Cardiology 60: 852-856, 1987.*
- Dolan, M. S. et al.: Quantification of aortic regurgitation by Doppler echocardiography: A practical approach. *American Heart Journal 129: 10141020, 1995*
- Gozzelino, G. et al.: The effect of heart rate on the slope and pressure half-time of the Doppler regurgitant velocity curve in aortic insufficiency. *Journal of the American Society of Echocardiography 9: 516-526, 1996.*

- Grayburn, P. A. et al.: Quantitative assessment of hemodynamic consequences of aortic regurgitation by means of continuous wave Doppler recordings. *Journal of the American College of Cardiology 10: 135-141, 1987.*
- Griffin, B.P. et al.: The effects of regurgitant orifice size, chamber compliance, and systemic vascular resistance on aortic regurgitant velocity slope and pressure half-time. *American Heart Journal 122: 1049-1056, 1991.*
- Griffin, B.P. et al.: Relationship of aortic regurgitant velocity slope and pressure half-time to severity of aortic regurgitation under changing haemodynamic conditions. *British Heart Journal 15: 681-685, 1994.*
- Labovitz, A. J. et al.: Quantitative evaluation of aortic insufficiency by continuous-wave Doppler echocardiography. *Journal of the American College of Cardiology 8: 1341-1347, 1986.*
- Le, M. et al.: Reappraisal of quantitative evaluation of pulmonary regurgitation and estimation of pulmonary artery pressure by continuous wave Doppler echocardiography. *Cardiology 86: 249-256, 1995.*
- Masuyama, T. et al.: Noninvasive evaluation of aortic regurgitation by continuous-wave Doppler echocardiography. *Circulation 73: 460-466, 1986.*
- Samstad, S. et al.: Half time of the diastolic aortoventricular pressure difference by continuous wave Doppler ultrasound: a measure of the severity of aortic regurgitation? *British Heart Journal 61: 336-343, 1989.*
- Teague, S.M. et al.: Quantification of aortic regurgitation utilizing continuous wave Doppler ultrasound. *Journal of the American College of Cardiology. 8: 592-599, 1986.*
- Wilkenshiff, U. M. et al.: Validity of continuous wave Doppler and colour Doppler in the assessment of aortic regurgitation. *European Heart Journal 15: 1227-1234, 1994.*

Colour Flow Doppler Imaging of Regurgitant Jets:
- Cape, E.G. et al.: Adjacent solid boundaries alter the size of regurgitant jets on Doppler color flow maps. *Journal of the American College of Cardiology 17: 1094-1102, 1991.*
- Chen, C. et al.: Impact of impinging wall jet on color Doppler quantification of mitral regurgitation. *Circulation 84: 712-720, 1991.*
- Dolan, M. S. et al.: Quantification of aortic regurgitation by Doppler echocardiography: A practical approach. *American Heart Journal 129: 1017, 1995.*
- Helmcke, F. et al.: Color Doppler assessment of mitral regurgitation with orthogonal planes. *Circulation 75: 175-183, 1987.*
- McCully, R.B. et al.: Overestimation of severity of ischemic/functional mitral regurgitation by color Doppler jet area. *American Journal of Cardiology 74: 790-793, 1994.*
- Perry, G.J et al.: Evaluation of aortic insufficiency by Doppler color flow mapping. *Journal of the American College of Cardiology. 9: 952-959, 1987.*

- Reynolds, T. et al.: The JH/LVOH method in the quantification of aortic regurgitation: how the cardiac sonographer may avoid an important potential pitfall. *Journal of the American Society of Echocardiography 4: 105-108, 1991.*
- Sahn, D.J.: Instrumentation and physical factors related to visualization of stenotic and regurgitant jets by Doppler color flow mapping. *Journal of the American College of Cardiology 12: 1354-1365, 1988.*
- Chambers, J.B.: Mitral pressure half-time: is it a valid measure of orifice area in artificial heart valves? *Journal of Heart Valve Disease 2: 571-577, 1993.*
- Chen, C. et al.: Reliability of the Doppler pressure half-time method for assessing effects of percutaneous mitral balloon valvuloplasty. *Journal of the American College of Cardiology 13:1309-1313,1989.*
- Come, P.C. et al.: Noninvasive assessment of mitral stenosis before and after percutaneous balloon mitral valvuloplasty. *American Journal of Cardiology 61:817-825,1988.*
- Gonzalez, M.A. et al.: Comparison of two-dimensional and Doppler echocardiography and intracardiac hemodynamics for quantification of mitral stenosis. *American Journal of Cardiology 60:327-332,1987.*
- Hatle, L. et al.: Noninvasive assessment of atrioventricular pressure half-time by Doppler ultrasound. *Circulation 60: 1096-1104, 1979.*
- Oh, J.K. et al.: Characteristic Doppler echocardiographic pattern of mitral inflow velocity in severe aortic regurgitation. *Journal of the American College of Cardiology. 14: 1712-1717, 1989.*
- Nakatani, S. et al. : Value and limitations of Doppler echocardiography in the quantification of stenotic mitral valve area: Comparison of the pressure half-time and continuity equation methods. *Circulation 11: 78-85, 1988.*
- Reid ,C. et al.: Mechanism of increase in mitral valve area and influence of anatomic features in double-balloon catheter balloon valvuloplasty in adults with mitral stenosis: A Doppler and two-dimensional echocardiographic study. *Circulation 76:628-636,1987.*
- Sagar, K.B. et al.: Doppler echocardiographic evaluation of Hancock and Bjork-Shiley prosthetic valves. Journal of the American College of Cardiology 7: 681-687, 1986.
- Smith, M.D. et al.: Comparative accuracy of two-dimensional echocardiography and Doppler pressure half-time methods in assessing the severity of mitral stenosis in patients with and without prior commissurotomy. *Circulation 73: 100-107, 1986.*
- Smith, M.D. et al.: Measurement of mitral pressure half-time in patients with curvilinear spectral patterns. (Abstract) *Circulation 78: II - 78, 1998.*
- Smith, M.D. et al.: Value and limitations of Doppler pressure half-time in quantifying mitral stenosis: A comparison with micromanometer catheter recordings. *Am Heart J 121:480-488,1991.*
- Stamm, R.B., Martin, R.P.: Quantification of pressure gradients across stenotic valves by Doppler ultrasound. *Journal of the American College of Cardiology 2: 707-718, 1983.*
- Tabbalat, R.A., Haft, J.I.: Effect of severe pulmonary hypertension on the calculation of mitral valve area in patients with mitral stenosis. *Am Heart J 121:488-493,1991.*
- Thomas, J.D. et al.: Inaccuracy of mitral pressure half-time immediately after percutaneous mitral valvotomy. *Circulation 78: 980-993, 1988.*
- Thomas, J.D. et al.: Doppler pressure half-time: a clinical tool in search of theoretical justification. *Journal of the American College of Cardiology 10: 923-929, 1987.*
- Wilkins, G.T. et al.: Validation of continuous-wave Doppler echocardiographic measurement of mitral and tricuspid prosthetic valve gradients: A simultaneous Doppler-catheter study. *Circulation 74: 786-795, 1986.*

Proximal Isovelocity Surface Area for Calculation of the Mitral Valve Area:

- Aguilar, J.A. et al.: Calculation of the mitral valve area with the proximal convergent flow method with Doppler-color in patients with mitral stenosis. (English abstract only) *Arch Inst Cardiol Mex 64:257-263,1994.*
- Centamore, G. et al.: Validity of the proximal isovelocity surface area color Doppler method for calculating the valve area in patients with mitral stenosis: Comparison with the two-dimensional echocardiographic method. (English Abstract only) *G Ital Cardiol 22:1201-1210,1992.*
- Deng, Y-B. et al.: Estimation of mitral valve area in patients with mitral stenosis by the flow convergence region method: Selection of aliasing velocity. *Journal of the American College of Cardiology 24:683-689,1994.*
- Rifkin, R.D. et al.: Comparison of proximal isovelocity surface area method with pressure half-time and planimetry in the evaluation of mitral stenosis. *Journal of the American College of Cardiology 26:458-465,1995.*
- Rodriguez, L. et al.: Validation of the proximal flow convergence method: Calculation of orifice area in patients with mitral stenosis. *Circulation 88:1157-1165,1993.*
- Simpson, I.A., Sahn, D.J.: Quantification of valvular regurgitation by Doppler echocardiography. *Circulation (supplement) 84: I-188-I-192, 1991.*
- Spain, M.G. et al.: Quantitative assessment of mitral regurgitation by Doppler color flow imaging: angiographic and hemodynamic correlations. *Journal of the American College of Cardiology 13: 585-590, 1989.*
- Tribouilloy, C. et al.: Assessment of severity of aortic regurgitation by M-mode colour Doppler flow imaging. *European Heart Journal 12: 352-356, 1991.*
- Willems, T.P. et al.: Reproducibility of color Doppler flow quantification of aortic regurgitation. *Journal of the American Society of Echocardiography. 10: 899-903, 1997.*

Regurgitant Fractions:

- Dujardin, K.S. et al.: Grading of mitral regurgitation by quantitative Doppler echocardiography. *Circulation 96: 3409-3415, 1997.*

- Enriquez-Sarano, M. et al.: Quantitative Doppler assessment of valvular regurgitation. *Circulation 87: 841-848, 1993.*
- Goldberg, S.J., Allen, H.D.: Quantitative assessment by Doppler echocardiography of pulmonary or aortic regurgitation. *American Journal of Cardiology 56: 131-135, 1985.*
- Kitabatake, A., et al.: A new approach to noninvasive evaluation of aortic regurgitant fraction by two-dimensional Doppler echocardiography. *Circulation 72:523-529,1985*
- Marx, G.R. et al.: Noninvasive assessment of hemodynamic responses to exercise in pulmonary regurgitation after operations to correct pulmonary outflow obstruction. *American Journal of Cardiology 61: 595-601, 1988.*
- Nishimura, R.A. et al.: Semiquantitation of aortic regurgitation by different Doppler echocardiographic techniques and comparison with ultrafast computed tomography. *American Heart Journal 124: 995-1001, 1992.*
- Reimold, S.C. et al.: Aortic flow velocity patterns in chronic aortic regurgitation: implications for Doppler echocardiography. *Journal of the American Society of Echocardiography 9: 675-683, 1996.*
- Rokey, R., et al.: Determination of regurgitant fraction in isolated mitral or aortic regurgitation by pulsed Doppler two-dimensional echocardiography. *Journal of the American College of Cardiology 7:1273-1278,1986.*
- Touche, T. et al.: Assessment and follow-up of patients with aortic regurgitation by an updated Doppler echocardiographic measurement of the regurgitant fraction in the aortic arch. *Circulation 72: 819-824, 1985.*
- Tribouilloy, C., et al.: Noninvasive measurement of pulsed Doppler echocardiography in isolated pure mitral regurgitation. *British Heart Journal 66:290-294,1991.*
- Xie, G. et al.: A simplified method for determining regurgitant fraction by Doppler echocardiography in patients with aortic regurgitation. *Journal of the American College of Cardiology 24: 1041-1045, 1994.*

Effective Regurgitant Orifice Area:
- Bargiggia, G.S., et al.: A new method for quantitation of mitral regurgitation based on color flow Doppler imaging of flow convergence proximal to regurgitant orifice. *Circulation 84:1481-1489,1991.*
- Cape, E.G. et al.: Cardiac motion can alter proximal isovelocity surface area calculations of regurgitant flow. Journal of the American College of Cardiology 22: 1730-1737, 1993.
- Chen, C., et al.: Noninvasive estimation of regurgitant flow rate and volume in patients with mitral regurgitation by Doppler color mapping of accelerating flow field. *Journal of the American College of Cardiology 21:374-383,1993.*
- Dujardin, K.S. et al.: Grading of mitral regurgitation by quantitative Doppler echocardiography. *Circulation 96: 3409-3415, 1997.*
- Enriquez-Sarano, M. et al.: Color flow imaging compared with quantitative Doppler assessment of severity of mitral regurgitation: influence of eccentricity of jet and mechanism of regurgitation. *Journal of the American College of Cardiology 21: 1211-1219, 1993.*
- Enriquez-Sarano, M. et al.: Effective regurgitant orifice area: a noninvasive Doppler development of an old hemodynamic concept. *Journal of the American College of Cardiology 23: 443-451, 1994.*
- Enriquez-Sarano, M., et al.: Effective mitral regurgitant orifice area: Clinical use and pitfalls of the proximal isovelocity surface area method. *Journal of the American College of Cardiology 25:703-709,1995.*
- Enriquez-Sarano, M. et al.: Changes in effective regurgitant orifice throughout systole in patients with mitral valve prolapse. *Circulation 92: 2951-2958, 1995.*
- Grayburn, P.A., Peshock, R.M.: Noninvasive quantification of valvular regurgitation. *Circulation 94: 119-121, 1996.*
- Grossman, G. et al.: Comparison of the proximal flow convergence method and the jet area method for the assessment of the severity of tricuspid regurgitation. *European Heart Journal 19: 652-659, 1998.*
- Mele, D. et al.: Proximal jet size by Doppler color flow mapping predicts severity of mitral regurgitation. *Circulation 91: 746-754, 1995.*
- Recusani, F., et al.: A new method for quantification of regurgitant flow rate using color Doppler flow imaging of the flow convergence region proximal to a discrete orifice: An in vitro study. *Circulation 83:594-604,1991.*
- Reimold, S.C. et al.: Effective aortic regurgitant orifice area: description of a method based on the conservation of mass. *Journal of the American College of Cardiology 18: 761-768, 1991.*
- Rivera, J.M., et al.: Quantification of mitral regurgitation with the proximal flow convergence method: A clinical study. *American Heart Journal 124: 1289-1296,1992.*
- Riveria, J.M., et al.: Quantification of tricuspid regurgitation by means of the proximal flow convergence method: A clinical study. *American Heart Journal 127:1354-1362,1994.*
- Riveria, J.M., et al.: Effective regurgitant orifice area in tricuspid regurgitation: Clinical implementation and follow-up study. *American Heart Journal 128:927-933,1994.*
- Rossi, A. et al.: Rapid estimation of regurgitant volume by the proximal isovelocity surface area method in mitral regurgitation: can continuous-wave Doppler echocardiography be omitted? *Journal of the American Society of Echocardiography 11: 138-148, 1998.*
- Seiler, C. et al.: Quantitation of mitral regurgitation using the systolic/diastolic pulmonary venous flow velocity ratio. *Journal of the American College of Cardiology 31: 1383-1390, 1998.*

- Shiota, T. et al.: New echocardiographic windows for quantitative determination of aortic regurgitation volume using color Doppler flow convergence and vena contracta. *American Journal of Cardiology 83: 1064-1068, 1999.*

- Simpson, I.A. et al.: Current status of flow convergence for clinical applications: is it a leaning tower of "PISA"? *Journal of the American College of Cardiology 27: 504-509, 1996.*

- Tribouilloy, C.M. et al.: Application of the proximal flow convergence method to calculate the effective regurgitant orifice area in aortic regurgitation. *Journal of the American College of Cardiology 32: 1032-1039, 1998.*

- Utsunomiya, T., et al.: Doppler color flow mapping of the proximal isovelocity surface area: A new method for measuring volume flow rate across a narrowed orifice. *Journal of the American Society of Echocardiography. 4:338-348,1991.*

- Utsunomiya, T. et al.: Doppler color flow "Proximal Isovelocity Surface Area" method for estimating volume flow rate: effects of orifice shape and machine factors. *Journal of the American College of Cardiology 17: 1103-1111, 1991.*

- Vandervoort, P.M. et al.: Application of color Doppler flow mapping to calculate effective regurgitant orifice area. *Circulation 88: 1150-1156, 1993.*

- Xie, G-Y, et al.: Quantification of mitral regurgitant volume by the color Doppler proximal isovelocity surface area method: A clinical study. *Journal of the American Society of Echocardiography. 8:48-54,1995.*

- Yamachika, S. et al.: Usefulness of color Doppler proximal isovelocity surface area method in quantitating valvular regurgitation. *Journal of the American Society of Echocardiography. 10: 159-168, 1997.*

- Yoshida, K. et al.: Value of acceleration flow signals proximal to the leaking orifice in assessing the severity of prosthetic mitral valve regurgitation. *Journal of the American College of Cardiology 19: 333-338, 1992.*

Chapter 14
Doppler Assessment of Left Ventricular Systolic and Diastolic Function

Doppler parameters which can be used in the assessment of left ventricular systolic function include the calculation of the stroke volume and cardiac output, and the dP/dt. Left ventricular diastolic function can be assessed from diastolic filling profiles while "global" left ventricular function (that is, systolic and diastolic function) can be evaluated by the index of myocardial performance.

Stroke Volume and Cardiac Output Calculations

Measurement of the stroke volume and cardiac output can be used in the assessment of systolic ventricular function. As previously mentioned, spectral Doppler velocity measurements, in conjunction with 2-D echocardiographic imaging, can be reliably used to noninvasively measure volumetric flow at specific locations within the heart and great vessels.

Studies validating Doppler-derived stroke volume and cardiac output with other techniques are tabulated in Appendix 12.

Theoretical Considerations:

The theoretical principles of volumetric flow calculations have been discussed in detail under "Volumetric Flow Calculations". Recall that the calculation of volumetric flow is based on a simple hydraulic principle which states that the flow rate (Q) through a tube of a constant diameter is directly proportional to the cross-sectional area (CSA) of the tube and the mean velocity of fluid moving through the tube (V) when the orifice CSA is fixed and the velocity is constant.

Calculation of volumetric flow within the heart becomes more complex because velocity is not constant (in the heart blood flow is pulsatile and changes with systole and diastole as well as throughout the flow period). Therefore, in this situation, volumetric flow can be calculated as the product of the "integrated" velocity over time and the CSA. Furthermore, two important assumptions are made in the calculation of volumetric flow within the heart: (1) that the CSA, which is most commonly derived from a single diameter measurement across a valve annulus or across vessel lumens, has a circular geometry, and (2) that flow is laminar and has a flat profile.

Calculation of the Stroke Volume, Cardiac Output and Cardiac Index:

The **stroke volume** is defined as the volume of blood ejected during one cardiac cycle and is calculated from the following equation:

(Equation 11.1)

$$SV = CSA \times VTI$$

where SV = stroke volume (cc)
VTI = distance a column of blood travels with each stroke (cm)
CSA = cross-sectional area (cm²)

The **cardiac output** is defined as the effective volume of blood ejected by either the right or left ventricle per unit of time. The cardiac output is usually measured as volume per minute; therefore, the cardiac output is a product of the stroke volume and the heart rate:

(Equation 9.11)

$$CO = \frac{SV \times HR}{1000}$$

where CO = cardiac output (L/min²)
SV = stroke volume (cc)
HR = heart rate (bpm)
= R-R interval x 60
1000 = conversion of millilitres (cc) to litres (L).

The **cardiac index** is simply the cardiac output indexed for the body surface area:

(Equation 9.12)

$$CI = \frac{CO}{BSA}$$

where CI = cardiac index (L/min/m²)
CO = cardiac output (L/min)
BSA = body surface area (m²)
= 0.007184 x (weight$^{0.425}$ [kg]) x (height$^{0.725}$ [cm])

Methods for Measuring Stroke Volume and Cardiac Output:

The stroke volume and cardiac output can be measured from any cardiac site using the CSA and VTI. Most commonly, the sites used in the calculation of the stroke volume and cardiac output include all four cardiac valves as well as the ascending aorta and main pulmonary artery. Methods of measurement of the CSA and VTI at each of these various sites is discussed below and summarised in Table 14.1.

Calculation of the Stroke Volume and Cardiac Output using the Left Ventricular Outflow Tract:

Cross-Sectional Area (CSA) Measurements:

The CSA area of the aortic annulus or LVOT is best derived from the diameter of the annulus measured from the parasternal long axis view of the left ventricle. From this view, the annulus diameter (D) is measured, by either 2-D or M-mode echocardiography, as the maximum distance between the hinge points of the anterior and posterior aortic cusps in early systole.

Table 14.1: Method of Measurement of the Cross-sectional Area and Velocity Time Integral for Calculation of the Stroke Volume and Cardiac Output from Various Sites.

Site	CSA Measurement		VTI Measurement	
	Echo View	Phase of Cardiac Cycle	Echo View	PW Sample Volume Position
Ascending aorta	PLAX (LV) at or above sinotubular junction	early systole	suprasternal view	ascending aorta at 3-5 cm toward Asc. Ao. (or CW Doppler)
Aortic annulus	PLAX	early systole	apical 4 chamber apical 5 chamber	LVOT - proximal (just below) AoV
Mitral Inflow:				
Method 1	apical 4 chamber	mid-diastole	apical 4 chamber	mitral annulus
Method 2	apical 4 chamber apical 2 chamber	mid-diastole	apical 4 chamber	mitral annulus
Method 3	PSAX (MV) + MV M-mode	diastole	apical 4 chamber	mitral leaflet tips
Tricuspid inflow	apical 4 chamber	mid-diastole	apical 4 chamber	tricuspid annulus
Pulmonary annulus	PLAX (RVOT) PSAX (RVOT)	early systole	PLAX (RVOT) PSAX (RVOT)	RVOT - proximal to PV
Pulmonary artery	PLAX (RVOT) PSAX (RVOT)	early systole	PLAX (RVOT) PSAX (RVOT)	distal to PV (at same level as diameter measurement)

Abbreviations: AoV = aortic valve; **Asc. Ao.** = ascending aorta; **CSA** = cross-sectional area; **CW** = continuous-wave Doppler; **LVOT** = left ventricular outflow tract; **MV** = mitral valve; **PLAX (LVOT)** = parasternal long axis view of the left ventricle; **PLAX (RVOT)** = parasternal long axis view of the right ventricular outflow tract; **PSAX (MV)** = parasternal short axis view at the level of the mitral valve; **PSAX (RVOT)** = parasternal short axis view at the level of the aorta; **PV** = pulmonary valve; **VTI** = velocity time integral.

Assuming a circular geometry of the aortic annulus, the CSA is calculated by:

(Equation 9.2)

$$Area = 0.785 \times D^2$$

Velocity Time Integral (VTI) Measurements:
The VTI for the LVOT is obtained from the apical five chamber or apical long axis views using PW Doppler. From either of these views, the PW sample volume is positioned just proximal to the aortic valve leaflets (within the LVOT). The VTI is measured by tracing the leading edge of the velocity spectrum.

A simplified method for the calculation of the VTI of the LVOT has been derived using the maximum velocity and the left ventricular ejection time. This simplified measurement is based on the principle that the peak velocity and the flow duration (time) are primary determinants of the VTI [50]; hence:

(Equation 14.1)

$$VTI = V_{max} \times LVET$$

where VTI = velocity time integral (cm)
Vmax = maximum velocity of the left ventricular outflow tract signal (cm/s)
LVET = left ventricular ejection time (s)

Calculation of the Stroke Volume and Cardiac Output using the Ascending Aorta:
Cross-Sectional Area (CSA) Measurements:
The CSA area of the ascending aorta is determined from diameter of the aortic root measured from the parasternal long axis view of the left ventricle. From this view, the diameter (D) is measured at or above the sinotubular junction in early systole by either 2-D or M-mode echocardiography. Assuming a circular geometry of the ascending aorta, the CSA is calculated by:

(Equation 9.2)

$$Area = 0.785 \times D^2$$

Velocity Time Integral (VTI) Measurements:
The VTI for the ascending aorta is obtained from the suprasternal window using either CW Doppler or PW Doppler. When using CW Doppler, the ultrasound beam is manipulated to ensure that the maximum velocity is obtained. When using the PW Doppler, the sample volume is positioned within the ascending aorta at a depth of between 3 to 5 cm. The VTI is measured by tracing the leading edge of the velocity spectrum.

Calculation of the Stroke Volume and Cardiac Output using the Main Pulmonary Artery:
Cross-Sectional Area (CSA) Measurements:
The CSA area of the main pulmonary artery (MPA) is determined from maximum diameter of this vessel as

50: Derias, S.L et al.: Circulation 72 (supplement III): III-351, 1985. (n = 41, r = 0.924, SEE = 1.6 cm, y = 0.64 x + 0.92).

measured from either the parasternal long axis or parasternal short axis views of the RVOT. From these views, the diameter (D) is measured across the vessel lumen in early systole. Assuming a circular geometry of the MPA, the CSA is calculated by:

(Equation 9.2)

$$Area = 0.785 \times D^2$$

Velocity Time Integral (VTI) Measurements:
The VTI for the MPA is obtained from either the parasternal long axis or parasternal short axis views of the RVOT using PW Doppler. The sample volume is positioned at the same location from which the diameter measurement is made. The VTI is measured by tracing the leading edge of the velocity spectrum.

Calculation of the Stroke Volume and Cardiac Output using the Right Ventricular Outflow Tract:
Cross-Sectional Area (CSA) Measurements:
The CSA area of the pulmonary annulus or right ventricular outflow tract (RVOT) is determined from the diameter of the annulus measured from either the parasternal long axis or parasternal short axis views of the RVOT. From these views, the annulus diameter (D) is measured as the maximum distance between the insertion of the anterior and posterior pulmonary leaflets in early systole. Assuming a circular geometry of the annulus, the CSA is calculated by:

(Equation 9.2)

$$Area = 0.785 \times D^2$$

Velocity Time Integral (VTI) Measurements:
The VTI for the RVOT is obtained from either the parasternal long axis or parasternal short axis views of the RVOT using PW Doppler. The sample volume is positioned just proximal to the pulmonary valve leaflets. The VTI is measured by tracing the leading edge of the velocity spectrum.

Calculation of the Stroke Volume and Cardiac Output using the Mitral Valve:
Cross-Sectional Area (CSA) Measurements:
Several methods have been described for the calculation of the CSA of the mitral valve including (1) measurement of the annulus diameter assuming a circular geometry, (2) measurement of the valve annulus in two planes and assuming an elliptical geometry, and (3) measurement of the valve area at the leaflet tips with correction of this area by the mean-to-maximum leaflet separation to derive a mean flow area (orifice method).

Method 1:
2-D echocardiographic calculation of the CSA of the mitral valve annulus can be determined from a single measurement of the valve annulus from the apical four

chamber view. From this view, the maximal diameter (D) is measured from the hinge points of the posterior and anterior mitral leaflets in the mediolateral plane. Since the area of the mitral annulus increases about 12% from end systole to end diastole [51], the diameter measurement should be performed in mid-diastole. Assuming that the annulus is circular, the CSA is derived by:

(Equation 9.2)

$$Area = 0.785 \times D^2$$

Method 2:
This method for the calculation of the CSA of the mitral valve was derived to account for the fact that the mitral valve annulus is elliptical in shape rather than circular. Determination of the CSA by this method requires that two measurements of the mitral annulus are made in perpendicular planes. Usually measurements of the mitral annulus are made from the apical four and two chamber views. Since the area of the mitral annulus increases about 12% from end systole to end diastole [51], the diameter should be measured in mid-diastole. Assuming that the annulus is elliptical in shape, the CSA is calculated by:

(Equation 11.2)

$$area = \frac{\pi}{4} a\, b$$

where area = area of an ellipse (cm²)
     a = annular diameter in one plane (cm)
     b = annular diameter in a plane perpendicular to [a] (cm)

Method 3:
This method for calculation of the mitral CSA is derived from both 2-D and M-mode echocardiography. Using this method, the maximum valve area is derived by planimetry of the largest mitral valve orifice from the parasternal short axis view. However, because the MVA does not maintain this maximal area throughout diastole, this value must be corrected. The correction factor is derived by the ratio of the mean-to-maximum diastolic mitral leaflet separation obtained by M-mode (Figure 14.1). Hence, the *mean mitral flow area* is derived from the product of the maximum valve area and the mean-to-maximum ratio. This method is commonly referred to as the mitral orifice method.

Technical Consideration:
In routine clinical practice, method (1) is considered to be method of choice for calculating the mitral CSA for stroke volume and cardiac output calculations due to its ease of measurement and relative accuracy (see Appendix 12).

51: Ormiston, J.A. et al.: Circulation 64: 113-120, 1981.

Velocity Time Integral (VTI) Measurements:
Measurement of the VTI for the mitral valve is obtained from the apical four chamber view using PW Doppler. Positioning of the sample volume is dependent upon the method used to determine the CSA. When the CSA is derived by either method (1) or method (2), the sample volume should be positioned at the level of the mitral annulus as there is less change in the CSA of flow at this level than at the leaflet tips. Thus, the flow profile is relatively flat.

When the CSA is derived by method (3), the sample volume should be positioned at the tips of the mitral leaflets.

For all methods, the VTI is measured tracing the modal velocity. The modal velocity reflects the dominant flow velocity at any given instant in time and is identified as the darkest velocity signal on the spectral Doppler display.

Calculation of the Stroke Volume and Cardiac Output using the Tricuspid Valve:
Cross-Sectional Area (CSA) Measurements:
2-D echocardiographic calculation of the CSA of the tricuspid valve annulus can be determined from a single measurement of the valve annulus from the apical four chamber view at mid-diastole. Assuming that the annulus is circular, the CSA is derived by:

(Equation 9.2)

$$Area = 0.785 \times D^2$$

Velocity Time Integral (VTI) Measurements:
Measurement of the VTI for the tricuspid valve is obtained from the apical four chamber view using PW Doppler. The sample volume should be positioned at the level of the tricuspid annulus. The VTI is measured tracing the modal velocity, which reflects the dominant flow velocity at any given instant in time, and is identified as the darkest velocity signal on the spectral Doppler display.

Technical Consideration:
The LVOT is the most common site for the calculation of the stroke volume and cardiac output because: (1) in most patients, the LVOT can be measured with greater ease and accuracy than any other area of the heart, (2) the LVOT can be measured in the axial plane of the transducer (axial resolution is generally better than the lateral resolution), (3) the LVOT diameter is nearly circular so that calculation of the CSA is more accurate and closer to the true area, (4) the CSA of the LVOT is constant throughout systole (atrioventricular valve areas are constantly changing during diastole), and (5) flow within the entrance of the LVOT has a flat flow profile.

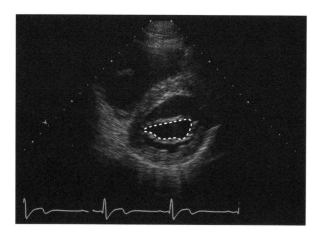

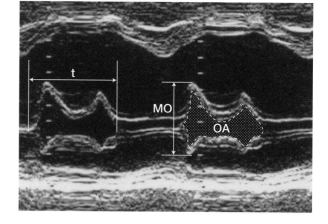

$$mean-to-maximal\ opening = \left(\frac{OA}{t}\right) \div MO$$

mean mitral flow area = mean-to-maximal opening x maximal valve area

Figure 14.1: Measurement of the Mean-to-Maximum Diastolic Mitral Leaflet Separation.
The maximal MVA can be measured from the parasternal short axis view by planimetry of the mitral valve orifice during diastole *(left)*. However, since the mitral valve does not maintain this maximal area throughout diastole, the maximal area must be corrected. Essentially, changes in the valve area are proportional to changes in anteroposterior diameter throughout diastole. The changes in the anteroposterior diameter can be depicted on the mitral M-mode trace *(right)*. By this technique, the ratio of mean-to-maximal opening can be derived. Three measurements are required to measure this ratio: (1) the *maximal opening (MO)* of the mitral valve, which is measured as the maximal separation of the anterior and posterior E points or A points (depending on which is larger); (2) the *opening area (OA)* enclosed by the two leaflets (*shaded area*); and (3) the *diastolic time interval (t)* which is measured as the distance between the D and C points of the mitral valve. From these measurements, the *mean opening* of the two leaflets is obtained dividing OA by t. The mean-to-maximal opening is then obtained by dividing the *mean opening* by the *maximal opening*. The *mean mitral flow area* is then derived by the product of the maximum valve area and the mean-to-maximum ratio. Variations to this technique have also been described [52, 53, 54].

52: Dittmann. H. et al.: Journal of the American College of Cardiology. 10: 818-823, 1987. 53: DeZuttere, D. et al.: Journal of the American College of Cardiology 11: 343-350, 1988. 54: Hoit, B.D. et al.: American Journal of Cardiology 62: 131-135, 1988

Normal Values for the Stroke Volume, Cardiac Output, and Cardiac Index:
The normal values for the stroke volume, cardiac output and cardiac index are listed in Table 14.2.

Method of Measurement of the Stroke Volume and Cardiac Output:
Below (boxed) is a "step-by-step" method for calculating the stroke volume and cardiac output using the left ventricular outflow tract.

Limitations to Stroke Volume and Cardiac Output Calculations:
Assumptions of Volumetric Flow Calculations:
Volumetric flow calculations are based on a simple

hydraulic formula that determines the volumetric flow rate through a cylindrical tube under steady flow conditions. Therefore, in applying this concept to the heart, the following assumptions are made: (1) flow is occurring in a rigid, circular tube, (2) there is a uniform velocity across the vessel, (3) the derived CSA is circular, (4) the CSA remains constant throughout the period of flow, and (5) the sample volume remains in a constant position throughout the period of flow. However, blood vessels are elastic, changing throughout the duration of flow within the cardiac cycle. In addition, annular diameters may change throughout the period of flow and, while the left and right ventricular outflow tracts assume a circular configuration, the same may not be said for the atrioventricular valves, which assume a more elliptical shape.

Table 14.2: Normal values for stroke volume, cardiac output and cardiac index

Parameter	Normal Range
Stroke Volume (cc)	75 - 100
Cardiac Output (L/min)	4 - 8
Cardiac Index (L/min/m²)	2.8 - 4.2 (mean 3.4)

Source: Schlant, R. and Alexander R.W.: <u>Hurst's. The Heart.</u> 8th Edition McGraw-Hill, Inc. pp: 141, 503, 1994

Error in VTI Measurements:
Technical errors in the VTI measurements include the following (1) *failure to optimise the Doppler velocity spectrum:* inadequate beam alignment with blood flow (a large angle θ) will lead to suboptimal Doppler signals and underestimation of the peak velocity, (2) *failure to correctly measure the VTI:* the modal velocity (darkest,

---

Method for determining the stroke volume using the left ventricular outflow tract

Step 1:   **measure the left ventricular outflow tract (LVOT) diameter:**
- from the parasternal long axis view of the LV during systole
- measured at the level of the aortic annulus
- measured from the inner edge to the inner edge of aortic cuspal insertion

Step 2:   **calculate the LVOT area:**
- assuming a circular shape of the LVOT, the LVOT area can be calculated:

$$CSA = 0.785 \times D^2$$

Step 3:   **measure the LVOT VTI:**
- from the apical five chamber view
- P-W Doppler sample volume is positioned in the centre of LVOT about 0.5 - 1.0 cm proximal to aortic valve
- VTI is traced along the leading velocity

Step 4:   **calculate the stroke volume (SV):**

$$SV \ (cc) = CSA \ (cm^2) \times VTI \ (cm)$$

Step 5:   **calculate the heart rate (HR):**
- measure the R-R interval using the ECG
- the HR is calculated by using the following formula :

$$HR \ (bpm) = 60 \div R\text{-}R$$

Step 6:   **calculate the cardiac output (CO):**

$$CO \ (L/\min) = \frac{SV \times HR}{1000}$$

brightest line) should be traced when measuring the VTI from the AV valves while the leading edge velocity should be measured when using the left or right ventricular outflow tracts or the aorta or pulmonary artery, and (3) *measuring too few beats:* for sinus rhythm it is recommended that 3 to 5 beats are measured and averaged while for atrial fibrillation, 8 to 10 beats should be measured and averaged.

Another error which may occur lies in the assumption that, when using PW Doppler, the sample volume position is constant. However, the sample volume position may vary with respiration and during the cardiac cycle. For example, when sampling the mitral annulus, the plane of the annulus moves apically during systole and posteriorly with diastole. Furthermore, respiratory variations in the flow profile are commonly seen in the Doppler velocity spectrum on the right-side of the heart.

Calculation of stroke volume and cardiac output is also based on the assumption that the flow profile measured is flat. While this assumption is essentially true in the outflow tracts and at the annulus of the semilunar valves, certain conditions exist whereby the flow profile is not uniform. For example, flow divergence occurs within a ventricular chamber or in a dilated aortic root. Furthermore, alterations in vessel geometry such as curvature of a vessel and asymmetry of the outflow tract, may cause the peak velocities to shift away from the centre of the lumen. And finally, the flow profile is not uniform in the presence of turbulent flow. Therefore, under these circumstances, the volumetric flow cannot be accurately calculated.

Error in Diameter Measurement:
Technical errors in the diameter measurement will be reflected in the calculation of the CSA and, hence, the volumetric flow. Technical errors which may occur include: (1) measurement of the diameter during the wrong phase of the cardiac cycle (measurement of CSA must be performed at the time of flow through that site), (2) inconsistent annulus measurement, (3) difficulty in measuring the RVOT (it is not possible to measure the pulmonary artery in the direction of axial resolution and it is often difficult to measure the left lateral border of the RVOT due to adjacent lung tissue), and (4) any error in the diameter measurement is magnified in the area calculation (recall that the CSA is derived by squaring the diameter [equation 9.2]).

Furthermore, calculations of the stroke volume and cardiac output assume that the CSA remains constant throughout the period of flow. Although this assumption is essentially true for the LVOT where the CSA of the annulus does not change significantly from diastole to systole [55], the same cannot be said for other regions of the heart. The CSA of the ascending aorta increases 2 to 11% during systole whereas the CSA of the pulmonary artery may increase up to 18% [56]. In addition, mitral annulus area, on average, increases 12% from end-systole to end-diastole [57].

Another error arises from the assumption that the flow area and the anatomic CSA of the vessel or annulus are identical.

Overestimation of the Cardiac Output with Valvular Regurgitation or Stenosis:
Valvular regurgitation:
There must be little or no regurgitation through the valve used to determine the cardiac output. For example, when there is aortic regurgitation, calculation of the cardiac output using the LVOT will include the regurgitant volume as well as forward stroke volume; thus, overestimating the cardiac output.

Valvular stenosis:
The stroke volume and cardiac output will also be overestimated if these measurements are calculated through a stenotic valve. In valvular stenosis, the gradients and, therefore, flow will be increased across the stenotic valve.

dP/dt in Left Ventricular Systolic Function Assessment
Indices obtained during the ejection phase of the cardiac cycle are commonly used to assess left ventricular systolic function. However, these indices are influenced by loading conditions of the heart. Indices obtained during the nonejection phase of the cardiac cycle are less dependent on loading conditions and have, therefore, been used in the assessment of left ventricular systolic function. The dP/dt is one such measurement. The peak positive dP/dt is a measure of the rate of rise of ventricular pressure during isovolumic contraction.

Until recently, the dP/dt was typically derived from the left ventricular pressure curve obtained at cardiac catheterisation. With the advent of Doppler echocardiography, the dP/dt can now be accurately measured noninvasively from the mitral regurgitant CW Doppler signal (see Appendix 13).

The velocity of the mitral regurgitant signal reflects the instantaneous pressure gradient between the left ventricle and left atrium during systole. Assuming that the left atrial pressure does not increase significantly during the isovolumic contraction phase, the rate of rise of the Doppler velocity reflects the rate of rise of left ventricular pressure.

Measurement of the dP/dt is performed by measuring the time interval between two arbitrary points on the mitral regurgitant velocity spectrum (usually between 1 and 3 m/s). Using the modified Bernoulli equation, the velocity can be converted to pressure; hence, the pressure difference between these two arbitrary points can be determined. For example, the pressure difference between 1 and 3 m/s is 32 mm Hg. Therefore, the dP/dt, which measures the change in pressure over time, is defined as the time it takes for the left ventricle to generate 32 mm Hg of pressure during the isovolumic

55: Ihlen, H. et al.: British Heart Journal 51: 54-60, 1984. 56: Greenfield, J.C. et al.: Circulation Research 10: 557-559 and 778-781, 1962. 57: Ormiston, J.A. et al.: Circulation 64: 113-120, 1981.

contraction time (Figure 14.2):

(Equation 14.2)

$$dP/dt = \frac{32}{\Delta t}$$

where dP/dt = rate of pressure rise over time
           (mm Hg/s)
    32   = the pressure difference between 1 m/s
           and 3 m/s using the modified
           Bernoulli equation:
           $(4 \times 3^2) - (4 \times 1^2) = 32$ mm Hg
    Δt = time period between 1 m/s and 3 m/s
           points (seconds)

The dP/dt can also be used in the assessment of right ventricular systolic function using the tricuspid regurgitant signal. When using the tricuspid regurgitant jet, the time interval between 0 and 2 m/s is usually measured. Hence, using the modified Bernoulli equation, the *pressure difference* between 0 and 2 m/s is 16 mm Hg. Therefore, the dP/dt, which measures the change in pressure over time, is derived from time it takes for the right ventricle to generate 16 mm Hg of pressure during the isovolumic contraction time.

Method of Measurement of the dP/dt:
Below (boxed), is the "step-by-step" method for calculation of the dP/dt from the mitral regurgitant Doppler signal.

Clinical significance of the dP/dt in the assessment of left ventricular systolic function.
In the setting of left ventricular systolic dysfunction, there is prolongation of the dP/dt (see Figure 14.3).

Values indicating the relationship between the dP/dt and left ventricular systolic function are listed in Table 14.3.

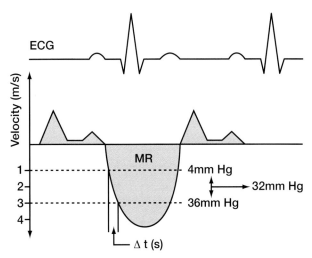

Figure 14.2: Measurement of the dP/dt from the Mitral Regurgitant Doppler Signal.
From the CW Doppler signal of the mitral regurgitant jet, the time interval between 1 and 3 m/s is measured in seconds. Using the modified Bernoulli equation, the velocity can be converted to pressure so that the *pressure difference* between 1 and 3 m/s can be determined: $(4 \times 3^2) - (4 \times 1^2) = 32$ mm Hg. Therefore, the dP/dt, which measures the change in pressure over time, is derived from time it takes for the left ventricle to generate 32 mm Hg of pressure during the isovolumic contraction time.

Method of calculating the dP/dt

Step 1:   **optimise the CW Doppler signal of the mitral regurgitant signal:**
      a) obtain complete Doppler spectrum
      b) best signal usually from apical window

Step 2:   **maximise Doppler envelope from zero baseline to 4 m/s:**
      a) move zero baseline upward
      b) reduce velocity scale
      c) increase sweep speed ($\geq$ 100 mm/s)

Step 3:   **calculate the dP/dt:**
      a) the rate of pressure rise (dP) is estimated using the modified Bernoulli equation and the time (dt) taken
          for the MR signal to change from 1 m/s to 3 m/s
      b) mark MR jet at 1 m/s
      c) mark MR jet at 3 m/s
      d) measure the time interval (dt) between these two points in seconds
      f) dP/dt is calculated from the following formula:
 	
      $dP/dt = \dfrac{32}{\Delta t}$

Table 14.3: Clinical significance of the dP/dt in the assessment of left ventricular systolic function.

Left Ventricular Systolic Function	dP/dt Values (mm Hg/sec)	Time taken for LV to generate 32 mm Hg
Normal	> 1,200	< 0.027 sec (27 ms)
Mild-moderate dysfunction	800 - 1,200	0.027 - 0.040 sec (27 ms - 40 ms)
Severe dysfunction	< 800	> 0.040 sec (40 ms)

Source: Nishimura, R.A. and Tajik, A.J.: Quantitative hemodynamics by Doppler echocardiography: A noninvasive alternative to cardiac catheterization. *Progress in Cardiovascular Disease 4: 332,1994.*

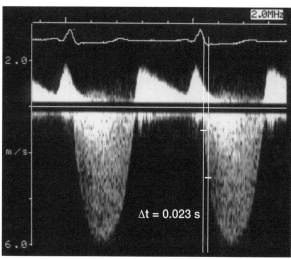

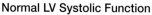

Normal LV Systolic Function

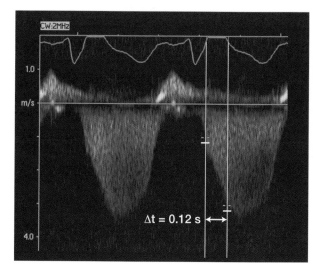

Poor LV Systolic Function

Figure 14.3: The Relationship between the dP/dt and Left Ventricular Systolic Function.
Left, This is measurement of the dP/dt of the mitral regurgitant signal in a patient with normal left ventricular (LV) systolic function. The time interval between 1 and 3 m/s is 0.023 s. Thus, the dP/dt is equal to 32 ÷ 0.023 or 1391 mm Hg/s.
Right, This is measurement of the dP/dt of the mitral regurgitant signal in a patient with a severe reduction in left ventricular systolic function. Observe the obvious prolongation of the ascending limb of the regurgitant signal during the isovolumetric contraction phase compared with the image on the left. The time interval between 1 and 3 m/s is 0.120 s. Thus, the dP/dt is equal to 32 ÷ 0.107 or 267 mm Hg/s.

Limitations of dP/dt in the Assessment of Left Ventricular Systolic Function:
Acute Mitral Regurgitation:
As mentioned, the CW Doppler signal of the mitral regurgitant jet reflects the instantaneous pressure gradient between the left ventricle and the left atrium during systole. The dP/dt is calculated based on the assumption that the left atrial pressure is insignificant during the pre-ejection period of ventricular contraction and that the atrium is compliant. However, in acute mitral regurgitation, the left atrium is noncompliant and the pressure in the atrium during isovolumic contraction may be elevated.

Inadequate Doppler signal:
Suboptimal Doppler signals of the mitral regurgitant jet may occur when there is poor alignment of the Doppler beam with the regurgitant jet direction. This is particularly problematic with eccentric jets. Under these circumstances, calculation of the dP/dt will be underestimated. Another problem which may affect the accuracy of this measurement is valve click artefact which may obscure the early mitral regurgitant Doppler profile.

Significant aortic stenosis or hypertension:
Patients with significant aortic stenosis or hypertension may have normal dP/dt even when there is impaired systolic performance.

Diastolic Function Assessment
Two-dimensional echocardiography has become the method of choice for the noninvasive evaluation of systolic ventricular function in patients with signs and symptoms of heart disease. More recently, the importance of diastolic function of the ventricle has been recognised as a contributing factor in the signs and symptoms of heart disease. In most cardiac disease processes, abnormalities of diastolic function often precede the development of systolic dysfunction. In fact, approximately 30% of patients congestive heart failure have normal systolic function [58].

Diastolic dysfunction of the left ventricle produces signs and symptoms of heart failure due to an elevation of left ventricular filling pressures which increases left atrial pressure. This increase in left atrial pressure is reflected back to the pulmonary circulation and causes symptoms of shortness of breath and signs of pulmonary congestion.

58: Dougherty, A.H. et al: American Journal of Cardiology 54:778-782, 1984.

Until recently, the assessment of diastolic function was only possible via invasive cardiac catheterisation. The evolution of Doppler echocardiography has now provided a means for the noninvasive evaluation of diastolic function and has, thus, become an integral addition to the routine echocardiographic examination.

This section aims to cover the basic concepts of diastolic function. For a more comprehensive review of the principles and practice of diastolic function assessment of the heart, readers are referred to the many excellent articles listed in the references at the end of this chapter.

Background:

The term "Diastole" originates from the Greek word that means "to draw asunder or expansion" of the heart. While many definitions of diastole exist, it is best defined as the time period beginning at the end of ventricular ejection (at the closure of the semilunar valves) and extending to the closure of the atrioventricular valves. Therefore, in simple terms, diastole refers to the filling of the ventricle while normal diastolic function refers to the ability of the ventricle to fill without an abnormal increase in diastolic pressure. Diastole, however, is far from simple. In fact, diastole is a complex process consisting of several interrelated events which ultimately result in filling of the ventricle during this period. Abnormalities or impairment of any one of these factors can alter diastolic function by increasing the resistance to filling of the ventricle. Therefore, in order to sustain filling and to maintain the cardiac output, this resistance to filling is compensated for by an increase in atrial pressures.

Essentially, diastolic function is primarily dependent upon two processes: (1) relaxation of the ventricle, and (2) compliance or stiffness of the ventricle. Like myocardial contraction, *relaxation* of the ventricle is an active and energy dependent process and largely modulates filling of the ventricle during early diastole. Following completion of relaxation, filling of the ventricle during mid and late diastole is governed by the *compliance* of the ventricle, which is defined as the change in pressure within the ventricle for a change in volume (dP/dv). Diastolic dysfunction occurs early in disease processes of the myocardium. Relaxation abnormalities occur first, followed later by changes in ventricular compliance.

Diastolic function of the left ventricle (LV) can be determined from the measurements of diastolic filling indices which are derived from the mitral inflow and pulmonary venous Doppler flow profiles. Diastolic function of the right ventricle can be determined from the measurements of diastolic filling indices which are derived from the tricuspid inflow, hepatic venous, and superior vena caval Doppler flow profiles.

While diastolic function of both the right or left ventricles can be assessed, this section will primarily concentrate on the assessment of the diastolic function of the left ventricle. Furthermore, it is important to remember that diastolic function reflects ventricular physiology and is NOT specific for any particular disease process.

> The following section aims to review the factors which contribute to the production of the Doppler flow profiles through each of these regions and does not discuss the techniques used to obtain these flow profiles. The technique for obtaining Doppler flow profiles through each of these regions is described in detail in: "The Spectral Doppler Examination".

Review of the phases of diastole of the mitral valve inflow:

In order to develop a comprehensive understanding of the complex processes of diastole as well as be able to interpret the Doppler findings, it is important to have a sound knowledge of the normal diastolic flow profiles and the properties that contribute to these flow profiles.

The period of diastole can be divided into four phases: (1) the isovolumic relaxation phase, (2) the early or rapid filling phase, (3) diastasis or the slow filling phase, and (4) the atrial filling phase. Each of these phases is depicted on the mitral inflow Doppler profile (Figure 14.4). Measurement of these indices is used in the assessment of diastolic function of the left ventricle.

1. Isovolumic relaxation phase:

This phase of diastole occurs immediately after ventricular ejection when both the mitral and the aortic valves are closed.

Immediately following ventricular ejection, myocardial relaxation occurs. This is a process whereby the myocardial cells return to their presystolic length and tension. Myocardial relaxation is a complex, active, energy-dependent process.

Relaxation of the LV causes the pressure within the ventricle to decrease rapidly. When the LV pressure falls below that of the aortic pressure, the ejection of blood into the aorta ceases and the aortic valve closes. At this stage, the mitral valve is also closed as the LV pressure is still greater than the left atrial (LA) pressure. Thus, during the isovolumic relaxation phase, the LV volume remains constant as there is no filling or emptying of the ventricle. Hence, the **isovolumic relaxation phase** is defined as the period between the closure of the aortic valve and the opening of the mitral valve.

The duration of relaxation (or the isovolumic relaxation time) is determined by several factors including: (1) cessation of excitation-contraction coupling, (2) loading conditions of the LV (preload or LA pressure), and (3) age (relaxation lengthens with advancing age).

The Normal Spectral Doppler Display:

The **isovolumic relaxation phase** is identified as the time interval between aortic valve closure and mitral valve opening and is, therefore, also referred to as the isovolumic relaxation time or IVRT. The IVRT is depicted when both the mitral inflow signal and the LVOT signal are displayed on the same spectral trace.

It is important to remember the measurement of the IVRT is not a measure of the rate of ventricular relaxation but rather a measurement of the time of isovolumic relaxation.

As mentioned, this interval is affected by a number of factors. Importantly, the IVRT is prolonged by a slowing of the relaxation rate of the ventricle. However, this interval is also affected by LA pressure (Figure 14.5).

2. Early and rapid filling phase:

Following the isovolumic relaxation phase, the pressure within the LV falls below that of the LA resulting in the mitral valve opening and the beginning of the early, rapid filling phase of the LV.

Early diastolic filling is primarily determined by four factors: (1) the rate of relaxation of the LV, (2) the elastic recoil of the ventricle (suction), (3) chamber compliance, and (4) the LA pressure. All of these factors together contribute to the driving pressure (pressure gradient) between the LA and LV which propels blood forward through the mitral valve into the LV.

As the LV fills in early diastole, the LV volume and, thus, the LV pressure increases. *At the same time*, the LA empties and the LA volume and pressure decreases. Hence, the diastolic pressure gradient between the LA and LV decreases. The rate at which the diastolic gradient between the LA and LV declines reflects the rate of LV filling and the rate of LA emptying. Normally, the rate of LV filling and LA emptying is rapid. Approximately 80% of LV filling occurs during this phase.

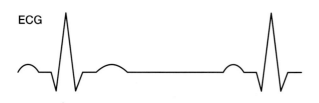

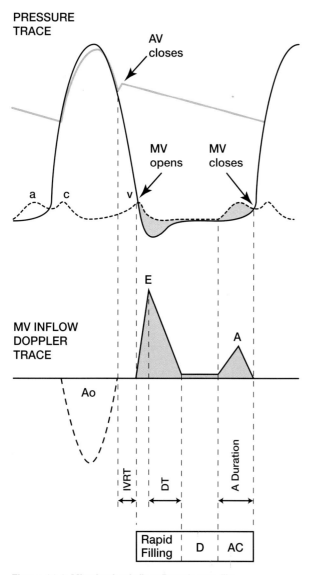

Figure 14.4: Mitral valve inflow Doppler profile.
This schematic illustrates the relationship between the mitral inflow Doppler signal and the cardiac cycle by comparing the pressure traces from the aorta, left ventricle and left atrium with the transmitral Doppler velocity trace (see text for details).
Abbreviations: AC = atrial contraction; **Ao** = aortic Doppler velocity curve; **AV** = aortic valve; **D** = diastasis; **DT** = deceleration time; **IVRT** = isovolumic relaxation time; **LA** = left atrium; **LV** = left ventricle; **mv** = mitral valve.

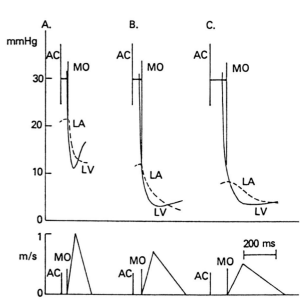

Figure 14.5: Effect of Left Atrial Pressure on the Left Ventricular Isovolumic Relaxation Time (IVRT).
In this schematic, only the early diastolic pressures of the left atrial (LA) and left ventricular (LV) pressure curves are displayed; furthermore, the rate of LV relaxation is assumed to be constant. The IVRT is the time interval between aortic valve closure and mitral valve opening (*AC-MO* interval).
A, When the LA pressures increase, the LV and LA pressures crossover earlier than normal and, thus, mitral valve also opens earlier than normal. Hence, the AC-MO interval becomes shorter and the early diastolic pressure gradient increases resulting in increased transmitral flow.
B, When LA pressure is normal, mitral valve opening occurs later and at a time with less rapid LV pressure decrease.
C, When the LA pressure is decreased, the LV and LA pressures crossover later than normal resulting in a prolongation of the AC-MO interval. Furthermore, there is a smaller transmitral pressure gradient and subsequent reduction in transmitral flow.
From Appleton, C.P et al.: The natural history of left ventricular filling abnormalities: Assessment by two-dimensional and Doppler echocardiography. *Echocardiography 9: 440, 1992.* Reproduced with permission from Futura Publishing Company, Inc.

The Normal Spectral Doppler Display:
The early, rapid filling phase creates the **peak E wave** of the mitral inflow Doppler trace. The rapidity of LV filling (or LA emptying) is reflected as a rapid and steady fall in the Doppler velocities throughout this early filling phase. This rate of decline in pressures and, thus, Doppler velocities is reflected by the **deceleration rate or slope**. Since the rate of deceleration is relatively linear, the deceleration slope of the Doppler velocity spectrum can be extrapolated to the zero baseline and the deceleration time can be derived. The deceleration time is measured as the interval between the peak E wave velocity and the point of deceleration extrapolated to the zero baseline. Note that the deceleration time rather than deceleration slope is measured because it is less affected by the peak E velocity (refer to Figure 14.6).

3. Diastasis:
Following the early, rapid filling phase, the pressures within the LA and LV begin to equalise. Despite this equilibrium of pressures, reduced blood flow continues across the mitral valve due to inertia. This phase of diastole is referred to as **diastasis**.
The duration of diastasis is essentially determined by the heart rate. Bradycardia demonstrates a longer period of diastasis while diastasis maybe totally absent with tachycardia.

The Normal Spectral Doppler Display:
On the Doppler spectral trace, the decreased flow during diastasis is reflected as low, uniform velocities close to the zero baseline.

4. Atrial filling phase:
The atrial filling phase occurs following atrial contraction. With atrial contraction there is a small increase in the LA-LV pressure gradient which results in a further bolus of blood being propelled into the LV. This phase of diastole contributes approximately 15 to 20% of total LV filling.

The Normal Spectral Doppler Display:
The atrial filling phase creates a second peak on the mitral inflow trace referred to as the **peak A wave**.

> **E at A:**
> Another measurement which may be obtained from the Doppler trace of mitral inflow is the "E at A" velocity. This velocity is a measure of the E wave velocity at the onset of atrial contraction. This variable becomes important with higher heart rates. When this velocity exceeds 20 cm/s, it indicates that the A wave velocity is significantly higher than it would be a slower heart rates. In these cases, the E/A ratio will be reduced and is not comparable with that which would be derived when the "E at A" is less than 20 cm/s [59].

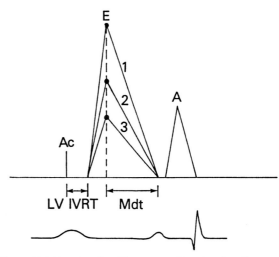

Figure 14.6: Deceleration Time versus Deceleration Slope.
This schematic illustrates that the mitral deceleration time (Mdt) is less velocity dependent than the deceleration slope (DS). Observe in this example that the Mdt is equal at all three peak E wave velocities. However, the DS, which is derived from the peak E wave velocity divided by the deceleration time, varies at each different peak E wave velocity.
Abbreviations: Ac = aortic valve closure; **LV IVRT** = left ventricular isovolumic relaxation time.
From Appleton, C.P et al.: The natural history of left ventricular filling abnormalities: Assessment by two-dimensional and Doppler echocardiography. *Echocardiography 9: 439, 1992.* Reproduced with permission from Futura Publishing Company, Inc.

Review of the phases of diastole of the pulmonary venous inflow:
As with all venous flow, pulmonary venous flow is continuous throughout the cardiac cycle; that is, flow occurs throughout diastole and systole. Normal pulmonary venous flow is characterised by three distinct waveforms: (1) systolic forward flow, (2) diastolic forward flow, and (3) atrial flow reversal (Figure 14.7).

1. Systolic forward flow:
Systolic forward flow occurs as a result of LA relaxation and the descent of the mitral annulus toward the cardiac apex with ventricular systole (corresponds to the x descent on the atrial pressure curve). Systolic forward flow is biphasic in approximately 37% of normal individuals [60].
In the presence of a biphasic S velocity, the first, early peak (S_1) is related to atrial relaxation. Atrial relaxation lowers the LA pressure promoting pulmonary venous return into the LA which increases the LA volume. The second peak (S_2) which occurs in mid to late systole is produced by an additional increase in LA volume as the mitral annulus descends toward the cardiac apex with ventricular systole.
Pulmonary venous systolic forward flow is also closely related to the LA pressure. When LA pressure is elevated, systolic filling from the pulmonary veins is reduced.

59: Appleton, C.P. et al.: Echocardiography 9: 437-457, 1992. 60: Klein, A.L. et al.: Mayo Clinic Proceedings 69:212-224,1994.

The Normal Spectral Doppler Display:
Systolic forward flow creates the systolic peak on the pulmonary venous Doppler trace and is referred to as the **S wave**.

2. Diastolic forward flow:
Diastolic forward flow occurs in diastole when there is an open conduit between the pulmonary veins, the LA, the open mitral valve, and the LV (corresponds to the y descent on the atrial pressure curve). Pulmonary venous diastolic flow essentially parallels that of the mitral E velocity and deceleration time.

The Normal Spectral Doppler Display:
Diastolic forward flow creates the diastolic peak on the pulmonary venous Doppler trace and is referred to as the **D wave**. Normally, diastolic forward flow velocity is slightly less than the systolic forward flow velocity.

3. Atrial flow reversal:
Atrial flow reversal (AR) refers to retrograde flow back into the pulmonary vein secondary to atrial contraction. With atrial contraction, blood is ejected from the LA into the LV and also backward into the pulmonary veins. The magnitude and duration of this flow reversal during atrial systole is determined by the transmitral and atriovenous pressure gradients which are influenced by LA systolic function, and LA and LV compliance.

The Normal Spectral Doppler Display:
Atrial flow reversal creates a retrograde peak on the pulmonary venous Doppler trace corresponding to atrial contraction (the P wave on the ECG).

Indices of Diastolic Function:
The indices which are commonly measured in the assessment of diastolic function are listed in Table 14.4. Factors affecting Doppler indices used in the assessment of diastolic function of the LV are listed in Table 14.5.

Normal Values:
Filling is progressively delayed in the aging ventricle as myocardial relaxation slows and wall thickness increases. For this reason, normal values of diastolic filling indices have been derived over various age groups (see Tables 14.6 and 14.7 and Figures 14.8 and 14.9).

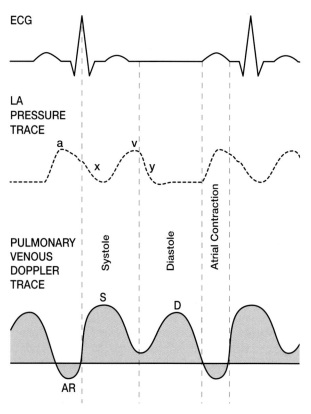

Figure 14.7: The Normal Pulmonary Venous Spectral Doppler Trace.
This schematic illustrates the relationship between the pulmonary venous Doppler signal and the cardiac cycle by comparing the pressure trace from the left atrium with the pulmonary venous Doppler velocity trace (see text for details).
Abbreviations: AR = atrial reversal; **D** = diastolic forward flow; **S** = systolic forward flow.

Table 14.4: Diastolic Function Indices.

Left Ventricle:	
Mitral Valve Inflow	peak E velocity
	peak A velocity
	E/A ratio
	A wave duration
	DT
	IVRT
Pulmonary Venous Inflow	peak S velocity
	peak D velocity
	peak atrial reversal velocity
	AR duration
Right Ventricle:	
Tricuspid Valve Inflow	peak E velocity
	peak A velocity
	E/A ratio
	DT
Hepatic Venous Inflow	peak S velocity
	peak D velocity
	peak AR velocity
Superior Vena Caval Flow	peak S velocity
	peak D velocity
	peak AR velocity

Table 14.5: Haemodynamic factors affecting transmitral and pulmonary venous flow profiles.

Doppler Index	LA Factors	LV Factors
Mitral E wave velocity *	LA pressure LA compliance	LV relaxation LV contractility LV compliance myocardial viscoelasticity interventricular interaction
Mitral A wave velocity **	LA pressure LA contractility PR interval	LV compliance pericardial constraint coronary perfusion myocardial viscoelasticity
Deceleration time	LA pressure	myocardial relaxation LV pressure LV compliance passive filling
IVRT	LA pressure	LV pressure rate of LV relaxation
Pulmonary venous systolic velocity	LA contractility LA relaxation LA pressure LA compliance LA size PR interval	LV contractility (mitral annular motion)
Pulmonary venous diastolic velocity *	LA pressure LA compliance	LV relaxation LV contractility LV compliance myocardial viscoelasticity interventricular interaction
Pulmonary venous atrial reversal velocity **	LA pressure LA contractility LA compliance PR interval	LV compliance pericardial restraint coronary perfusion myocardial viscoelasticity

*   Observe that the factors affecting the pulmonary venous diastolic velocity are the same as those which affect mitral E wave velocity.

** Observe that the factors affecting the pulmonary venous atrial reversal velocity are the same as those which affect mitral A wave velocity.

Table 14.6: Normal Values for Diastolic Function Indices in the Adult Population based on age < or > 50 years.

Doppler Parameters	Normal Values	
	Age 21 - 49 yrs	**Age ≥ 50 yrs**
Mitral Valve Inflow: [1]	**n = 61**	**n = 56**
Peak E wave (cm/s)	72 ± 14 (44 - 100)	62 ± 14 (34 - 90)
Peak A wave (cm/s)	40 ± 10 (20 - 60)	59 ± 14 (31 - 87)
E/A ratio	1.9 ± 0.6 (0.7 - 1.3)	1.1 ± 0.3 (0.5 - 1.7)
DT (ms)	179 ± 20 (139 - 219)	210 ± 36 (138-282)
IVRT (ms)	76 ± 11 (54 - 98)	90 ± 17 (56 – 124)
Pulmonary Venous Inflow: [1]	**n = 44**	**n = 41**
Peak S velocity (cm/s)	48 ± 9 (30 - 66)	71 ± 9 (53 – 89)
Peak D velocity (cm/s)	50 ± 10 (30 - 70)	38 ± 9 (20 – 56)
Peak AR velocity (cm/s)	19 ± 4 (11 - 27)	23 ± 14 (-5 – 51)
Tricuspid Valve Inflow: [2]	**n = 61**	**n = 56**
Peak E wave (cm/s)	51 ± 7 (37 - 65)	41 ± 8 (25 – 57)
Peak A wave (cm/s)	27 ± 8 (11 - 43)	33 ± 8 (17 – 49)
E/A ratio	2.0 ± 0.5 (1.0 - 3.0)	1.34 ± 0.4 (0.5 – 2.1)
DT (ms)	188 ± 22 (144 - 232)	198 ± 23 (152 – 244)
Superior Vena Cava: [2]	**n = 59**	**n = 53**
Peak S velocity (cm/s)	41 ± 9 (23 - 59)	42 ± 12 (18 – 66)
Peak D velocity (cm/s)	22 ± 5 (12 - 32)	22 ± 5 (12 – 32)
Peak AR velocity (cm/s)	13 ± 3 (7 - 19)	16 ± 3 (10 – 22)

* Normal reference values for Doppler measurements of diastolic function in two age groups of normal subjects. Data presented are mean value ± standard deviation (confidence interval).

Sources: (1) Klein, A.L. et al.: *Mayo Clinic Proceedings 69:218, 1994*; **(2)** Klein, A.L. et al.: *Cleveland Clinic Journal of Medicine 59:281, 1992.*

Table 14.7: Normal Values for Diastolic Function Indices in Children*.

Doppler Parameter	Age 3 – 8 yrs, n = 75	Age 9 – 12 yrs, n = 72	Age 13 – 17 yrs, n = 76
Mitral Valve Inflow:			
Peak E wave (cm/s)	92 ± 14	86 ± 15	88 ± 14
Peak A wave (cm/s)	42 ± 11	41 ± 9	39 ± 8
E/A ratio	2.4 ± 07	2.2 ± 0.6	2.3 ± 0.6
A duration (ms)	136 ± 22	142 ± 21	141 ± 22
DT (ms)	145 ± 18	157 ± 19	172 ± 22
IVRT (ms)	62 ± 10	67 ± 10	74 ± 13
Pulmonary Venous Inflow:			
Peak S velocity (cm/s)	46 ± 9	45 ± 9	41 ± 10
Peak D velocity (cm/s)	59 ± 8	54 ± 9	59 ± 11
Peak AR velocity (cm/s)	21 ± 4	21 ± 5	21 ± 7
AR duration (ms)	130 ± 20	125 ± 20	140 ± 28
PV AR/MV A duration	0.96 ± 0.19	0.88 ± 0.16	0.98 ± 0.23

* Normal reference values for Doppler measurements of diastolic function in three age groups of normal children. Data presented are mean value ± standard deviation.

Source: O'Leary, P.W. et al.: *Mayo Clinic Proceedings 73:616-628,1998.*

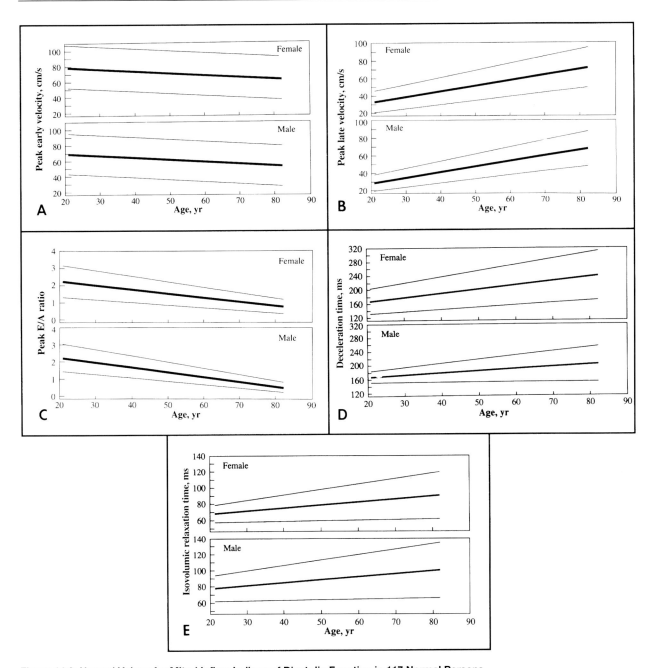

Figure 14.8: Normal Values for Mitral Inflow Indices of Diastolic Function in 117 Normal Persons.
Peak early velocity, peak late velocity, peak E/A ratio, deceleration time, and isovolumic relaxation time in female and male subjects are shown by increasing age.
Boldface lines = mean values; *lightface lines* = 95% confidence limits.
From Klein, A.L. et al.: Effects of age on left ventricular dimensions and filling dynamics in 117 normal persons. *Mayo Clinic Proceedings 69: 219, 1994*. Reproduced with permission from Mayo Clinic Proceedings.

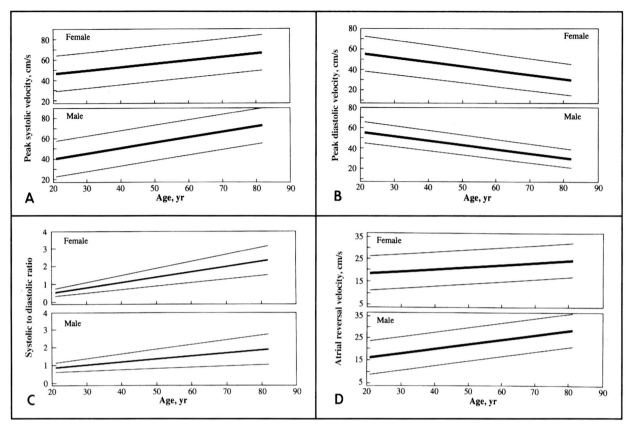

Figure 14.9: Normal Values for Pulmonary Venous Flow Indices of Diastolic Function in 85 Normal Persons.
Pulmonary venous peak systolic velocity, diastolic velocity, systolic to diastolic ratio, and atrial reversal velocity in female and male subjects are shown by increasing age.
Boldface lines = mean values; *lightface lines* = 95% confidence limits.
From Klein, A.L. et al.: Effects of age on left ventricular dimensions and filling dynamics in 117 normal persons. *Mayo Clinic Proceedings 69: 217, 1994*. Reproduced with permission from Mayo Clinic Proceedings.

Abnormal Diastolic Function:

Remember that diastolic dysfunction can occur in the presence or absence of systolic dysfunction. Doppler echocardiography can indirectly assess LV diastolic function by analysis of LV inflow (mitral inflow) and LA inflow (pulmonary venous flow). Right ventricular diastolic function can be primarily assessed by examination of right ventricular inflow (tricuspid inflow) and right atrial inflow (hepatic veins and superior vena cava).

The principal goals of the Doppler assessment of diastolic function are twofold: (1) to determine by noninvasive means whether or not abnormalities in LV relaxation and/or compliance are present, and (2) to define if the filling pressures are normal or elevated.

Diastolic filling abnormalities are broadly classified into three categories: (1) abnormal relaxation, (2) restrictive physiology (or filling), and (3) pseudonormalisation. The third category, the pseudonormal flow profile, is a transitional phase between abnormal relaxation and restrictive physiology and signifies increased filling pressure and decreased compliance. Each of these categories is discussed in detail below.

Abnormal Relaxation

As the term suggests, abnormal relaxation refers to impaired relaxation of the LV during diastole.

Doppler profile of abnormal relaxation:

Abnormal relaxation of the ventricle means that the LV relaxation occurs at a slower than normal rate. Therefore, because ventricular relaxation is slowed, the fall in ventricular pressure is also slowed so that the normal crossover between the LA and LV pressures is delayed. This delay in the crossover between the LA and LV pressures, delays the opening of the mitral valve and reduces the early transmitral pressure gradient. Therefore, abnormal relaxation results in prolongation of the IVRT and a reduction in the peak E wave velocity. In addition, the deceleration time (DT) is also prolonged. Prolongation of the DT occurs as a longer time is required for the LA and LV pressures to equilibrate because of the slower than normal fall in LV pressure. Furthermore, because early ventricular filling is reduced, there is an increase in compensatory filling with atrial contraction. Therefore, due to the reduction in the early diastolic filling velocity (peak E wave) and the increased filling velocity with atrial contraction (peak A wave), the E/A ratio is reduced.

The pulmonary venous Doppler profile is characterised by a decrease in the diastolic pulmonary venous forward flow (D wave) and predominant pulmonary venous forward flow during systole (S wave). This can be simply explained by considering the fact that there is reduced ventricular filling in early diastole. Therefore, it follows that there will be less filling of the atrium via the pulmonary veins during diastole. Furthermore, because atrial filling is reduced during diastole, there is a compensatory increase atrial filling with systole. The duration and magnitude of pulmonary venous AR may be normal or increased depending on the left ventricular end-diastolic pressure (see "Assessment of Left Ventricular Filling Pressures" later in the section).

Figure 14.10 illustrates the typical LV, LA and aortic pressure traces and the mitral inflow and pulmonary venous Doppler profiles seen with abnormal relaxation. Typical examples of cardiac disease that produce an abnormal relaxation profile include LV hypertrophy (hypertension and aortic stenosis), hypertrophic cardiomyopathy, myocardial ischaemia/infarction and infiltrative cardiomyopathies (during early stage of the disease).

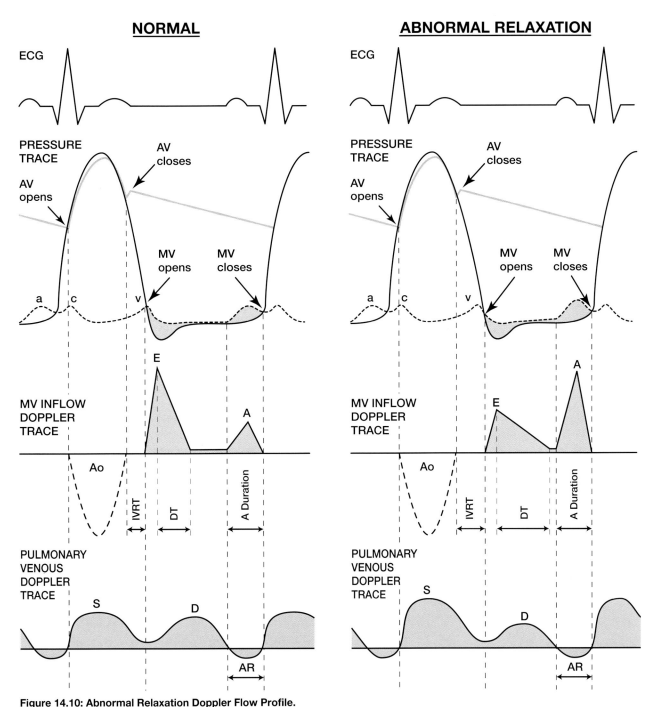

Figure 14.10: Abnormal Relaxation Doppler Flow Profile.
Left, This schematic illustrates the aortic, LV and LA pressure curves and the mitral inflow and pulmonary venous Doppler flow profiles under normal conditions. *Right,* This schematic illustrates the aortic, LV and LA pressure curves and the mitral inflow and pulmonary venous Doppler flow profiles seen with abnormal relaxation. Observe that with abnormal relaxation the following changes occurs: (1) prolongation of the IVRT, (2) reduced peak E wave velocity, (3) prolongation of the deceleration time, (4) increased peak A wave velocity, (5) reduced E/A ratio, (6) decreased pulmonary venous D velocity, and (7) increased pulmonary venous S velocity.

Restrictive Physiology or Filling

At this point, it is important to differentiate "restrictive cardiomyopathy" from "restrictive physiology or filling". Restrictive physiology or filling can be present in any heart disease or in a combination of diseases that produce decreased LV compliance and a subsequent marked increase in the LA pressure. Restrictive cardiomyopathy, on the other hand, refers to a myocardial disease process which impairs LV filling due to an increase in intrinsic myocardial stiffness.

Doppler profile of restrictive physiology:

As mentioned, the restrictive filling pattern occurs as a result of a severe reduction in LV compliance and a subsequent increase in ventricular filling pressures (LA pressure). It is important to note that myocardial relaxation is still impaired in these individuals but is now masked by the marked increase in LA pressure.

As for abnormal relaxation, ventricular relaxation is slowed so that the fall in ventricular pressure is also slowed. However, because LA pressure is greatly increased, the crossover between the LA and LV pressures is not delayed. In fact, mitral valve opening occurs earlier than normal. Therefore, the increased LA pressure increases the transmitral gradient in early diastole (increased peak E wave) and the early opening of the mitral valve results in shortening of the IVRT. Furthermore, increased early diastolic flow into the noncompliant ventricle results in a rapid increase in early LV diastolic pressure with rapid equalisation of LV and LA pressures. This results in shortening of the deceleration time and an increase in the left ventricular end-diastolic pressure (LVEDP). Finally, because of the high LVEDP, little or no filling occurs with atrial contraction (reduced or absent peak A wave). Therefore, due to the increase in the early diastolic filling velocity (peak E wave) and the decreased filling velocity with atrial contraction (peak A wave), the E/A ratio is increased (usually greater than 2.0).

The pulmonary venous Doppler profile is characterised by an increase in the diastolic pulmonary venous forward flow (D wave) and a reduction in forward flow during systole (S wave). This can be simply explained by considering the fact that there is rapid ventricular filling in diastole due to the elevated LA pressure and decreased LV compliance. Therefore, it follows that there must be increased filling of the atrium via the pulmonary veins during diastole. Furthermore, because atrial filling occurs predominantly during diastole, there is a decrease in atrial filling with systole.

Furthermore, because of the elevation in the LVEDP, atrial contraction into a stiff, noncompliant ventricle, results in increased blood flow into the pulmonary veins. This results in increased flow reversal into the pulmonary veins during atrial contraction (AR velocity). In addition, the duration of flow reversal with atrial contraction (AR wave) is longer than that for the mitral A wave. This phenomenon is explained by the elevated LVEDP.

The length of the mitral A wave is essentially determined by the LVEDP so that the mitral A wave ends when the LVEDP reaches the LA pressure. Therefore, when the LVEDP is increased, there is an early crossover of LA and LV pressures which shortens the mitral A wave duration. The pulmonary venous AR duration, however, is governed by the LA and pulmonary venous pressures and is not directly affected by the LVEDP. It is important to note that it is the *difference* between the durations of the mitral A wave and the pulmonary venous AR wave that is relevant and not the absolute durations of each.

Diastolic mitral and/or tricuspid regurgitation may be present in those patients with restrictive physiology. Diastolic mitral and/or tricuspid regurgitation is indicative of a marked increase in ventricular diastolic pressure that exceeds the atrial pressure resulting in reversal of flow through the AV valves during diastole.

Figure 14.11 illustrates the typical LV, LA and aortic pressure traces and mitral inflow and pulmonary venous Doppler profiles seen with restrictive physiology.

Restrictive filling is associated with greater filling pressures, more symptoms and a worsened prognosis. Typical examples of cardiac disease that produce restrictive physiology include decompensated congestive heart failure, advanced restrictive cardiomyopathy, severe coronary artery disease, constrictive pericarditis, and acute, severe aortic regurgitation.

Pseudonormalisation

In most cardiac diseases, a transition from abnormal relaxation to restrictive physiology can be seen. During this transitional phase, the transmitral inflow may resemble a normal diastolic filling profile. This profile is a result of decreased LV compliance in conjunction with a moderate increase in LA pressure superimposed on an abnormal relaxation profile. This pattern is referred to as "pseudonormalisation" to indicate that although LV filling appears normal there are significant abnormalities of LV diastolic function.

Doppler profile of pseudonormalisation:

Pseudonormalisation occurs when there is an underlying impairment of relaxation together with worsening ventricular compliance. In this situation, the mitral inflow Doppler profile may appear normal. Recall that with abnormal relaxation of the ventricle, ventricular relaxation and the fall in ventricular pressure occurs at a slower than normal rate. With pseudonormalisation, there is also a concurrent increase in the LA pressure. This increase in LA pressure results in a higher driving pressure across the mitral valve. Therefore, the abnormally low mitral E velocity that is typical of abnormal relaxation may increase to reach normal level. Furthermore, if there is also a decrease in the effective compliance of the ventricle, ventricular pressure rises more rapidly in early diastole and the abnormally long deceleration time that is typically seen with abnormal relaxation shortens. The end result is a "normal" mitral inflow curve.

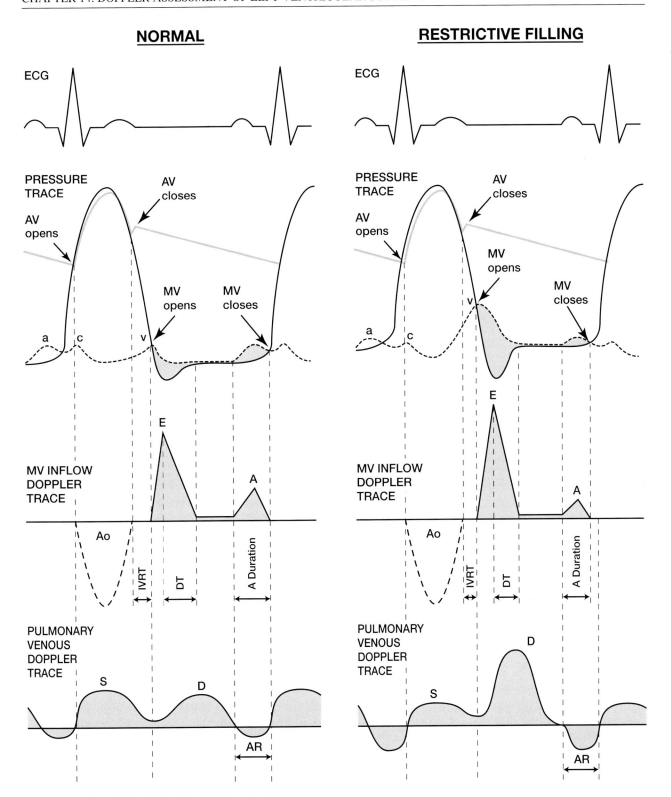

Figure 14.11: Restrictive Filling Doppler Flow Profile.
Left, This schematic illustrates the LV and LA pressure curves and the mitral inflow and pulmonary venous Doppler flow profiles under normal conditions. *Right,* This schematic illustrates the LV and LA pressure curves and the mitral inflow and pulmonary venous Doppler flow profiles seen with restrictive physiology. Observe that with restrictive physiology the following changes occurs: (1) shortening of the IVRT, (2) increased peak mitral E wave velocity, (3) shortening of the deceleration time, (4) decreased peak mitral A wave velocity, (5) shortening of the mitral A wave duration when compared to the pulmonary venous AR duration, (6) increased E/A ratio, (7) increased pulmonary venous D velocity, (8) decreased pulmonary venous S velocity, and (9) increased pulmonary atrial reversal velocity.

Pseudonormalisation is, thus, difficult to differentiate from normal using the mitral inflow Doppler profile alone. The simplest method which can be employed in the recognition of a pseudonormal filling pattern is obtained from the pulmonary venous Doppler trace. In particular, patients with a pseudonormal filling pattern have an elevated LVEDP. As described previously in restrictive physiology, elevation of the LVEDP can be identified by: (1) an increase in flow reversal into the pulmonary veins with atrial contraction and/or (2) by shortening of the duration of the mitral A wave compared with pulmonary venous AR duration with atrial contraction (Figure 14.12).

Figure 14.13 summarises the typical findings associated with the different diastolic flow profiles described above.

Other Methods used to Identify a Pseudonormal Filling Pattern.

While the pulmonary venous flow profile can be used to unmask a pseudonormal flow profile, pulmonary venous flow may be difficult to measure or obtain. Fortunately, there are several other methods which can be used to identify a pseudonormal filling pattern. These methods include: (1) the recognition of other ancillary findings, (2) the Valsalva manoeuvre, (3) colour M-mode Doppler flow propagation velocities, and (4) Doppler tissue imaging. Each of these methods is discussed below.

1. Other ancillary findings:

In patients with abnormal LV size, systolic dysfunction, or increased wall thickness, abnormal relaxation is expected. Therefore, a normal E/A ratio is suggestive of an elevation in the LA pressure which is masking the abnormal relaxation. The presence of an increased LA size also suggests elevation in the LA and diastolic LV pressures.

2. Valsalva manoeuvre:

The pseudonormal flow profile on mitral inflow is produced when there is abnormal relaxation and an elevation of the LA pressure. The Valsalva manoeuvre can be used to unmask abnormal relaxation by reducing the LA pressure (Figure 14.14).

The Valsalva manoeuvre is performed by instructing the patient to suspend breathing at the end of normal inspiration and then to strain down without breathing at expiration. An adequate Valsalva manoeuvre is defined as a 10% reduction in the maximal E velocity from baseline [61].

3. Colour M-Mode Propagation Velocity:

Conventional pulsed-wave Doppler permits the determination of time, direction and velocity at a single spatial location which is depicted by the sample volume. Colour M-mode Doppler, on the other hand, allows the acquisition of information about velocity, time and space along the entire line of the M-mode cursor. Using this technique, it is possible to accurately assess the transmitral flow propagation velocity from the mitral annulus across the cavity of the LV (Figure 14.15).

Recent studies have demonstrated that the rate of transmitral flow propagation velocity reflects changes in the rate of LV relaxation. Furthermore, this propagation slope appears relatively independent of preload. For these reasons, this modality may prove useful in the identification of patients with pseudonormal mitral inflow (Figure 14.16).

Significance of the flow propagation velocity:

The normal flow propagation velocity is 0.84 ± 0.11 m/s (ranges from 0.68 to 1.05 m/s) [62].

Abnormal relaxation results in significant slowing of this velocity. Pseudonormalisation can be identified when the flow propagation velocity is less than 0.50 m/s [63].

4. Doppler Tissue Imaging:

Conventional Doppler echocardiography permits the determination of the velocity and direction of blood flow through the heart and great vessels throughout the cardiac cycle as a function of time. Doppler tissue imaging (DTI), on the other hand, records systolic and diastolic Doppler velocities within the myocardium and at the corners of the mitral annulus.

Theoretical considerations:

Before discussing the role of DTI in the assessment of diastolic function of the LV, it is important to recognise the principal differences between conventional PW Doppler and DTI. Firstly, conventional Doppler echocardiography sets filters to detect signals within the ranges of intracardiac blood flow velocities (15 to 100 cm/s). Secondly, the amplitude of signals arising from moving blood cells is fairly low (0 to 15 dB). However, myocardial Doppler signals have important acoustic differences compared with blood (Figure 14.17). Firstly, myocardial wall motion velocity is much slower than blood flow velocity (usually less than 10 cm/s). Secondly, the Doppler signal intensity of wall motion is much greater than that of the Doppler signals arising from red blood cells (greater than 40 dB). For these reasons, adjustments must be made to record low-velocity, high-intensity myocardial signals. Current DTI settings measure velocities in a range of 0.2 to 40 cm/s and detect amplitudes of greater than 20 dB.

DTI velocities may be displayed as either spectral PW Doppler velocities or colour-encoded M-mode or 2-D mode. However, for the purpose of diastolic function assessment, DTI velocities are best displayed as spectral PW Doppler velocities because this modality provides high temporal and velocity range resolution as well as displaying quantitative velocity information.

61: Dumesnil, J.G et al.: American Journal of Cardiology 68: 517, 1991. 62: Brun, P. et al.: Journal of the American College of Cardiology 20:420-432,1992. 63: Scalia, G.M. and Burstow, D.J.: Circulation 100 (suppl):I-295, 1999.

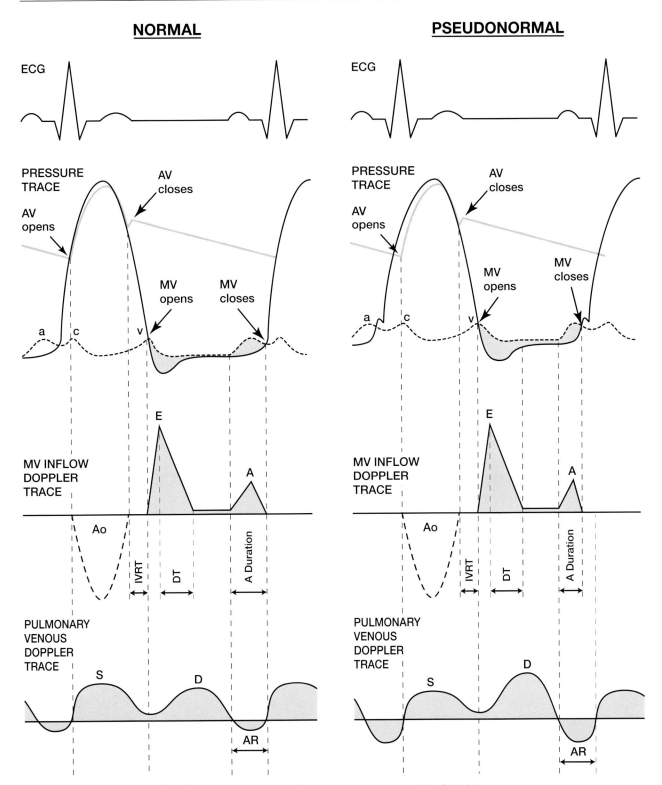

Figure 14.12: Recognition of the Pseudonormal Flow Profile using Pulmonary Venous Doppler.

Left, This schematic illustrates the LV and LA pressure curves and the mitral inflow and pulmonary venous Doppler flow profiles under normal conditions. Observe that: (1) the duration of the mitral A velocity is dependent on the point of crossover of the LA and LV pressure traces following atrial contraction, and (2) in the pulmonary veins, atrial contraction leads to a small amount of blood being displaced retrograde into the pulmonary veins (the velocity of this retrograde flow is relatively small as the majority of blood in the LA is propelled forward into the LV).

Right, This schematic illustrates the LV and LA pressure curves and the mitral inflow and pulmonary venous Doppler flow profiles seen with pseudonormalisation. Observe that when LV compliance decreases, there is an abnormal increase in the LVEDP. Therefore, following atrial contraction, the increase in LV pressure is greater than the increase in LA pressure. This results in the early termination of the mitral A wave due to the earlier than normal crossover of the LVEDP and LA pressures. Furthermore, atrial contraction into a stiff, noncompliant ventricle results in an increase in the retrograde flow velocity into the pulmonary veins as forward flow into the LV is impeded because of the abnormal increase in LVEDP. The duration of flow reversal into the pulmonary veins with atrial contraction is not affected by the increased LVEDP and, therefore, continues throughout atrial systole exceeding the duration of the mitral A wave.

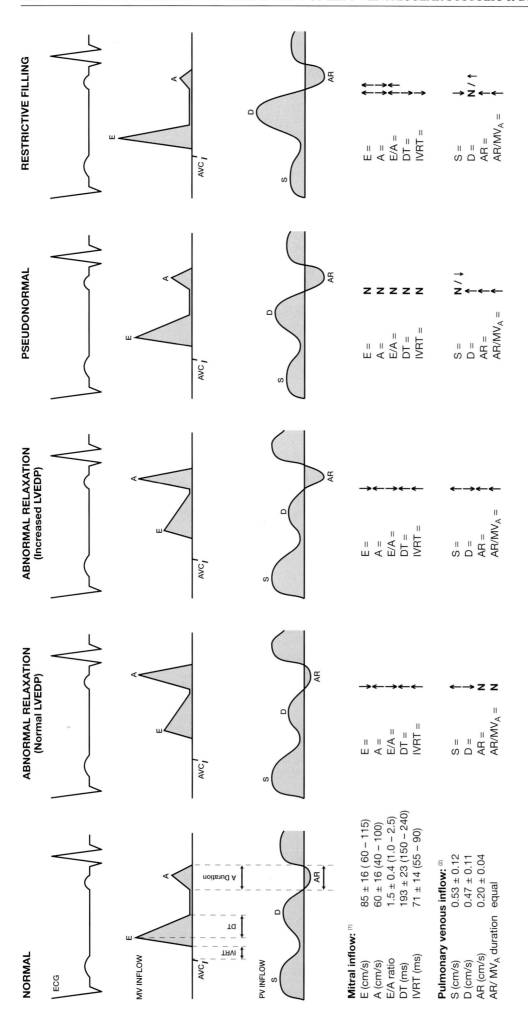

Figure 14.13: Schematic illustration of the transmitral and pulmonary venous Doppler flow profiles seen in different diastolic filling patterns.
Observe that with abnormal relaxation, the LVEDP may be either normal or elevated. An elevated LVEDP is suggested when there is: (1) an increase in the pulmonary venous AR velocity with atrial contraction, and/or (2) by an increase in the AR/MV$_A$ duration with atrial contraction (due to shortening of the duration mitral A wave).

Sources for normal values: (1) Appleton, C.P. et al.: *Journal of the American College of Cardiology 11:757-768, 1988*; (2) Masuyama, T. et al.: *American Journal of Cardiology 67: 1396-1404, 1991.*

Abbreviations: AR/MV$_A$ = pulmonary venous AR velocity to mitral atrial velocity ratio; **AVC** = aortic valve closure; **DT** = deceleration time; **IVRT** = isovolumic relaxation time; **LVEDP** = left ventricular end-diastolic pressure; **MV** = mitral valve; **PV** = pulmonary venous.

NORMAL   PSEUDONORMAL

BASELINE   **BASELINE**

VALSALVA   **VALSALVA**

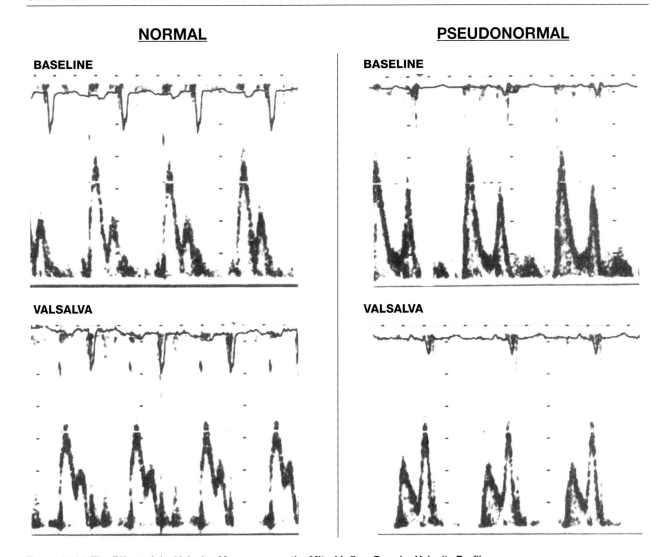

Figure 14.14: The Effect of the Valsalva Manoeuvre on the Mitral Inflow Doppler Velocity Profile.

Upper left panel, This is a transmitral flow profile at rest and *bottom left* is the transmitral flow profile during the Valsalva manoeuvre in a patient without evidence of heart disease. Observe that in patients with normal LV relaxation and normal LA pressure, a reduction in venous return during the Valsalva manoeuvre results in an overall decrease of LV filling velocities without significant change in the E/A ratio. That is, there is a fall in both the E and A velocities with the E/A ratio remaining greater than 1.0.

Upper right panel, This is a transmitral flow profile at rest and *bottom right* is the transmitral flow profile during the Valsalva manoeuvre in a patient with coronary artery disease. Observe that in this patient with a pseudonormal filling profile, a decrease in venous return with the Valsalva manoeuvre produces a reduction in the mitral E velocity (as in the normal patient) without a corresponding decrease in A velocity. This is because early atrial emptying is abnormal. Therefore, due to reduced emptying in early diastole, emptying with atrial contraction will actually increase. This results in a marked decrease of the E/A ratio less than 1.0.

From Dumesnil, J.G. et al.: Use of Valsalva manoeuvre to unmask left ventricular diastolic function abnormalities by Doppler echocardiography in patients with coronary artery disease or systemic hypertension. *American Journal of Cardiology 68:515-519, 1991.* Reproduced with permission from Excerpta Medica Inc.

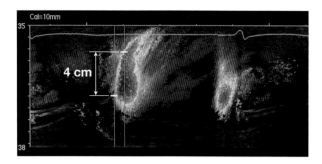

Figure 14.15: Measurement of Colour M-Mode Doppler Flow Propagation of Mitral Inflow.
Using colour M-mode Doppler it is possible to visualise the propagation of flow along the entire length of the ventricle throughout diastole. The mitral inflow propagation velocity is a measurement of the slope of propagation of the first clearly demarcated isovelocity line during early filling from the level of the mitral annulus plane to a distance of 4 cm into the LV cavity. For optimal demarcation of the first aliased velocity, the baseline is adjusted to alias at 50% to 75% of the peak transmitral pulsed-wave Doppler velocity or to about 40 cm/s.

NORMAL

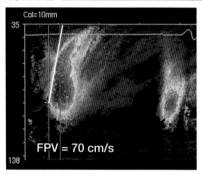
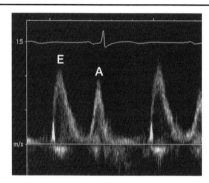
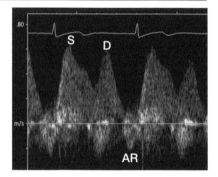

ABNORMAL RELAXATION

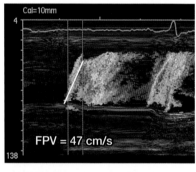
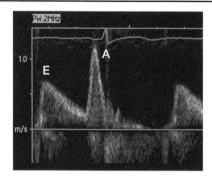
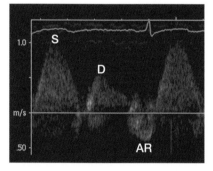

PSEUDONORMALISATION

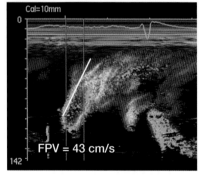
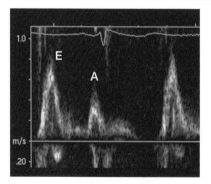
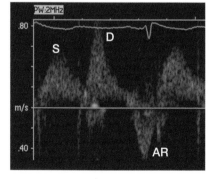

Figure 14.16: Application of Colour M-Mode Doppler in the differentiation of Normal from Pseudonormal Mitral Filling Pattern.
The propagation slope of mitral inflow has been shown to be inversely related to the rate of relaxation. Therefore, the velocity of mitral inflow propagation is lower in patients with abnormal relaxation and pseudonormalisation compared with normal subjects. This example illustrates flow propagation velocities, transmitral inflow Doppler velocities, and pulmonary venous Doppler velocities in three representative cases: normal LV function (*top row*), abnormal relaxation profile (*middle row*), and pseudonormal (*bottom row*). Observe that despite the normal appearance of the mitral inflow Doppler signal in the case of pseudonormalisation (*bottom row*), the flow propagation velocity is significantly reduced. Therefore, reduction of the flow propagation velocity allows easy identification of the pseudonormal profile from the normal flow profile.
Abbreviations: A = mitral atrial velocity; **AR** = pulmonary venous atrial reversal velocity; **D** = pulmonary venous diastolic forward flow; **E** = mitral early diastolic velocity; **FPV** = flow propagation velocity; **S** = pulmonary venous systolic forward flow.

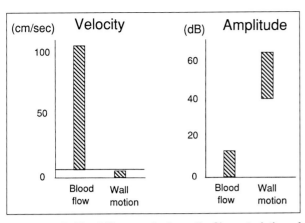

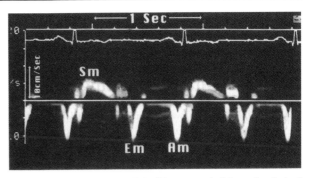

Figure 14.18: Myocardial Velocities recorded from the Apical View.

From the apical view, the myocardial velocity is comprised of three distinct components: (1) an apically directed systolic component **(Sm)**, (2) an atrially directed early myocardial lengthening velocity **(Em)**, and (3) an atrially directed late diastolic myocardial lengthening velocity **(Am)**. Less prominent biphasic velocities are seen during isovolumic contraction and relaxation as well.

From Pai, R.G. and Gill, K.S.: Amplitudes, durations, and timings of apically directed left ventricular myocardial velocities: I. Their normal pattern and coupling to ventricular filling and ejection. *Journal of the American Society of Echocardiography 11: 106, 1998.* Reproduced with permission from Mosby Inc., St. Louis, MO, USA.

Figure 14.17: The Difference in Acoustic Characteristics of the Myocardial Wall Motion and Blood Flow.

Left, Observe that wall motion velocity of myocardium is much lower than blood flow velocity.

Right, In contrast, the Doppler signal amplitude of myocardial wall motion is much greater than that of blood flow.

From Miyatake, K. et al.: New method for evaluating left ventricular wall motion by color-coded tissue Doppler imaging: In vitro and in vivo studies. *Journal of the American College of Cardiology 25:718, 1995.* Reproduced with permission from the American College of Cardiology.

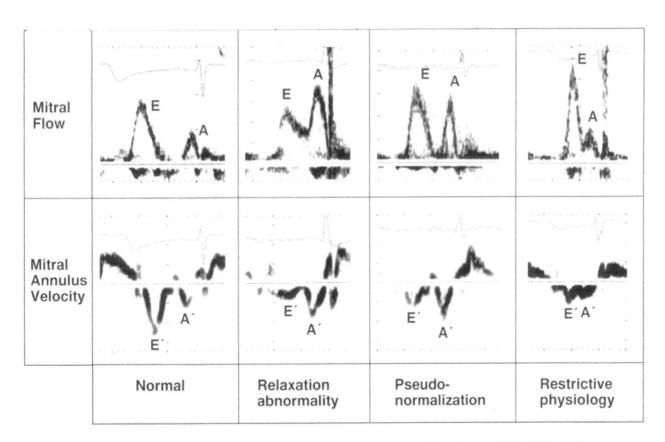

Figure 14.19: Application of Mitral Annular DTI in the differentiation of Normal from Pseudonormal Mitral Filling Pattern.

This example illustrates conventional transmitral inflow Doppler velocities and mitral annulus velocities in four representative cases: normal, abnormal relaxation, pseudonormal, and restrictive physiology. Observe that despite the normal appearance of the mitral inflow Doppler signal in the case of pseudonormalisation, the mitral annulus velocity is typical of the abnormal relaxation pattern (markedly reduced E' or Em); thus, the mitral annulus velocity allows easy identification of the pseudonormal profile from normal.

From Sohn, D-W. et al.: Assessment of mitral annulus velocity by Doppler tissue imaging in the evaluation of left ventricular diastolic function. *Journal of the American College of Cardiology 30:479, 1997.* Reproduced with permission from the American College of Cardiology.

Myocardial velocities can be recorded by placing the PW Doppler sample volume at the lateral corner of the mitral annulus from the apical four chamber view. Myocardial velocities may also be recorded from the septal side of the mitral annulus in a similar manner. When recorded from the apical views, the myocardial velocity is composed of three components (Figure 14.18). These components include: (1) an apically directed systolic myocardial velocity (**Sm**), (2) an early diastolic atrially directed myocardial velocity (**Em**), and (3) a late diastolic atrially directed myocardial velocity (**Am**). In addition to these three distinct velocities, less prominent biphasic velocities can be seen between the Sm and Em waves during LV isovolumic relaxation period and between Am and Sm waves during the isovolumic contraction period.

Since the velocity of annular motion reflects shortening and lengthening of the myocardial fibres along a longitudinal plane, it has been suggested that the early diastolic velocity recorded at the septal or lateral corner of the mitral annulus can provide an index of LV relaxation which is not affected by the LA pressure. In particular, it has been suggested that the Em can be used in the differentiation between normal and pseudonormal filling profiles (Figure 14.19).

Clinical Significance:
Several studies have reported normal values for the mitral annulus velocities (Table 14.8). Values of the mitral Em velocity have also been reported separating abnormal relaxation, pseudonormal, and restrictive physiology from normal (Table 14.9).

Assessment of Elevated Left Ventricular Filling Pressures
As already mentioned, elevation of LV filling pressures can also be derived from the transmitral and pulmonary venous Doppler velocities. Simplistically, elevation in LA pressure is reflected during early diastole while

elevation in the LVEDP is reflected during late diastole. In patients with pseudonormalisation and restrictive physiology, both LA pressure and the LVEDP are elevated. However, in patients with abnormal relaxation, the LVEDP can be either normal or elevated. Therefore, it is important to be able to identify those patients with abnormal relaxation who also have an increased LVEDP. The best method for the evaluation of the LVEDP is from the comparison between the duration of the mitral A wave and the pulmonary venous AR wave.

The length of the mitral A wave is determined by the LVEDP. Essentially, the mitral A wave ends when the LVEDP exceeds the LA pressure. The duration of the pulmonary venous AR wave, however, is governed by the pressure difference between the LA and the pulmonary veins.

Under normal circumstances, atrial contraction results in increased pressure within the LA. This results in a pressure gradient between the LA and LV as well as between the LA and pulmonary veins. Normally, the pressure gradient between the LA and LV is greater than that between the LA and pulmonary veins and, thus, the amount and duration of transmitral flow (mitral A wave) exceeds reversed flow into the pulmonary veins (pulmonary venous AR wave).

When there is a decrease in LV compliance and elevated filling pressures, the pressure increase in the LV is larger and more rapid following atrial contraction. This results in the early crossover of pressures between the LA and the LV at end-diastole and effectively shortens the duration of the positive transmitral pressure gradient and, thus, transmitral flow with atrial contraction. *At the same time*, the increased pressure rise in the LA results in a larger velocity of backward flow into the pulmonary veins (increased pulmonary venous AR wave). The duration of the pulmonary venous AR wave also exceeds that of the mitral A wave since the mitral A wave duration is shortened.

Table 14.8: Normal values for the mitral annulus velocities derived by DTI.

Author (Year)	Pt No.	Sampling Site	Em velocity (cm/s)	Am velocity (cm/s)	Sm velocity (cm/s)
Sohn 1997 [1]	59	septal side	10.0 ± 1.3	9.5 ± 1.5	-
Nagueh 1997 [2]	34	lateral side	12 ± 2.8	8.4 ± 2.4	10 ± 1.5
Farias 1999 [3]	27	average *	16.0 ± 3.8	11.0 ± 2.1	9.7 ± 1.9

* averaged values obtained at the basal lateral, septal, inferior and anterior myocardial segments of the mitral annulus from the apical four-chamber and two-chamber views.

Sources: (1) Sohn, D-W. et al.: *Journal of the American College of Cardiology* 30:474-480, 1997. **(2)** Nagueh, S.F. et al.: *Journal of the American College of Cardiology* 30:1527-1533, 1997. **(3)** Farias, C.A. et al.: *Journal of the American Society of Echocardiography* 12:609-617, 1999.

Table 14.9: Values of the mitral Em velocity derived by DTI separating abnormal relaxation, pseudonormal, and restrictive physiology from normal.

Author (Year)	Sampling Site	Normal	Abnormal Relaxation	Pseudonormal	Restrictive Physiology
Nagueh 1997 [1]	lateral side	12 ± 2.8	5.8 ± 1.5	5.2 ± 1.4	-
Farias 1999 [2]	average *	16.0 ± 3.8	7.5 ± 2.2	7.6 ± 2.2	8.1 ± 3.5

Sources: (1) Nagueh, S.F. et al.: *Journal of the American College of Cardiology* 30:1527-1533, 1997. **(2)** Farias, C.A. et al.: *Journal of the American Society of Echocardiography* 12:609-617, 1999.

Table 14.10: Value of a difference between the mitral A wave duration and pulmonary venous atrial reversal duration as a predictor of elevated left ventricular end-diastolic pressure.

Author (Year)	Pt No.	PVa-A dur (ms)	LVEDP (mm Hg)	Sensitivity	Specificity
Rossvoll (1993) [1]	45	> 0	> 15	85 %	79 %
Appleton (1993) [2]	65	> 20	> 12	74 %	> 95 %
Cecconi (1996) [3]	101	A dur/PVa ≤ 0.9	≥ 15	79 %	96 %
			≥ 20	90 %	90 %
Yamamoto (1997) [4]	87	> 0	≥ 20	82 %	92 %
Yamamoto (1997) [5]	82	0	≥ 15	73 %	83 %
		25		46 %	97 %
		0	≥ 20	100 %	43 %
		25		71 %	93 %
O'Leary (1998) [6]	186	≥ 29	≥ 18	90 %	86 %
Sohn (1999) [7]	43	> 0	≥ 20	67 %	85 %

Abbreviations: LVEDP = left ventricular end-diastolic pressure; **Pt No.** = patient numbers; **PVa-A dur** = pulmonary venous atrial reversal duration to mitral A velocity duration.
Sources: (1) Rossvoll, O. and Hatle, L.K.: *Journal of the American College of Cardiology 21:1687-1696, 1993*: patient population: 19 patient = LVEDP < 15 mm Hg; 26 patients = LVEDP > 15 mm Hg; **(2)** Appleton, C.P. et al.: *Journal of the American College of Cardiology 22:1972-1982,1993*: patient population: 39 patients = LVEDP ≤ 12 mm Hg; 26 patients = LVEDP > 12 mm Hg; **(3)** Cecconi, M. et al.: *Journal of the American Society of Echocardiography 9:241-250,1996*: patient population: 64 patients = LVEDP ≤ 12 mm Hg; 17 patients = LVEDP 13 to 19 mm Hg; 20 patients = LVEDP ≥ 20 mm Hg.; **(4)** Yamamoto, K. et al.: *Journal of the American Society of Echocardiography 10:52-59,1997*: patient population: 50 patients = LVEDP < 20 mm Hg; 27 patients = LVEDP ≥ 20 mm Hg; **(5)** Yamamoto, K. et al.: *Journal of the American College of Cardiology 30: 1819-1826, 1997*; **(6)** O'Leary, P.W. et al.: *Mayo Clinic Proceedings 73:616-628,1998*: patient population: 162 normal children (mean age 10.6 years); 24 children with elevated LVEDP ≥ 18 mm Hg (mean age 10.6 years); **(7)** Sohn, D-W., et al.: *Journal of the American Society of Echocardiography 12:106-112,1999*: patient population: 14 patients = LVEDP < 20 mm Hg; 29 patients = LVEDP ≥ 20 mm Hg;

Based on these findings, elevation of the LVEDP can be identified when there is: (1) an increase in the pulmonary venous AR velocity greater than 35 cm/s [64], or (2) when the duration of the pulmonary venous AR wave exceeds the mitral A wave duration (see Table 14.10).

Physiological and Technical Influences on Diastolic Function:
Several physiological and technical factors can affect diastolic filling profiles. Recognition of the effect of these factors on diastolic filling profiles is crucial to the accurate interpretation of the various diastolic filling abnormalities.

Loading conditions:
Loading conditions (preload and afterload) affect the transmitral flow profile. In particular, changes in loading conditions in normal patients may "mimic" an impaired relaxation pattern.
Preload is defined as the LV volume at end-diastole and is essentially equivalent to the LA pressure. Alterations to preload such as an increase or decrease in preload can alter the diastolic filling profiles (Figure 14.20).
Preload reduction, which occurs with the administration of nitroglycerine, effectively reduces the LA pressure. The decrease in LA pressure reduces the early filling gradient between the LA and LV. This results in a decreased mitral E wave velocity and, therefore, a decrease in the mitral E/A ratio. Furthermore, because of the reduced early diastolic gradient between the LA and LV, a longer time is required for the LV pressure to increase and for the LA to empty; hence, the deceleration time is prolonged.

An increase in preload, which occurs with fluid loading, increases the pressure gradient between the LA and LV in early diastole. This results in an increase in the mitral E wave velocity and, to a lesser degree, the A wave velocity. In addition, as a consequence of increased early filling of the LV, the LV pressure rises more rapidly during early diastole resulting in a more rapid deceleration of flow and shortening of the deceleration time. Furthermore, there is also a decrease in the IVRT due to earlier crossover of the LA and LV pressure traces.

Afterload:
Afterload of the LV is defined as the resistance to ejection of blood from the ventricle to the systemic circulation. In other words, afterload is the systemic vascular resistance. Alterations to afterload can alter the diastolic filling profiles (Figure 14.20).
Changes in afterload primarily affects the rate of LV relaxation with subsequent changes in the transmitral inflow curve. An increase in afterload prolongs ventricular relaxation. Hence, the crossover of pressures between the LV and LA occurs later. This results in a smaller initial driving pressure between the LV and LA and a reduction in the peak mitral E wave velocity. Furthermore, there is also a decreased rate of fall in the gradient between the LA and LV because of continued delayed myocardial relaxation resulting in prolongation of the deceleration time. Finally, because there is less filling in early diastole there will be greater filling with atrial contraction (increased A wave velocity).
Note that an increase in afterload produces the same effect as a decrease in preload.

64: Nishimura, R.A. et al.: Circulation 81: 1488-1497, 1990.

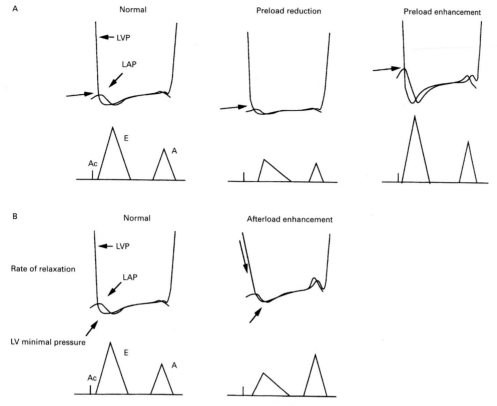

Figure 14.20: Effect of Loading Conditions on the Mitral Inflow Doppler Trace.
A, This example demonstrates the effect of *preload* on the transmitral Doppler trace. An acute decrease in preload or LA pressure reduces the transmitral pressure gradient in early diastole and, therefore, the mitral E velocity is decreased. The resultant decrease in early diastolic filling of the ventricle is associated with a slower increase in LV pressure which prolongs the deceleration time. A decreased preload for atrial contraction also reduces the mitral A velocity. The opposite effects occur with preload enhancement (increased LA pressure).
B, This example demonstrates the effect of *afterload* on the transmitral Doppler trace. An acute increase in afterload is associated with: (1) increased LV end-diastolic volume, (2) a slowed rate of LV relaxation, and (3) increased preload. Thus, early diastolic filling and the mitral E velocity are decreased owing to impaired relaxation and elastic recoil. Left ventricular relaxation continues into mid or even late diastole, LV filling continues to be impaired and mitral deceleration time is prolonged. Mitral A velocity is increased by increased atrial preload at the time of atrial contraction.
From Yamamoto, K. et al.: Analysis of left ventricular diastolic function. *Heart (supplement 2) 75:30, 1996*. Reproduced with permission from the BMJ Publishing Group.

Heart rate and rhythm:

Optimal assessment of the mitral inflow signal requires a biphasic transmitral flow signal. Heart rate and rhythm may affect the appearance of this biphasic signal.

Sinus tachycardia: In the presence of tachycardia, there is shortening of the diastolic filling period which results in an increase in the mitral A wave velocity relative to the mitral E velocity. As heart rate increases further, the diastolic filling time shortens further and atrial contraction may occur before early filling is completed. In this instance, the mitral E and A velocities may fuse to produce a single signal. Furthermore, when the mitral E and A waves overlap, it is difficult to compare the difference between the mitral A wave duration and the pulmonary venous flow reversal duration with atrial contraction (Figure 14.21). In fact, the pulmonary venous AR duration may measure shorter than the mitral A wave duration instead of longer even when the LVEDP is greater than 20 mm Hg (false negative result). However, in this instance, the end of flow is important in predicting an elevation of the LVEDP (see Figure 14.22).
The pulmonary venous flow profile is particularly useful

in the assessment of diastolic function in patients who exhibit E/A fusion. In this instance, abnormal relaxation pattern can be identified when the pulmonary venous S velocity exceeds that of the pulmonary venous D velocity; conversely, restrictive physiology is seen when the pulmonary venous S velocity is less than the pulmonary venous D velocity.

Atrial fibrillation: In patients with atrial fibrillation, the accelerated heart rate and the cycle-to-cycle variability of atrial fibrillation (AF) reduces the value of transmitral flow velocities. Furthermore, in patients with AF, there is blunting of systolic flow. Recall that the systolic component of the pulmonary venous flow profile is dependent, in part, on LA relaxation.
In patients with atrial fibrillation, there is no effective LA relaxation; thus, the first systolic component of the pulmonary venous trace is lost. As a result, the pulmonary venous S velocity is always smaller than that of the pulmonary venous D velocity.

Atrioventricular dissociation: The atrioventricular sequence alters the mitral A velocity and, hence, the E/A

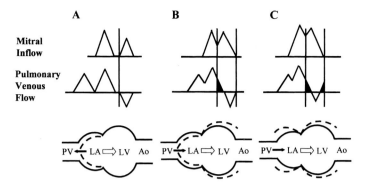

Figure 14.21: The Effects of Heart Rate on the Durations of the Mitral A Wave and the Pulmonary Venous Atrial Reversal Duration.

A. This diagram displays the mitral and pulmonary venous Doppler traces when the mitral E and A waves are separated.

B. When the mitral E and A waves overlap, the pulmonary venous AR wave starts later than the beginning of the mitral A wave.

C. When LA contraction occurs early enough to allow the LA relaxation to be present before early LV filling is completed, pulmonary venous systolic forward flow starts earlier than the end of the mitral A wave.

Abbreviations: Ao = aorta; **LA** =, left atrium; **LV** = left ventricle; **PV** = pulmonary venous.

From Sohn, D-W, et al.: Estimation of LV end-diastolic pressure with the difference in pulmonary venous and mitral A durations is limited when mitral E and A waves are overlapped. *Journal of the American Society of Echocardiography. 12: 109, 1999*. Reproduced with permission from Mosby, Inc., St. Louis, MO, USA.

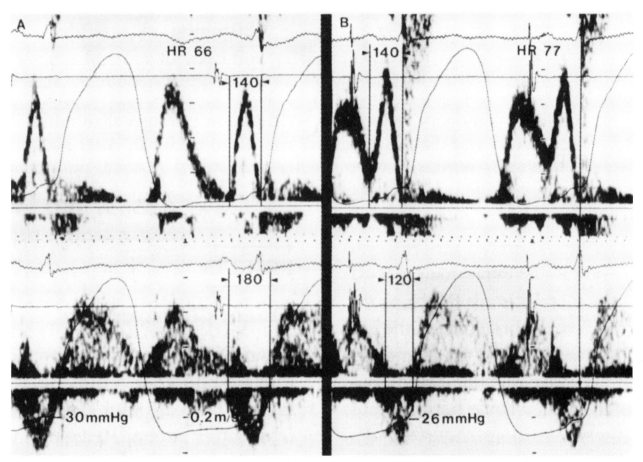

Figure 14.22: The Effects of Heart Rate on the Durations of the Mitral A Wave and the Pulmonary Venous Atrial Reversal Duration in a Patient with an Elevated Left Ventricular End-Diastolic Pressure.

The transmitral flow profile appears at the top and the pulmonary venous flow profile appears at the bottom.

A. At baseline (heart rate of 66 bpm and a LVEDP of 30mm Hg), the pulmonary venous AR duration was longer than the mitral A wave duration (180 ms versus 140 ms), therefore,correctly indicating an elevation in the LVEDP.

B. After pacing (heart rate 77 bpm and a LVEDP off 26 mm Hg), the absolute duration of the pulmonary venous AR duration was shorter than the mitral A wave duration (120 ms versus 140 ms). Observe however that the pulmonary venous AR duration ends later than the mitral A wave duration.

From Sohn, D-W, et al.: Estimation of left ventricular end-diastolic pressure with the difference in pulmonary venous and mitral A durations is limited when mitral E and A waves are overlapped. *Journal of the American Society of Echocardiography. 12: 109, 1999*. Reproduced with permission from Mosby, Inc., St. Louis, MO, USA.

ratio. Furthermore, an abnormally long or short PR interval also influences the mitral inflow velocities. If the PR interval is abnormally long, it produces an effect similar to that of sinus tachycardia. Recall that with sinus tachycardia, the diastolic filling time shortens such that atrial contraction occurs before early filling is completed.

Likewise, when there is a long PR interval, the mitral A wave velocity is augmented because atrial contraction occurs during the early filling phase. This results in the fusion of the mitral E and A velocities.

Conversely, when the PR interval is abnormally short, the mitral A velocity is abbreviated because atrial contraction is interrupted by ventricular systole and an abrupt rise in LV systolic pressure.

Second and third degree atrioventricular heart block: In the presence of second- and third-degree atrioventricular heart block, the mitral E and A velocities and the pulmonary venous S and D velocities vary according to the timing of atrial contraction in relation to ventricular systole.

If atrial activation and contraction occur during ventricular systole, the mitral E velocity will increase. If atrial contraction occurs before the completion of rapid filling phase, the mitral A velocity will increase. If atrial contraction occurs in late systole just before ventricular contraction, the mitral A wave magnitude will be diminished. If atrial contraction occurs during the rapid diastolic filling phase, a single summation velocity will occur.

In addition, activation of the LV from left bundle branch block, VVI pacing or post ventricular ectopics may cause prolongation of relaxation resulting in a decreased mitral E velocity and prolongation of the deceleration time.

Pacemaker Rhythm: As mentioned above, VVI pacing may produce an abnormal relaxation pattern due to abnormal depolarisation of the left ventricle during systole. Furthermore, pacemaker rhythm may result in abnormalities to the pulmonary venous flow profile; in particular, the pulmonary venous AR wave (Figure 14.23).

Left ventricular systolic function:
Recall that the systolic component of the pulmonary venous flow profile is dependent on LA relaxation and the descent of the mitral annulus toward the cardiac apex with ventricular systole. During ventricular systole, the mitral annulus moves downward and rightward. This leads to an increase in the LA area and a decrease in LA pressure which results in increased pulmonary venous flow into the LA. Therefore, when LV systolic function is impaired, the pulmonary venous S wave velocity may be decreased due to reduced motion of the mitral valve annulus.

Valvular abnormalities:
The transmitral flow profile can be significantly influenced by the presence of left-sided valvular abnormalities.

Aortic regurgitation: In patients with severe aortic regurgitation, there may be a rapid increase in the LVEDP. This rapid increase in LVEDP results in a rapid equalisation between the LA and LV pressures. Therefore, the pressure gradient between the LA and LV will decrease sharply resulting in shortening of the deceleration time.

Mitral regurgitation: The transmitral flow profile may be affected by the presence of mitral regurgitation depending on its severity. In patients with significant mitral regurgitation and normal LV systolic function, the mitral E wave increases while the deceleration time and IVRT are shortened.

Furthermore, one of the variables which is used in the recognition of restrictive physiology includes a reduction in the pulmonary venous S velocity. However, in patients with severe mitral regurgitation, the LA pressure is increased during systole, thus, reducing the pressure gradient between pulmonary veins and LA. Hence, the pulmonary venous S wave velocity may also be decreased in patients with significant mitral regurgitation in the absence of restrictive physiology.

Mitral stenosis and prosthetic mitral valves: Coexistent mitral stenosis or a mitral valve prosthesis prohibits any interpretation of diastolic function of the LV. This is because of the intrinsic pressure gradient between the LA and LV in these situations.

Effects of age on diastolic filling parameters:
As previously mentioned, age is an important variable which affects the interpretation of diastolic filling profiles. Abnormalities of LV diastolic function have been described as part of the normal aging process resulting from intrinsic myocardial changes and hypertrophy of the

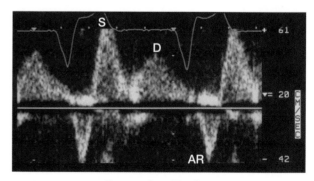

Sinus Rhythm   Pacemaker Rhythm

Figure 14.23: Abnormalities to the pulmonary venous Doppler profile with pacemaker rhythm.
The two examples displayed above were obtained from the same patient in sinus rhythm (left) and in with pacemaker rhythm (right).
Left, Observe that when the patient is in sinus rhythm, the pulmonary venous S wave is of a slightly higher velocity than the pulmonary venous D wave. Also note that the pulmonary venous AR velocity is very low.
Right, Observe that in the presence of pacemaker rhythm the pulmonary venous S wave velocity is significantly greater than the pulmonary venousD wave velocity. Also note that the AR velocity is markedly increased. This is because atrial contraction is occurring during systole against the closed mitral valve (observe the timing of the AR wave compared to the ECG).

LV. Due to these changes in myocardial relaxation and compliance with aging, different diastolic filling patterns are expected for different age groups (Figure 14.24).

In the normal, young individual, LV elastic recoil is vigorous and myocardial relaxation is swift. As a result approximately 85 - 95% of LV filling occurs in early diastole and only a small proportion of filling occurs with atrial contraction (5 - 15%).

With aging, there is a gradual decrease in the rate of myocardial relaxation and elastic recoil and, therefore, the LV pressure decline and filling becomes slower. With a normal LA pressure, the pressure crossover between the LV and LA (that is, mitral valve opening) occurs later and the early transmitral pressure gradient is decreased. Hence, the IVRT becomes longer and the mitral E velocity decreases with increasing age. Furthermore, the reduced filling in early diastole retards the equilibrium between the LV and LA resulting in prolongation of the deceleration time. Because early filling of the LV is reduced, the contribution from atrial contraction becomes significant. This results in a gradual increase in the mitral A velocity with aging.

Pulmonary venous flow velocities show similar changes with aging. Since the pulmonary venous flow in diastole parallels the early mitral inflow, it follows that if the mitral E velocity decreases with age, the pulmonary venous D velocity also decreases with advancing age. To compensate for this reduction in diastolic filling, systolic forward flow becomes more prominent. Note that the mitral inflow and pulmonary venous flow profiles in young individuals may be similar to that of the restrictive filling pattern. In these individuals, the mechanism producing this filling pattern is vigorous, normal relaxation rather than the high-driving pressure that occurs with restrictive physiology. Furthermore, the pulmonary venous D velocity may be greater than the pulmonary venous S velocity in normal young persons. In addition, there may also be shortening of the mitral A wave duration. However, when compared to the pulmonary venous AR duration, the mitral A wave duration should equal to or slightly longer than the pulmonary venous AR wave. In patients with restrictive physiology, the reverse is true (the mitral A wave duration is shorter than the pulmonary venous AR wave).

Respiratory cycle: Normally there is minimal changes in the mitral inflow pattern (< 10%) and mild changes in the tricuspid inflow patterns (less than 30%) throughout respiration.

On the right side of the heart, during inspiration, a fall in intrathoracic pressure increases venous return to the right heart, which in turn, slightly decreases early LV diastolic inflow velocities and increases right ventricular filling.

Respiratory variation of Doppler flows may be helpful in the diagnosis of constrictive pericarditis and cardiac tamponade [65 + 66].

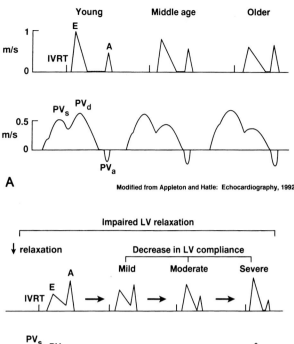

Figure 14.24: The Expected Normal Mitral Inflow and Pulmonary Venous Inflow in Normal Young, Middle-Aged, and Older Subjects.

The upper panel (A) illustrates the expected normal mitral inflow Doppler profile which can be seen in normal young, middle-aged, and older subjects. The lower panel (B) illustrates the expected normal pulmonary venous inflow Doppler profile which can be seen in normal young, middle-aged, and older subjects.

In younger individuals, the majority of LV filling occurs in early diastole which is reflected on the mitral inflow and pulmonary venous Doppler traces. Observe that the mitral E velocity is predominant and the deceleration time (DT) and isovolumic relaxation time (IVRT) are relatively short while the pulmonary venous systolic (PV_s) and diastolic (PV_d) velocities are almost equal. With advancing age, LV relaxation slows leading to a decline in early filling of the LV and an increase in filling with atrial contraction. As a result, the mitral E and the PV_d velocities decrease and the IVRT, DT and the mitral A and PV_s velocities all increase.

From Oh, J.K. et al.: The noninvasive assessment of left ventricular diastolic function with two-dimensional Doppler echocardiography. *Journal of the American Society of Echocardiography* 10:251,1997. Reproduced with permission from Mosby, Inc., St. Louis, MO, USA.

Angle of ultrasound beam:

The angle at which the ultrasound beam interrogates blood flow is crucial to the accurate display and measurement of Doppler signals. Recall that optimal Doppler signals are obtained when blood flow is parallel to the ultrasound beam. When angles of greater than 30 degrees between the ultrasound beam and blood direction are used, the velocity is greatly underestimated.

Therefore, to minimise this potential problem and to maximise diastolic flow velocities, the Doppler sample

65: Burstow, D.J. et al.: Mayo Clinic Proceedings 64: 312-324, 1989. 66: Oh, J.K et al.: Journal of the American College of Cardiology 23: 154-162, 1994.

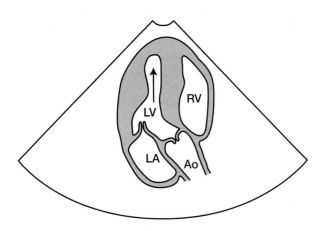
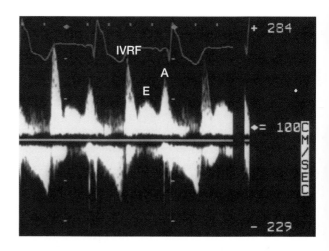

Figure 14.25: Isovolumic Relaxation Flow.
Isovolumic relaxation flow occurs between two regions of the LV because of marked asynchrony in LV relaxation (left). This flow is most commonly directed from the base of the heart to the apex during the isovolumic relaxation flow period (right) in patients with intracavity gradients caused by LV hypertrophy, vigorous LV systolic function, and near cavity obliteration in systole. It is important to recognise this flow and not to confuse it for the mitral E wave velocity.

must be aligned parallel to blood flow direction. This can be facilitated utilising CFI to ascertain blood flow direction (especially for pulmonary venous inflow signals).

Isovolumic relaxation flow:
Flow does not usually occur during the isovolumic relaxation period. During this phase of the cardiac cycle, both the mitral and aortic valves are closed and there is no filling or emptying of the LV. However, in patients with a hyperdynamic or hypertrophic ventricle, flow may occur during this period. In these instances, flow occurs because of early relaxation of the apex of the ventricle relative to the base (Figure 14.25). This effectively creates an intraventricular pressure gradient between the base of the heart and the ventricular apex. Isovolumic relaxation flow may be confused for the mitral E velocity; however, this flow can be distinguished from the mitral E velocity by examining the timing of flow with the ECG.

Sample volume position and size:
Transmitral flow velocities are typically obtained by placing the PW Doppler sample volume at the tips of the mitral leaflets. It is important to note that the sample volume location directly affects the shape of the mitral inflow profile (Figure 14.26). The highest Doppler velocities are recorded when the sample volume is placed at the tips of the mitral valve due to the "funnel" shape of the mitral valve in diastole. Furthermore, the E/A ratio may be higher when measured at the tips of the mitral valve compared with the ratio recorded at the level of the mitral annulus. The deceleration time is also greatest at the tips.

Filter settings:
The lowest possible filter settings should be used to ensure that a full and complete Doppler spectrum is obtained. In addition, low filter settings improve the

measurement of flow durations. Filters may need to be increased when measuring the IVRT. To increase the accuracy of measuring the IVRT, both the closing click of the aortic valve and the opening click of the mitral valve should be identified.

Poor acoustic windows:
Poor acoustic windows due to patient body habitus or chronic obstructive airway disease (COAD) limit the usefulness of transthoracic echocardiography in the assessment of diastolic function.

Measurement of the mitral A and pulmonary venous AR durations:
Direct measurement of the mitral A wave and pulmonary venous AR durations may be difficult. In particular, it may be difficult to identify the start of flow. In this instance, the relative durations between these two signals can be approximated by identifying the end of atrial flow to the ECG (Figure 14.27).

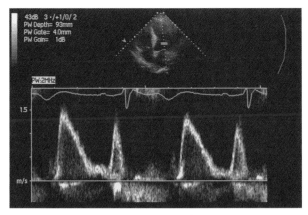

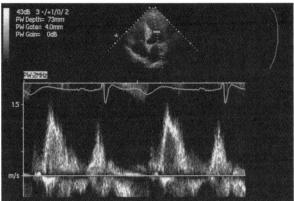

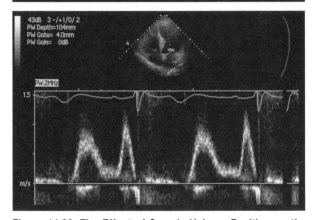

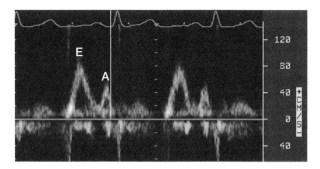

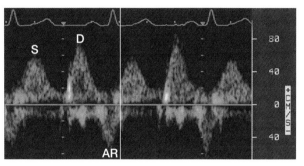

Figure 14.27: Termination of Flow Velocities following Atrial Contraction.

In some cases it may be difficult to identify the beginning of flow on the mitral A wave, pulmonary venous AR wave, or both. In these circumstances, the relationship of flow durations may be approximated by determining the discontinuation of flow referenced to the ECG.

The mitral inflow profile appears at the top and the pulmonary venous flow profile appears at the bottom.

Observe that in this case, the mitral A wave terminates much earlier than the pulmonary venous flow reversal when compared to the QRS complex of the ECG.

Figure 14.26: The Effect of Sample Volume Position on the Transmitral Doppler Signal.

The Doppler velocity spectrum of mitral inflow changes with the alteration of sample volume position.

Top, This example depicts the typical Doppler spectrum seen when the sample volume is positioned at the tips of the mitral valve leaflets.

Middle, This example illustrates the typical Doppler spectrum seen when the sample volume is positioned too far into the LV. Observe the "feathering" of the Doppler trace which reflects the greater diameter and less laminar flow in the mid ventricle compared with flow between the mitral leaflets.

Bottom, This example illustrates the typical Doppler spectrum seen when the sample volume is at the level of the mitral annulus. Observe that the peak velocities are lower and the relationship between the E wave and the A wave has changed such that the E wave velocity decreases proportionally more than the A wave velocity (reduced E/A ratio).

Note: When assessing LV diastolic function and filling parameters, the sample volume is placed at the tips of the mitral valve leaflets. When calculating the stroke volume through the mitral valve, the sample volume is placed at the level of the mitral annulus.

Index of Myocardial Performance (IMP)

There are many parameters that can be used to assess either systolic or diastolic ventricular function; however, systolic and diastolic dysfunction may coexist. Left ventricular systolic dysfunction is seen when there is a decrease in the ejection fraction, prolongation of the pre-ejection period and a shortening of the ejection phases of the cardiac cycle. Left ventricular diastolic dysfunction is seen when there are alterations in the pattern of the inflow velocity profile as well as prolongation of the relaxation phase of the cardiac cycle.

The index of myocardial performance (IMP) is a relatively new index that reflects the "global" myocardial performance and incorporates both the elements of systole and diastole. This index can be used as a predictor of clinical outcome (survival) and functional status (symptoms). This index is particularly useful in the assessment of conditions where systolic and diastolic dysfunction coexist such as in patients with (1) dilated cardiomyopathy, (2) amyloidosis, (3) pulmonary hypertension, (4) right ventricular infarction, and (5) right ventricular dysplasia.

The IMP is simply the ratio between the isovolumic contraction time (ICT), the isovolumic relaxation time (IVRT), and the ejection time (ET):

(Equation 14.3)

$$IMP = \frac{(ICT + IVRT)}{ET}$$

The principal advantage of this new technique is that this measurement can be derived from two simple measurements that can be easily measured during a complete Doppler examination. Furthermore, this measurement is relatively independent of heart rate and other loading conditions such as blood pressure, right ventricular and pulmonary artery pressure, AV valve regurgitation as well as ventricular dilatation. Two methods for measuring this index have been described (Figures 14.28 and 14.29).

Clinical Significance of the IMP:

The normal IMP for the left ventricle is 0.37 ± 0.05 [66] while the normal IMP for the right ventricle is 0.28 ± 0.04 [67].

With "global" ventricular dysfunction, the IMP increases due an increase in both the ICT and IVRT as well as shortening of the ejection time (see Table 14.11).

METHOD 1

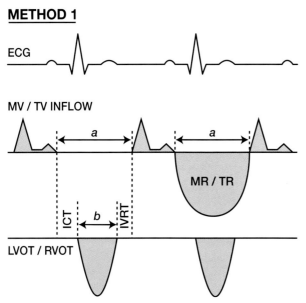

METHOD 2

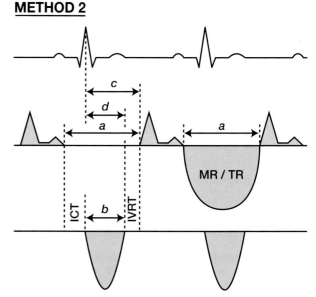

Figure 14.28: Calculation of the Index of Myocardial Performance.
The index of myocardial performance (IMP) is the ratio between the isovolumic contraction time (ICT), the isovolumic relaxation time (IVRT), and the ejection time (ET): **IMP = (ICT + IVRT) + ET**. There are two methods for measuring this index.
Method 1: Calculation of the IMP using this method requires measurement of the following intervals: (1) *interval a:* the interval between cessation to onset of AV valve flow <u>OR</u> the duration of the AV valve regurgitant signal, and (2) *interval b:* the ejection time which is obtained by measuring the duration of flow within the outflow tract. Observe that *interval a* incorporates the ICT, ET and IVRT. Therefore, the sum of the ICT and IVRT can be simply derived by subtracting the ET *(interval b)* from *interval a:* **(ICT + IVRT) = a - b**. Therefore:
$IMP = (a - b) \div b$.
Method 2: Using this method, four intervals are measured: (1) *interval a:* the interval between cessation to onset of atrioventricular valve flow <u>OR</u> the duration of the AV valve regurgitant signal, (2) *interval b: the* ejection time which is obtained by measuring the duration of flow within the outflow tract, (3) *interval c:* the interval from the R wave of the ECG to AV valve opening, and (4) *interval d:* the interval from the R wave of the ECG to aortic/pulmonary valve closure. The IVRT can be derived by subtracting *interval d* from *interval c:* IVRT = c - d. As mentioned above, *interval a* incorporates the ICT, the ET and the IVRT; therefore, the ICT can be derived by subtracting *interval b* and the IVRT from *interval a:* **ICT = (a - b) - IVRT**. Therefore:
$IMP = [(a - b) - (c - d)] \div (b)$

66: Durjardin, K.S. et al.: American Journal of Cardiology 82: 1071-1076,1998.   67: Tei, C. et al.: Journal of the American Society of Echocardiography 9:838-847,1996.

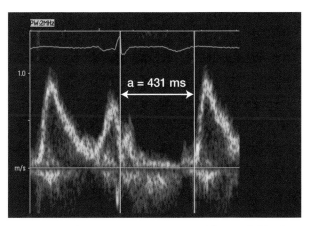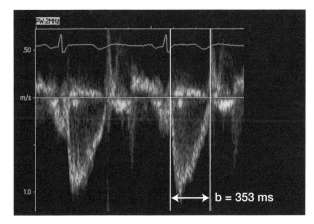

Figure 14.29: Calculation of the Index of Myocardial Performance.
This is an example demonstrating how the IMP can be measured from the mitral inflow PW Doppler signal *(left)* and the LVOT PW Doppler signal *(right)*. The index of myocardial performance (IMP) is the ratio between the isovolumic contraction time (ICT), the isovolumic relaxation time (IVRT), and the ejection time (ET). The (ICT + IVRT) is calculated by measuring the interval between cessation to onset of mitral valve flow (interval a); in this example, this interval equals 431 ms. The (ET) is measured as the interval from the beginning of flow in the outflow tract (interval b); in this example, this interval is 353 ms. Therefore:

$$IMP = (a - b) \div b$$
$$= (431 - 353) \div 353$$
$$= 0.22$$

Method of Measurement of the Index of Myocardial Performance:
Below is a "step-by-step" method for calculating the index of myocardial performance.

Method of calculating the Index of Myocardial Performance (IMP)

Step 1.   using pulsed-wave Doppler, optimise the Doppler signal of the mitral / tricuspid valve inflow signal:
    a) obtain complete Doppler spectrum
    b) best signal usually from apical window
    c) measure the interval from cessation to onset of AV valve inflow *(interval a)*

    <u>OR</u> using continuous-wave Doppler, optimise the Doppler signal of the mitral / tricuspid regurgitant flow signal:
    a) obtain complete Doppler spectrum
    b) best signal usually from apical window
    c) measure the interval from the beginning to the end of AV regurgitant flow signal *(interval a)*

Step 2.   using pulsed-wave Doppler, optimise the Doppler signal of the right / left ventricular outflow tract:
    a) for LVOT - use the apical 5 chamber view
    b) for the RVOT - use the parasternal views
    c) measure the ejection time of this signal *(interval b)*

Step 3.   calculate IMP:

    a) Method 1:

$$IMP = \frac{(a - b)}{b}$$

    b) Method 2:

      ● **IVRT** can be measured as the period from the R wave of the ECG to cessation of flow through the outflow tract *(interval d)* minus the period from the R wave of the ECG to the onset of AV inflow *(interval c)*

      ● **ICT** can be measured as the interval from cessation to onset of AV inflow *(interval a)* minus the ejection time *(interval b)* minus the IVRT

$$IMP = \frac{\left[(a - b) - (c - d)\right]}{b}$$

Table 14.11: Clinical Significance of the Index of Myocardial Performance and Ventricular Function.

Ventricular Function	IMP
Normal	< 0.40
Mild	0.40 - 0.50
Moderate	0.60 - 0.90
Severe	≥ 1.0

Sources: Tei, C. et al.: *Journal of the American Society of Echocardiography 9:838-847, 1996.* Tei, C. et al.: *Journal of Cardiology 26:357-366, 1995.*

Limitations of the IMP:
Arrhythmias:
Arrhythmias such as atrial flutter/fibrillation and atrioventricular heart block affect the inflow profiles through the atrioventricular valves.

Organic valvular disease:
Where there is secondary myocardial dysfunction due to valvular dysfunction, the IMP index may be influenced by abnormal haemodynamics related to valvular dysfunction rather than from ventricular dysfunction.

Loading conditions:
Loading conditions may alter this index (although studies to date have found that there is no correlation between heart rate, blood pressure, right ventricular systolic and diastolic pressure, pulmonary artery diastolic pressure or the degree of atrioventricular valve regurgitation).

References and Suggested Reading:
Stroke Volume and Cardiac Output calculations:
- Ascah, K.J. et al.: Doppler-echocardiographic assessment of cardiac output. *Radiological Clinics of North America 23: 659-670, 1985.*
- Bouchard, A. et al.: Measurement of left ventricular stroke volume using continuous wave Doppler echocardiography of the ascending aorta and M-mode echocardiography of the aortic valve. *Journal of the American College of Cardiology 9: 75-83, 1987.*
- Calafiore, P. and Stewart, W.J.: Doppler echocardiographic quantitation of volumetric flow rate. *Cardiology Clinics 8: 191-202, 1990.*
- De Zuttere, D. et al.: Doppler echocardiographic measurement of mitral flow volume: validation of a new method in adult patients. *Journal of the American College of Cardiology 11: 343-350, 1988.*
- Derias, S.L. et al.: Simplified Doppler method for determining stroke volume and cardiac output from the aortic annulus without computer assistance. *Circulation 72 (supplement III): III-351, 1985.*
- Dittmann, H. et al.: Influence of sampling site and flow area on cardiac output measurements by Doppler echocardiography. *Journal of the American College of Cardiology 10: 818-823, 1987.*
- Dubin, J. et al.: Comparative accuracy of Doppler echocardiographic methods for clinical stroke volume determination. *American Heart Journal 120: 116-123, 1990.*
- Fisher, D.C. et al.: The mitral valve orifice method for noninvasive two-dimensional echo Doppler determinations of cardiac output. *Circulation 67: 872-877, 1983.*
- Fisher, D.C. et al.: The effect of variations on pulsed Doppler sample site on calculation of cardiac output: an experimental study in open-chest dogs. *Circulation 67: 370-376, 1983.*
- Gillam, L.D. et al.: Which cardiac valve provides the best Doppler estimate of cardiac output in humans. *Circulation 72 (supplement III): III-99, 1985.*
- Greenfield, J.C. and Griggs, D.M.: Relation between pressure and diameter in main pulmonary artery of man. *Circulation Research 10: 557-559, 1962.*
- Greenfield, J.C. and Patel, D.J.: Relation between pressure and diameter in the ascending aorta of man. *Circulation Research 10: 778-781, 1962.*
- Hoit, B.D. et al.: Calculating cardiac output from transmitral volume using Doppler and M-mode echocardiography. *American Journal of Cardiology 62: 131-135, 1988.*
- Huntsman, L.L. et al.: Noninvasive Doppler determination of cardiac output in man. *Circulation 67: 593-602, 1983.*
- Ihlen, H. et al.: Determination of cardiac output by Doppler echocardiography. *British Heart Journal 51: 54-60, 1984.*
- Labovitz, A.J. et al.: The effects of sampling site on the two-dimensional echo-Doppler determination of cardiac output. *American Heart Journal 109: 327-332, 1985.*

- Lewis, J.F. et al.: Pulsed Doppler echocardiographic determination of stroke volume and cardiac output: clinical validation of two methods using the apical window. *Circulation 70: 425-431, 1984.*
- Loutfi, H. and Nishimura, R.A.: Quantitative evaluation of left ventricular systolic function by Doppler echocardiographic techniques. *Echocardiography 11: 305-314, 1994.*
- Meijboom, E.J. et al.: A two-dimensional Doppler echocardiographic method for calculation of pulmonary and systemic blood flow in a canine model with a variable-sized left-to-right extracardiac shunt. *Circulation 68: 437-445, 1983.*
- Meijboom, E.J. et al.: A Doppler echocardiographic method for calculating volume flow across the tricuspid valve: correlative laboratory and clinical studies. *Circulation 71: 551-556, 1985.*
- Nishimura, R.A. et al.: Noninvasive measurement of cardiac output by continuous-wave Doppler echocardiography: initial experience and review of the literature. *Mayo Clinic Proceedings 59: 484-489, 1984.*
- Ormiston, J.A. et al.: Size and motion of the mitral valve annulus in man. I. A two-dimensional echocardiographic method and findings in normal subjects. *Circulation 64: 113-120, 1981.*
- Otto, C.M. et al.: Experimental validation of Doppler echocardiographic measurement of volume flow through the stenotic aortic valve *Circulation 78: 435-441, 1988.*
- Rivera, J.M. et al.: Value of proximal regurgitant jet size in tricuspid regurgitation. *American Heart Journal 131: 742-747, 1996.*
- Stewart, W.J. et al.: Variable effects of changes in flow rate through the aortic, pulmonary and mitral valves on valve area and flow velocity: impact on quantitative Doppler flow calculations. *Journal of the American College of Cardiology 6: 653-662, 1985.*
- Valdes-Cruz, L.M. et al.: A pulsed Doppler echocardiographic method for calculating pulmonary and systemic blood flow in atrial level shunts: validation studies in animals and initial human experience. *Circulation 69: 80-86, 1984.*
- Zhang, Y. et al.: Doppler echocardiographic measurement of cardiac output using the mitral orifice method. *British Heart Journal 53: 130-136, 1985.*
- Zoghbi, W.A. and Quinones, M.A.: Determination of cardiac output by Doppler echocardiography: a critical appraisal. *Herz 11: 258-268, 1986.*

dP/dt in the Assessment of Left Ventricular Systolic Function:
- Anconina, J. et al.: Noninvasive estimation of right ventricular dP/dt in patients with tricuspid valve regurgitation. *American Journal of Cardiology 71: 1495-1497, 1993.*
- Bargiggia, G.S. et al.: A new method for estimating left ventricular dP/dt by continuous wave Doppler-echocardiography. *Circulation 80: 1287-1292, 1989.*

- Chen, C. et al.: Noninvasive estimation of the instantaneous first derivative of left ventricular pressure using continuous-wave Doppler echocardiography. *Circulation 8: 2101-2110, 1991.*
- Chung, N. et al.: Noninvasive measurement of left ventricular dP/dt by Doppler echocardiography. *Journal of the American College of Cardiology 15: 140A, 1990.*
- Chung, N. et al.: Measurement of left ventricular dP/dt by simultaneous Doppler echocardiography and cardiac catheterisation. *Journal of the American Society of Echocardiography 5: 147-152, 1992.*
- Ge, Z. et al.: A simultaneous study of Doppler-echo and catheterization in noninvasive assessment of the left ventricular dP/dt. *Clinical Cardiology 16: 422-428, 1993.*
- Loutfi, H. and Nishimura, R.A.: Quantitative evaluation of left ventricular systolic function by Doppler echocardiographic techniques. *Echocardiography 11: 305-314, 1994.*
- Murillo, A. et al.: Assessment of right ventricular function by Doppler ultrasound: A simplified noninvasive method for estimating dP/dt. *Circulation (supplement II) 78: II-650, 1988.*
- Neumann, A. et al.: Comparison of Doppler vs catherization derived dP/dt in dilated cardiomyopathy. *Circulation (supplement II) 80: II-170, 1989.*

Diastolic Function Assessment:
- Appleton, C.P. et al.: Demonstration of restrictive ventricular physiology by Doppler echocardiography. *Journal of the American College of Cardiology 11:757-768, 1988.*
- Appleton, C.P et al.: Relation of transmitral flow velocity patterns to left ventricular diastolic function: New insights from a combined hemodynamic and Doppler echocardiographic study. *Journal of the American College of Cardiology 12: 426-440, 1988.*
- Appleton, C.P. et al.: The natural history of left ventricular filling abnormalities: Assessment by two-dimensional and Doppler echocardiography. *Echocardiography 9: 437-457, 1992.*
- Appleton, C.P.: Doppler assessment of left ventricular diastolic function: the refinement continues. *Journal of the American College of Cardiology 21: 1697-1700, 1993.*
- Appleton, C.P., et al.: Estimation of left ventricular filling pressures using two-dimensional and Doppler echocardiography in adult patients with cardiac disease. Additional value of analyzing left atrial size, left atrial ejection fraction and the difference in duration of pulmonary venous and mitral flow velocity at atrial contraction. Journal of the *American College of Cardiology 22: 1972-1982, 1993.*
- Appleton, C.P. et al.: Doppler evaluation of left and right ventricular diastolic function: A technical guide for obtaining optimal flow velocity recordings. *Journal of the American Society of Echocardiography 10:271-291, 1997.*

- Basnight, M.A. et al.: Pulmonary venous flow velocity: Relation to hemodynamics, mitral flow velocity and left atrial volume, and ejection fraction. *Journal of the American Society of Echocardiography 4: 547-558, 1991.*

- Burstow, D.J. et al.: Cardiac tamponade: Characteristic Doppler observations. *Mayo Clinic Proceedings 64: 312-324, 1989.*

- Cecconi, M. et al.: Doppler echocardiographic evaluation of left ventricular end-diastolic pressure in patients with coronary artery disease. *Journal of the American Society of Echocardiography 9: 241-250, 1996.*

- Choong, C.Y. et al.: Preload dependence of Doppler-derived indexes of left ventricular diastolic function in humans. *Journal of the American College of Cardiology 10: 800-808, 1987.*

- Cohen, G.I. et al.: A practical guide to assessment of ventricular diastolic function using Doppler echocardiography. *Journal of the American College of Cardiology 27: 1753-1760, 1996.*

- Ding, Z.P. et al.: Effect of sample volume location on Doppler-derived transmitral inflow velocity values. *Journal of the American Society of Echocardiography 4: 451-456, 1991.*

- Dougherty, A.H. et al.: Congestive heart failure with normal systolic function. *American Journal of Cardiology 54: 778-782, 1984.*

- Dumesnil, J.G. et al.: Use of Valsalva maneuver to unmask left ventricular diastolic function abnormalities by Doppler echocardiography in patients with coronary artery disease or systemic hypertension. *American Journal of Cardiology 68:515-519, 1991.*

- Gardin, J.M. et al.: Effect of imaging view and sample volume location on evaluation of mitral flow velocity by pulsed Doppler echocardiography. *American Journal of Cardiology 57: 1335-1339, 1986.*

- Geelhood, B.J. and Pai, R.G.: Doppler tissue imaging: Principles and clinical applications. *Cardiac Ultrasound Today: Volume 4, Lesson 10, 1998.*

- Grodecki, P.V. and Klein, A.L.: Pitfalls in the echo-Doppler assessment of diastolic dysfunction. *Echocardiography 10: 213-234, 1993.*

- Hurrell, D.G. et al.: Utility of preload alteration in assessment of left ventricular filling pressure by Doppler echocardiography: A simultaneous catheterization and Doppler echocardiographic study. *Journal of the American College of Cardiology 30: 459-467, 1997.*

- Jaeyer, K.W., et al: Doppler characteristics of late diastolic flow in the left ventricular outflow tract. *Journal of the American Society of Echocardiography 3:179,1990.*

- Klein, A.L. et al.: Effect of age on pulmonary venous flow velocities in normal subjects. *Journal of the American College of Cardiology 13: 50A, 1989.*

- Klein, A.L. et al.: Influence of age and phase of respiration on right ventricular diastolic function in normal subjects. *Journal of the American Society of Echocardiography 3: 237,1990.*

- Klein, A.L. Tajik, A.J.: Doppler assessment of pulmonary venous flow in healthy subjects and in patients with heart disease. *Journal of the American Society of Echocardiography 4:379-392, 1991.*

- Klein, A.L. and Cohen, G.L.: Doppler echocardiographic assessment of constrictive pericarditis, cardiac amyloidosis, and cardiac tamponade. *Cleveland Clinic Journal of Medicine 59: 278-290, 1992.*

- Klein, A.L. et al.: Effects of age on left ventricular dimensions and filling dynamics in 117 normal persons. *Mayo Clinic Proceedings 69:212-224,1994.*

- Mantero, A. et al.: Effect of sample volume location on Doppler-derived transmitral inflow velocity values in 288 normal subjects 20 to 80 years old: An echocardiographic, two-dimensional color Doppler cooperative study. *Journal of the American Society of Echocardiography 11: 280-288, 1998.*

- Masuyama, T. et al.: Pulmonary venous flow velocity pattern as assessed with transthoracic pulsed Doppler echocardiography in subjects without cardiac disease. *American Journal of Cardiology 67: 1396-1404, 1991.*

- Miyaguchi, K., et al.: Dependency of the pulsed Doppler-derived transmitral filling profile on the sampling site. *American Heart Journal 122:142,1991.*

- Nishimura, R.A. et al.: Assessment of diastolic function of the heart: Background and current applications of Doppler echocardiography. Part 1. Physiologic and pathologic features. *Mayo Clinic Proceedings 64: 71-81, 1989.*

- Nishimura, R.A. et al.: Assessment of diastolic function of the heart: Background and current applications of Doppler echocardiography. Part 11. Clinical studies. *Mayo Clinic Proceedings 64: 181-204, 1989.*

- Nishimura, R.A. et al.: Relation of pulmonary vein to mitral flow velocities by transoesophageal Doppler echocardiography. Effect of different loading conditions. *Circulation 81: 1488-1497, 1990.*

- Nishimura, R.A. et al.: Noninvasive Doppler echocardiographic evaluation of left ventricular filling pressures in patients with cardiomyopathies: A simultaneous Doppler and cardiac catheterization study. *Journal of the American College of Cardiology 28: 1226-1233, 1996.*

- Nishimura, R.A. and Appleton, C.P.: "Diastology": Beyond E and A. *Journal of the American College of Cardiology 27: 372-374, 1996.*

- Oh, J.K et al.: Diagnostic role of Doppler echocardiography in constrictive pericarditis. *Journal of the American College of Cardiology 23: 154-162, 1994.*

- Oh, J.K. et al.: The noninvasive assessment of left ventricular diastolic function with two-dimensional Doppler echocardiography. *Journal of the American Society of Echocardiography 10: 246–270,1997.*

- O'Leary, P.W. et al.: Diastolic ventricular function in children: A Doppler echocardiographic study establishing normal values and predictors of increased ventricular end-diastolic pressure. *Mayo Clinic Proceedings 73: 616-628,1998.*

- Pai, R.G. and Buech, G.C.: Newer Doppler measures of left ventricular diastolic function. *Clinical Cardiology 19: 277-288, 1996.*
- Rakowski, H. et al.: Canadian consensus recommendations for the measurement and reporting of diastolic dysfunction by echocardiography. *Journal of the American Society of Echocardiography 9: 736-760, 1996.*
- Rossvoll, O. and Hatle, L.K.: Pulmonary venous flow velocities recorded by transthoracic Doppler ultrasound: Relation to left ventricular diastolic pressures. *Journal of the American College of Cardiology 21: 1687-1696, 1993.*
- Sasson, Z. et al.: Intraventricular flow during isovolumic relaxation: Description and characterization by Doppler echocardiography. *Journal of the American College of Cardiology 10:539-546, 1987.*
- Sohn, D-W. et al.: Estimation of left ventricular end-diastolic pressure with the difference in pulmonary venous and mitral A durations is limited when mitral E and A waves are overlapped. *Journal of the American Society of Echocardiography 12:106-112, 1999.*
- Yamamoto, K. et al.: Analysis of left ventricular diastolic function. *Heart (supplement 2):75:27-35, 1996.*
- Yamamoto, K. et al.: Assessment of left ventricular end-diastolic pressure by Doppler echocardiography: Contribution of duration of pulmonary venous versus mitral flow velocity curves at atrial contraction. *Journal of the American Society of Echocardiography 10:52-59, 1997.*
- Yamamoto, K. et al.: Determination of left ventricular filling pressure by Doppler echocardiography in patients with coronary artery disease: Critical role of left ventricular systolic function. *Journal of the American College of Cardiology 30: 1819-1826, 1997.*

Doppler Tissue Imaging and Diastolic Function:
- Farias, C.A. et al.: Assessment of diastolic function by tissue Doppler echocardiography: Comparison with standard transmitral and pulmonary venous flow. *Journal of the American Society of Echocardiography 12:609-617, 1999.*
- Miyatake, K. et al.: New method for evaluating left ventricular wall motion by color-coded tissue Doppler imaging: In vitro and in vivo studies. *Journal of the American College of Cardiology 25: 717-724, 1995.*
- Naguesh, S.F. et al.: Doppler tissue imaging: A noninvasive technique for evaluation of left ventricular relaxation and estimation of filling pressures. *Journal of the American College of Cardiology 30: 1527-1533, 1997.*
- Pai, R.G. and Gill, K.S.: Amplitudes, durations, and timings of apically directed left ventricular myocardial velocities: I. Their normal pattern and coupling to ventricular filling and ejection. *Journal of the American Society of Echocardiography 11: 105-111, 1998.*
- Pai, R.G. and Gill, K.S.: Amplitudes, durations, and timings of apically directed left ventricular myocardial velocities: II. Systolic and diastolic asynchrony in patients with left ventricular hypertrophy. *Journal of the American Society of Echocardiography 11: 112-118, 1998.*
- Sohn, D-W. et al.: Assessment of mitral annulus velocity by Doppler tissue imaging in the evaluation of left ventricular diastolic function. *Journal of the American College of Cardiology 30: 474-480, 1997.*

Colour M-Mode Propagation and Diastolic Function:
- Brun, P. et al.: Left ventricular flow propagation during early filling is related to wall relaxation: A color M-mode Doppler analysis. *Journal of the American College of Cardiology 20:420-432, 1992.*
- Garcia, M.J. et al.: Color M-mode Doppler flow propagation velocity is a relatively preload-independent index of left ventricular filling. *Journal of the American Society of Echocardiography 12: 129-137, 1999.*
- Garcia, M.J. et al.: An index of early left ventricular filling that combined with pulsed Doppler peak E velocity may estimate capillary wedge pressure. *Journal of the American College of Cardiology 29: 448-454, 1997.*
- Scalia, G.M. and Burstow, D.J.: Color M-Mode and Doppler-derived Tau as practical advances in clinical diastology: The TAUCOM project. *Circulation 100 (suppl): I-295, 1999.*
- Takatsuji, H. et al.: A new approach for evaluation of left ventricular diastolic function: Spatial and temporal analysis of left ventricular filling flow propagation by color M-mode Doppler echocardiography. *Journal of the American College of Cardiology 27: 365-371, 1996.*

Index of Myocardial Performance:
- Dujardin, K.S. et al.: Prognostic value of a Doppler index combining systolic and diastolic performance in idiopathic-dilated cardiomyopathy. *American Journal of Cardiology 82: 1071-1076, 1998.*
- Tei, C. et al.: New index of combined systolic and diastolic myocardial performance: A simple and reproducible measure of cardiac function - A study in normals and dilated cardiomyopathy. *Journal of Cardiology 26:357-366, 1995.*
- Tei, C. et al.: New non-invasive index of combined systolic and diastolic ventricular function. *Journal of Cardiology 26:135-136, 1995.*
- Tei, C. et al.: Doppler echocardiographic index for assessment of global right ventricular function. *Journal of the American Society of Echocardiography 9:838-847, 1996.*
- Tei, C. et al.: Doppler index combining systolic and diastolic myocardial performance: clinical value in cardiac amyloidosis. *Journal of the American College of Cardiology 28: 658-664, 1996.*

Appendixes

Appendix 1
Studies validating QP:QS calculations derived by Doppler methods compared with other techniques.

First Author (Year)	Pt. No.	QP Site	QS Site	Reference Standard	r	SEE	Regression Equation
Sanders (1983) [1]	22	MPA	Asc Ao	Fick	0.85	-	N/A
Meijboom (1983) [2]	26 *	MVO	RVOT	EM flow meter	0.96	0.21	DOPP = 0.913 x + 0.147
Kitabatake (1984) [3]	22	RVOT	LVOT	Fick	0.92	-	CATH = 1.11 x - 0.30
Valdes-Cruz (1984) [4]	10	MPA	Asc Ao	EM flow	0.96	0.28	DOPP = 0.845 x + 0.227
Vargas Barron (1984) [5]	4 (PDA) 6 (ASD) 11 (VSD)	MVO MPA MVO	RVOT MVO Asc Ao	Fick, dye dilution or radionulcide scintigraphy	0.85	0.48	DOPP = 0.681 x + 0.49
Cloez (1988) [6]	42	MPA	Asc Ao	Fick	0.93	0.23	DOPP = 0.80 x + 0.39
Dittmann (1988) [7]	16	RVOT	LVOT	Fick	0.82	0.54	N/A
Kurokawa (1988) [8]	16	MVO	LVOT	Dye dilution	0.97	0.23	DOPP = 0.96 x + 0.16

* Animal model, extracardiac shunt.

Sources: (1) Sanders, S.P. et al.: *American Journal of Cardiology 51: 953-956, 1983*; (2) Meijboom, E.J. et al.: *Circulation 68: 437-445, 1983*; (3) Kitatabake, A. et al.: *Circulation 69: 73-79, 1984*; (4) Valdes-Cruz, L.M. et al.: *Circulation 69: 80-86, 1984*; (5) Vargas Barron, J. et al.: *Journal of the American College of Cardiology 3: 169-178, 1984*; (6) Cloez, J-L. et al.: *Journal of the American College of Cardiology 11: 825-830, 1988*; (7) Dittman, H. et al.: *Journal of the American College of Cardiology 11: 338-342, 1988*; (8) Kurokawa, S. et al.: *American Heart Journal 116: 1033-1044, 1988*.

Appendix 2
Studies Validating Doppler-Derived Pressure Gradients by Simultaneous and Nonsimultaneous Cardiac Catheterisation Studies in Obstructive, Regurgitant and Shunt Lesions.

First Author Year	Pt. No.	Study Group	Type	r	SEE (mm Hg)	Regression Equation
Hatle (1979) [1]	18	MS	S	0.92 (ΔP_{mean})	-	N/A
	7	MS + MR	S	0.82 (ΔP_{mean})	-	N/A
Stamm (1983) [2]	26	AS		0.94 (ΔP_{p-p})	-	N/A
	27		NS	0.85 (ΔP_{mean})	-	N/A
		MS				
			NS			
Lima (1983) [3]	16	PS	NS	0.98 (ΔP_{max})	6.5	DOPP = 1.04 x – 6.99
Kosturakis (1984) [4]	14	PS (11), AS (3), S (9)		0.91 (ΔP_{p-p})	8.8	N/A
Yock (1984) [5]	54	TR		0.93 (ΔP_{max})	8	DOPP = 1.00 x – 1.0
Simpson (1985) [6]	24	AS		0.98 (ΔP_{max})	-	N/A
Currie (1985) [7]	100	AS	(S)	0.92 (ΔP_{max})	15	CATH = 0.97 x +10.3
				0.93 (ΔP_{mean})	10	CATH = 0.98 x + 5.2
				0.91 (ΔP_{p-p})	14	N/A
Currie (1985) [8]	111	TR	(S)	0.96 (ΔP_{max})	7	DOPP = 0.88 x + 2.2
Masuyama (1986) [9]	31	PR	(NS)	0.94 (ΔP_{max})	3	DOPP = 0.70 x + 1
Murphy (1986) [10]	28	VSD	(S)	0.96 (ΔP_{max})	-	DOPP = 1.15 x - 8.60
Smith (1986) [11]	33	AS	(S)	0.93 (ΔP_{max})	9	DOPP = 0.84 x + 5.7
				0.95 (ΔP_{mean})	6	DOPP = 0.82 x + 5.9
				0.85 (ΔP_{p-p})	12	DOPP = 0.72 x + 28.4
Currie (1986) [12]	62	LVOTO †	(S)	0.95 (ΔP_{max})	11	DOPP = 0.92 x + 11
				0.95 (ΔP_{mean})	8	DOPP = 0.94 x + 21
				0.92 (ΔP_{p-p})	13	N/A
	38	RVOTO ‡	(S)	0.96 (ΔP_{max})	9	DOPP = 0.92 x + 11
				0.93 (ΔP_{mean})	8	DOPP = 0.94 x + 21
				0.95 (ΔP_{p-p})	10	N/A
	100	all lesions	(S)	0.95 (ΔP_{max})	10	DOPP = 0.93 x + 0.5
				0.94 (ΔP_{mean})	8	DOPP = 0.93 x + 1.8
Nishimura (1988) [13]	23	MR(11),	(S)	0.98 (ΔP_{max})	8	DOPP = 1.0 x - 7.4
		AR(12)	(S)	0.94 (ΔP_{mean})	6	DOPP = 0.95 x - 1.2
Ge (1992) [14]	54	MR	(S)	0.91 (ΔP_{max})	6	DOPP = 0.955 x + 2.316
Ge (1992) [15]	64	VSD	(S)	0.98 (ΔP_{max})	6.3	DOPP = 1.04 x - 3.36
Ge (1993) [16]	47	MR	(S)	0.96 (ΔP_{max})	3.9	DOPP = 0.946 x + 4.740
	25	AR	(S)	0.90 (ΔP_{max})	4.4	DOPP = 0.912 x + 5.929
Nishimura (1994) [17]	17	MS	(S)	0.97 (ΔP_{mean})	-	DOPP = 0.98 x - 0.07
Lei (1995) [18]	17	PR (peak diastolic)	(S)	0.95 (ΔP_{max})	7	DOPP = 0.97 x - 13
		PR(end diastolic)	(S)	0.94 (ΔP_{max})	5	DOPP = 0.83 x - 2

Abbreviations: ΔP_{max} = maximal catheter and Doppler pressure gradients; ΔP_{mean} = mean catheter and Doppler pressure gradients; ΔP_{p-p} = peak-to-peak catheter gradient and maximal instantaneous Doppler pressure gradient; **AR** = aortic regurgitation; **AS** = aortic stenosis; **DOPP** = Doppler gradient; **LVOTO** = left ventricular outflow tract obstruction; **MS** = mitral stenosis; **MR** = mitral regurgitation; **N/A** = not available; **NS** = non-simultaneous; **PR** = pulmonary regurgitation; **Pt. No.** = patient number; **r** = correlation coefficient; **RVOTO** = right ventricular outflow tract obstruction; **S** = simultaneous; **SEE** =   standard error of the estimate; **TR** = tricuspid regurgitation.
† left ventricular outflow tract lesions included valvular aortic stenosis (52), discrete subvalvular stenosis (4), bulboventricular foramen obstruction (4), and hypertrophic obstructive cardiomyopathy (2).
‡ right ventricular outflow tract lesions included pulmonary artery band (17), valvular pulmonary stenosis (12), infundibular stenosis (5), conduit obstruction (3), supravalvular stenosis (1).

Sources: (1) Hatle, L. et al.: *Circulation 60:1096-1104,1979*; **(2)** Stamm, R.B., Martin, R.P., *Journal of the American College of Cardiology 2:707,718,1983*; **(3)** Lima, C.O. et al., *Circulation 67:866-871,1983*; **(4)** Kosturakis, D. et al., *Journal of the American College of Cardiology 3:1256-1262,1984*; **(5)** Yock, P.G., Popp, R.L., *Circulation 70:657-662,1984*; **(6)** Simpson, I.A. et al., *British Heart Journal 53:636-639,1985*; **(7)** Currie, P.J. et al., *Circulation 71:1162-1169,1985*; **(8)** Currie, P.J. et al, *Journal of the American College of Cardiology 6:750-756,1985*; **(9)** Masuyama, T. et al., *Circulation 74:484-492,1986*; **(10)** Murphy, .D.J. et al., *American Journal of Cardiology 57:428-432,1986*; **(11)** Smith, M.D. et al., *American Heart Journal 111:245-252,1986*; **(12)** Currie, P.J. et al., *Journal of the American College of Cardiology 7:800-806,1986*; **(13)** Nishimura, R.A., Tajik, A.J., *Journal of the American College of Cardiology 11:317-321,1988*; **(14)** Ge, Z. et al., *International Journal of Cardiology 37:243-251,1992*; **(15)** Ge, Z. et al., *American Heart Journal 124:176-182,1992*; **(16)** Ge, Z-M. et al.: *Clinical Cardiology 16:863-870,1993*; **(17)** Nishimura, R.A. et al., *Journal of the American College of Cardiology 24:152-158,1994*; **(18)** Lei, M-H. et al., *Cardiology 86: 249-256, 1995*.

Appendix 2 (continued)
Studies Validating Doppler-Derived Pressure Gradients by Invasive Pressure Measurement in Prosthetic Heart Valves.

First Author (Year)	Pt. No.	Valve Type (Size and Position)	r	SEE (mm Hg)	Regression Equation
Sagar (1986) [1]	19	Hancock & B-S (27-33 mm, mitral)	0.933 (ΔP_{mean})	2.5	CATH = 1.086 x − 1.624
	11	Hancock & B-S (23-27 mm, aortic)	0.937 (ΔP_{mean})	7.4	CATH = 1.32 x − 7.446
Wilkins (1986) [2]	13	S-E, B-S, porcine (27-33 mm, mitral)	0.96 (ΔP_{mean})	-	CATH = 1.07 x + 0.28
	8	Porcine only (27-33 mm, mitral)	0.96 (ΔP_{mean})	-	CATH = 1.06 x + 0.55
	5	S-E (3) + B-S (2) (27-33 mm, mitral)	0.93 (ΔP_{mean})	-	CATH = 1.06 x − 0.04
Burstow (1989) [3]	42	Mixed † (all)	0.94 (ΔP_{max}) 0.96 (ΔP_{mean})	6 3	DOPP = 1.09 x − 3.3 DOPP = 1.03 x − 1.2
	20	Mixed † (21-31 mm, aortic)	0.94 (ΔP_{max}) 0.94 (ΔP_{mean})	6 3	DOPP = 1.12 x − 3.9 DOPP = 1.01 x − 0.34
	12 ‡	Mixed † (25-34 mm, mitral)	0.96 (ΔP_{max}) 0.97 (ΔP_{mean})	2 1.2	DOPP = 1.22 x − 3.1 DOPP = 1.1 x − 0.7
Baumgartner (1990) [4]	IV	St. Jude (19-27 mm, aortic)	0.98 (ΔP_{max}) 0.98 (ΔP_{mean})	3.5 1.9	DOPP = 1.42 x + 5.5 DOPP = 1.6 x + 2.2
		Hancock (19-27 mm, aortic)	0.99 (ΔP_{max}) 0.98 (ΔP_{mean})	1.9 1.4	DOPP = 1.0 x + 3.1 DOPP = 1.1 x + 0
Stewart (1991) [5]	IV	Hancock, C-E, I-S (19-27 mm, aortic)	0.94-0.99 (ΔP_{max}) 0.78-0.98 (ΔP_{mean})	- -	N/A N/A
Baumgartner (1992) [6]	IV	St. Jude (19-27 mm, aortic)	0.99 (ΔP_{max}) 0.98 (ΔP_{mean})	3.1 2.0	DOPP = 1.76 x + 1.3 DOPP = 1.75 x + 0.68
		Medtronic-Hall (20-27 mm, aortic)	0.99 (ΔP_{max}) 0.99 (ΔP_{mean})	0.8 0.5	DOPP = 1.01 x + 1.2 DOPP = 1.06 x + 0.4
		Starr-Edwards (21-27 mm, aortic)	0.98 (ΔP_{max}) 0.97 (ΔP_{mean})	2.9 2.0	DOPP = 1.65 x + 1.4 DOPP = 1.58 x + 0.3
		Hancock (19-27 mm, aortic)	0.99 (ΔP_{max}) 0.99 (ΔP_{mean})	2.7 1.5	DOPP = 1.14 x + 2.2 DOPP = 1.02 x + 1.6

Abbreviations: ΔP_{max} = maximal catheter and Doppler pressure gradients; ΔP_{mean} = mean catheter and Doppler pressure gradients; ΔP_{p-p} = peak-to-peak catheter gradient and maximal instantaneous Doppler pressure gradient; **B-C** = Braunwald-Cutter; **B-S** = Bjork-Shiley; **C-E** = Carpentier-Edwards; **D-M** = Dura-Mater; **DOPP** = Doppler gradient; **H-M** = Hall-Medtronic; **I-S** = Ionescu-Shiley; **IV** = in vitro; **r** = correlation coefficient; **N/A** = not available; **S-C** = Smeloff-Cutter; **S-E** = Starr-Edwards; **SEE** = standard error of the estimate.
† Aortic valve prostheses: S-E (9), B-S (3), St Jude (2), B-C (1), H-M (1), Sorin (1), Hancock (3)
Mitral valve prostheses: S-E (6), B-S (4), Hancock (2), B-C (2), H-M (1), S-C (1), I-S (1), C-E (1), D-M (1)
Pulmonary valve prosthesis: I-S (1)
Tricuspid valve prosthesis: B-C (1)
‡ left atrial pressure measures by the trans-septal technique.

Sources: (**1**) Sagar, K.B. et al., *Journal of the American College of Cardiology 7:681-687,1986*; (**2**) Wilkins, G.T. et al., *Circulation 74:786-795,1986*; (**3**) Burstow, D.J. et al., *Circulation 80:504-514,1989*; (**4**) Baumgartner, H. et al., *Circulation 82:1467-1475,1990*; (**5**) Stewart, S.F.C. et al., *Journal of the American College of Cardiology 18:769-779,1991*; (**6**) Baumgartner, H. et al., *Journal of the American College of Cardiology 19:324-332,1992*.

Appendix 3
Normal Prosthetic Valve Haemodynamics by Doppler Echocardiography.

A. Normal Aortic Valve Prosthesis Haemodynamics.

Valve Type	Number	Peak Velocity *(m/s)	Mean Gradient* (mm Hg)
Heterograft	214	2.4 ± 0.5	13.3 ± 6.1
Ball and Cage	160	3.2 ± 0.6	23.0 ± 8.8
Bjork-Shiley	141	2.5 ± 0.6	13.9 ± 7.0
St Jude	44	2.5 ± 0.6	14.4 ± 7.7
Allograft	30	1.9 ± 0.4	7.7 ± 2.7
Medtronic-Hall	20	2.4 ± 0.2	13.6 ± 3.3
Total	**609**	**2.6 ± 0.7**	**15.8 ± 8.3**

Source: Connolly, H.M. et al., *Journal of the American College of Cardiology 17: 69A, 1991.*
* mean ± one standard deviation

B. Normal Mitral Valve Prosthesis Haemodynamics.

Valve Type	Number	Peak Velocity *(m/s)	Mean Gradient*(mm Hg)
Ball-cage	161	1.8 ± 0.3	4.9 ± 1.8
Bjork-Shiley	79	1.7 ± 0.3	4.1 ± 1.6
Heterograft	150	1.6 ± 0.3	4.1 ± 1.5
St Jude	66	1.6 ± 0.4	4.0 ± 1.8
Total	**456**	**1.7 ± 0.3**	**4.4 ± 1.7**

Source: Lengyel, M. et al., *Circulation 82 (suppl III): 43,1990.*
* mean ± one standard deviation.

C. Normal Tricuspid Valve Prosthesis Haemodynamics.

Valve Type	Number	Peak Velocity * (m/s)	Mean Gradient* (mm Hg)
Ball-cage	35	1.3 ± 0.2	3.2 ± 0.8
Heterograft	43	1.3 ± 0.2	3.2 ± 1.1
St Jude	7	1.2 ± 0.3	2.7 ± 1.1
Bjork-Shiley	1	1.3	2.2
Total	**86**	**1.3 ± 0.2**	**3.1 ± 1.0**

Source: Connolly, H.M. et al., *Journal of the American College of Cardiology 17: 69A, 1991.*
* mean ± one standard deviation.

Appendix 4

Studies validating pulmonary artery pressure estimation by Doppler echocardiography compared with cardiac catheterisation.

First Author (Year)	Pt. No.	Doppler Method		r	SEE (mm Hg)	Regression Equation
Hatle (1981) [1]	45	RVSP	= RVIVRT & nomogram¶	0.89	-	N/A
Kitabatake (1983) [2]	33	$\log_{10}$ MPAP = 0.0068 (A_cT) + 2.1		-0.88	-	N/A
		$\log_{10}$ MPAP = -2.8 (A_cT/RVET) + 2.4		-0.90	-	N/A
Yock (1984) [3]	62	RVSP	= 4 $(V_{TR})^2$ + JVP	0.95	7	DOPP = 1.00 x - 1.0
Marx (1985) [4]	25	RVSP	= BP_{sys} - 4 $(V_{VSD})^2$	0.92	9.9	DOPP = 0.92 x + 4.7
Currie (1985) [5]	41	RVSP	= 4 $(V_{TR})^2$ + JVP	0.90	8	N/A
Comparative study	48	RVSP	= regression equation †	0.89	9	N/A
(total of 111 patients)	48	RVSP	= 4 $(V_{TR})^2$ + 10	0.89	8	N/A
Murphy (1986) [6]	14	RVSP	= BP_{sys} - 4 $(V_{VSD})^2$	0.93	-	N/A
Masuyama (1986) [7]	31	PAEDP	= 4 $(V_{PR})^2$ + RAP	0.94	4	DOPP = 0.74 x + 1
	30	M PAP	= 4 $(V_{PR})^2$	0.92	5	DOPP = 0.70 x - 2
Debastini (1987) [8]	45	MPAP	= 79 - (0.45 x RVAcT)**	- 0.87	8.3	N/A
Chan (1987) [9]	36	RVSP	= 4 $(V_{TR})^2$ + 14	0.87	8	N/A
	36	RVSP	= 4 $(V_{TR})^2$ + JVP	0.89	7.4	N/A
	44	MPAP	= 79 - (0.45 x RVA_cT)‡	0.66	10	N/A
Comparative study	26	MPAP	= 79 - (0.45 x RVA_cT)§	0.85	7	N/A
(total of 50 patients)	11	RVSP	= RVIVRT & nomogram¶	0.87	11	N/A
Stevenson (1989) [10]	50	RVSP	= 4 $(V_{TR})^2$ + 7	0.96	6.9	N/A
		RVSP	= RVIVRT & nomogram¶	0.97	5.4	N/A
		$\log_{10}$ MPAP = -2.8 (A_cT/RVET) + 2.4		0.94	7.7	N/A
Comparative study		PAEDP	= 4 $(V_{PR})^2$ + RAP	0.96	4.5	N/A
Lee (1989) [11]	17	PAEDP	= 4 $(V_{PR})^2$ + JVP or CVP	0.94	-	DOPP = 0.95 X - 1.0
Ge (1993) [12]	26	PASP	= BP_{sys} - 4 $(V_{PDA})^2$	0.94	10.3	DOPP = 0.91 x + 3.50
Ge (1993) [13]	66	PASP	= BP_{sys} - 4 $(V_{VSD})^2$	0.97	8.2	DOPP = 1.012 x - 2.904
		RVSP	= BP_{sys} - 4 $(V_{VSD})^2$	0.97	7.6	DOPP = 1.035 x - 3.627
Lei (1995) [14]	32	MPAP	= 4 $(V_{PR})^2$	0.94	8	DOPP = 0.78 x - 8

Abbreviations: A_cT = right ventricular acceleration time; **BP_{diast}** = diastolic blood pressure; **BP_{sys}** = systolic blood pressure; **CVP** = central venous pressure; **DOPP** = Doppler-derived pressure; **JVP** = jugular venous pressure; **N/A** = not available; **MPAP** = mean pulmonary artery pressure; **PAEDP** = end-diastolic pulmonary artery pressure; **PASP** = pulmonary artery systolic pressure; **r** = correlation coefficient; **RAP** = right atrial pressure; **RVET** = right ventricular ejection time; **RVIVRT** = right ventricular isovolumic relaxation time; **RVSP** = right ventricular systolic pressure; **SEE** = standard error of the mean; **V_{PR}** = pulmonary regurgitant velocity; **V_{TR}** = tricuspid regurgitant velocity; **V_{VSD}** = ventricular septal defect velocity; **V_{PDA}** = patent ductus arteriosus velocity.

† derived regression equation based on mean jugular venous pressure < or > 20 cm to estimate mean right atrial pressure (JVP < 20 cm assumes RAP = 15 mm Hg; JVP > 20 cm, assumes RAP > 15 mm Hg). Derived regression equation as follows:
RVSP = 4 $(V_{TR})^2$ + 14   (RAP = 15 mm Hg)
RVSP = [4 $(V_{TR})^2$ x 1.1] + 20   (RAP > 15 mm Hg)

‡ using all heart rates (38 - 180 beats/minute)
** when RVA_cT was 120 ms or less
§ using heart rates between 60 - 100 beats/minute
¶ Burstin's nomogram[15]

Sources: (1) Hatle, L., et al., *British Heart Journal 45:157-165,1981*; **(2)** Kitabatake, A., et al., *Circulation 68:302-309,1983*; **(3)** Yock, P.G., Popp, R.L., *Circulation 70: 657-662, 1984*; **(4)** Marx, G.R., et al., *Journal of the American College of Cardiology 6:1132-1137,1985*; **(5)** Currie, P.J. et al., *Journal of the American College of Cardiology 6: 750-756, 1985*; **(6)** Murphy, D.J. et al., *American Journal of Cardiology 57: 428-432, 1986*; **(7)** Masauyama, T., et al., *Circulation 74: 484-492, 1986*; **(8)** Debastini, A. et al., *American Journal of Cardiology 59: 662-668, 1987*; **(9)** Chan, K-L., et al., *Journal of the American College of Cardiology 9:549-554,1987*; **(10)** Stevenson, J.G., *Journal of the American Society of Echocardiography 2:157-171,1989*; **(11)** Lee, R .T., et al., *American Journal of Cardiology 64:1366-1370,1989*; **(12)** Ge, Z., et al., *American Heart Journal 125:263-266,1993*; **(13)** Ge, Z., et al., *American Heart Journal 125:1073-1081,1993*; **(14)** Lei, M-H., et al., *Cardiology 86:249-256,1995*; **(15)** Burstin, L.: *British Heart Journal 29:393-404,1967*.

Appendix 4 (continued)

Studies validating left atrial and left ventricular pressure estimation by Doppler echocardiography compared with cardiac catheterisation.

First Author (Year)	Pt. No.	Doppler Method			r	SEE (mm Hg)	Regression Equation
Grayburn (1987) [1]	31	LVEDP	$= BP_{diast}$	$- 4 (V_{AR-ED})^2$	0.84	5.5	DOPP = 0.90 x + 4.60
Gorscan (1991) [2]	35	LAP	$= BP_{sys}$	$- 4 (V_{MR})^2$	0.88	4	CATH = 0.88 x + 3.3
Ge (1992) [3]	54	LAP	$= BP_{sys}$	$- 4 (V_{MR})^2$	0.93	2.9	DOPP = 0.935 x + 0.656
Ge (1993) [4]	47	LAP	$= BP_{sys}$	$- 4 (V_{MR})^2$	0.945	2.69	DOPP = 0.901 x + 1.103
	25	LVEDP	$= BP_{diast}$	$- 4 (V_{AR-ED})^2$	0.854	2.65	DOPP = 1.20 x + 2.159

Abbreviations: BP_{diast} = diastolic blood pressure; BP_{sys} = systolic blood pressure; **CATH** = catheter-derived pressure; **DOPP** = Doppler-derived pressure; **LAP** = mean left atrial pressure; **LVEDP** = left ventricular end-diastolic pressure; **r** = correlation coefficient; **SEE** = standard error of the mean; V_{AR-ED} = end-diastolic aortic regurgitant velocity; V_{MR} = peak mitral regurgitant velocity.

Sources: (**1**) Grayburn, P.A. et al., *Journal of the American College of Cardiology 10:135-141,1987*; (**2**) Gorscan ,J. et al., *American Heart Journal 121: 858-863,1991*; (**3**) Ge, Z. et al., *International Journal of Cardiology 37:243-251, 1992*; (**4**) Ge, Z. et al., *Clinical Cardiology. 16:863-870, 1993*.

Appendix 5
Normal Intracardiac Pressures of Normal Recumbent Adults.

Pressure	Mean (mm Hg)	Range (mm Hg)
Right atrium: mean	4	1 - 8
Left atrium: mean	7	4 - 12
Pulmonary artery: systolic end-diastolic mean	24 10 16	15 - 28 5 - 16 10 - 22
Right ventricle: systolic end-diastolic	24 4	15 – 28 0 - 8
Left ventricle: systolic end-diastolic	130 7	90 – 140 4 – 12
Systemic arterial: systolic diastolic mean	130 70 85	90 - 140 60 – 90 70 - 105

Source: Alexander, R.W., Schlant, R.C., and Fuster, V.: Hurst's. The Heart. 9th Edition. pp: 114, 1998. McGraw-Hill Inc.

Appendix 6

Studies validating valve area derived by the continuity equation in native valve stenosis (compared with the Gorlin equation) and prosthetic heart valves (compared to the actual valve area).

First Author (Year)	Pt. No.	Valve Lesion /Valve Prosthesis (Size and Position)	r	SEE (cm^2)	Regression Equation
Robson (1984) [1]	17	MS	0.79	0.21	N/A
Skjaerpe (1985) [2]	16	AS	0.89	0.12	DOPP = 0.74 x + 0.21
Zoghbi (1986) [3]	39	AS	0.94	0.16	CATH = 1.05 x - 0.05
Otto (1986) [4]	48	AS	0.86	-	DOPP = 0.96 x + 0.19
Teirstein (1986) [5]	30	AS	0.88	0.17	N/A
Come (1987) [6]	40	Pre-BAV	0.77	0.13	N/A
		Post-BAV	0.85	0.16	N/A
Nishimura (1988) [7]	55	Pre-BAV	0.72	0.10	DOPP = 0.54 X + 0.26
		Post-BAV	0.61	0.17	DOPP = 0.49 X + 0.47
Oh (1988) [8]	100	AS	0.83	0.19	DOPP = 0.76 x + 0.16
Nakatani (1988) [9]	41	MS	0.91	0.24	DOPP = 0.84 x + 0.15
Karp (1988) [10]	35	MS	0.84	0.20	N/A
Nakatani (1988) [11]	12	Pre-BMV	0.83	-	N/A
Otto (1988) [12]	103	AS	0.87	0.34	DOPP = 0.92 x + 0.16
Danielson (1989) [13]	100	AS	0.96	-	DOPP = 0.85 X + 0.08
Stoddard (1989) [14]	41	Pre-BAV	0.84	0.08	N/A
		Post-BAV	0.87	0.10	N/A
Rothbart (1990) [15]	22	Bioprosthesis (19-29 mm, aortic)	0.93 † / 0.78 ‡	- / -	N/A / N/A
Chafizadeh (1991) [16]	67	St. Jude (19-31 mm, aortic)	0.83 † / 0.87 ‡	-	N/A / N/A
Baumgartner (1992) [17]	IV	St. Jude (19-27 mm, aortic)	0.99	0.08	DOPP = 0.54 x + 0.24
		Medtronic-Hall (20-27 mm, aortic)	0.97	0.10	DOPP = 0.81 x + 0.08
		Hancock (19-27 mm, aortic)	0.93	0.10	DOPP = 0.80 x + 0.06
Mohan (1994) [18]	43	Bjork-Shiley (25-29 mm, mitral)	0.86	0.12	N/A
Bitar (1995) [19]	40	St. Jude (23-33 mm, mitral)	0.68	-	DOPP = 0.31 x + 0.42

Abbreviations: AS = aortic stenosis; **BAV** = balloon aortic valvuloplasty; **BMV** = balloon mitral valvuloplasty; **CATH** = catheter-derived valve areas; **cm^2** = centimetres squared; **DOPP** = Doppler-derived valve areas; **IV** = in vitro (compared with catheter-derived areas); **N/A** = not available; **mm** = millimetres; **MS** = mitral stenosis; **r** = correlation coefficient; **SEE** = standard error of the estimate.

† continuity equation valve area using the LVOT diameter
‡ continuity equation valve area using prosthetic valve sewing ring (valve size)

Sources: (1) Robson, D.J., Flaxman, J.C., *European Heart Journal 5:660-,1984*; **(2)** Skjaerpe, T. et al.:, *Circulation 72:810-818,1985*; **(3)** Zoghbi, W.A. et al., *Circulation 73:452-459,1986*; **(4)** Otto, C.M. et al., *Journal of the American College of Cardiology 7:509-517,1986*; **(5)** Teirstein, P. et al., *Journal of the American College of Cardiology 8:1059-1065,1986*; **(6)** Come, P.C. et al., *Journal of the American College of Cardiology 10:115-124,1987*; **(7)** Nishimura, R.A. et al., *Circulation 78:791-799,1988*; **(8)** Oh, J.K. et al., *Journal of the American College of Cardiology 11:1227-1234,1988*; **(9)** Nakatani, S. et al., *Circulation 77:78,1988*; **(10)** Karp, K. et al., *J Cardiovascular Ultrasonography 7:293,1988*; **(11)** Nakatani, S. et al., *Circulation 78:II-487,1988*; **(12)** Otto, C.M. & Pearlman, A.S.: *Archives of Internal Medicine 148: 2553- 2560, 1988*; **(13)** Danielson, R. et al., *American Journal of Cardiology 63:1107-1111,1989*; **(14)** Stoddard, M.F. et al., *Journal of the American College of Cardiology 14:1218-1228,1989*; **(15)** Rothbart, R.M. et al., *Journal of the American College of Cardiology 15:817-824,1990*; **(16)** Chafizadeh, E.R., Zoghbi, W.A., *Circulation 83:213-223,1991*; **(17)** Baumgartner, H. et al., *Circulation 85:2273-2283,1992*; **(18)** Mohan, J.C. et al. *International Journal of Cardiology 43:321-326,1994*; **(19)** Bitar, J.N. et al., *American Journal of Cardiology 76:287-293,1995*.

Appendix 7

Studies validating mitral valve area derived by the pressure half-time compared with the valve area calculated by the Gorlin equation at cardiac catheterisation in mitral valve stenosis and in prosthetic mitral valves.

First Author (Year)	Pt. No.	Study Population	r	SEE (cm2)	Regression Equation
Hatle (1985) [1]	20	MS	0.87	-	N/A
Stamm (1983) [2]	27	MS (incl. prior SMC in 8)	0.87	0.18	N/A
Smith (1986) [3]	37	MS	0.85	0.22	DOPP = 0.84 X + 0.17
	35	Prior SMC	0.90	0.14	DOPP = 0.63 X + 0.39
Sagar (1986) [4]	12	Hancock & B-S MVR	0.978	0.096	CATH = 1.093 x + 0.085
Wilkins (1986) [5]	8	Porcine MVR	0.65	-	CATH = 0.55 x + 0.61
Gonzalez (1987) [6]	14	Pure MS	0.95	0.11	DOPP = 0.78 x + 0.28
	19	Pure MS + MS/MR	0.90	0.11	N/A
Reid (1987) [7]	12	Pre-BMV	0.80	0.4	DOPP = 0.65 X + 0.32
Come (1988) [8]	37	Pre-BMV	0.51	-	N/A
Abascal (1988) [9]	17	Pre-BMV	0.75	-	CATH = 0.60 x + 0.38
Nakatani (1988) [10]	21	Pure MS	0.90	0.28	DOPP = 0.73 x + 0.26
Chen (1989) [11]	18	Pre-BMV	0.81	0.11	CATH = 0.88 x + 0.1
Smith (1991) [12]	37	MS (SR and 0-1+ MR)	0.84	0.13	DOPP = 0.64 x + 0.35
	17	MS (AF and 0-1+ MR)	0.76	0.26	DOPP = 0.89 x + 0.28
Tabbalat (1991) [13]	33	MS (PAP < 70 mm Hg)	0.85	0.27	DOPP = 0.76 x + 0.28

Abbreviations: AF = atrial fibrillation; **BMV** = balloon mitral valvuloplasty; **B-S** = Bjork-Shiley prosthetic valve; **CATH** = catheter-derived valve area; **DOPP** = Doppler-derived valve area; **incl.** = including; **N/A** = not available; **MR** = mitral regurgitation; **MS** = mitral stenosis; **MVR** = mitral valve replacement; **PAP** = pulmonary artery pressure; **r** = correlation coefficient; **SEE** = standard error of the estimate; **SMC** = surgical mitral commissurotomy; **SR** = sinus rhythm.

Sources: (1) Hatle, L., and Angelsen, B.: <u>Doppler Ultrasound in Cardiology. Physical Principles and Clinical Applications</u>. 2nd Edition *Lea and Febiger, 1985, p 118-122*; **(2)** Stamm, R.B., Martin, R.P, *Journal of the American College of Cardiology 2: 707-718, 1983*; **(3)** Smith, M.D. et al., *Circulation 73: 100-107, 1986*; **(4)** Sagar, K.B. et al., *Journal of the American College of Cardiology 7: 681-687, 1986*; **(5)** Wilkins, G.T. et al., *Circulation 74: 786-795, 1986*; **(6)** Gonzalez, M.A. et al., *American Journal of Cardiology 60:327-332,1987*; **(7)** Reid ,C. et al., *Circulation 76:628-636,1987*; **(8)** Come, P.C. et al., *American Journal of Cardiology 61:817-825,1988*; **(9)** Abascal, V. et al., *Journal of the American College of Cardiology 12:606-615,1988*; **(10)** Nakatani, S. et al., *Circulation 11: 78-85, 1988*; **(11)** Chen, C. et al., *Journal of the American College of Cardiology 13:1309-1313,1989*; **(12)** Smith, M.D. et al., *Am Heart J 121:480-488,1991*; **(13)** Tabbalat, R.A., Haft, J.I., *Am Heart J 121:488-493,1991*.

Appendix 8
Studies validating mitral valve area estimation using the proximal isovelocity surface area method.

First Author (Year)	Pt. No.	Reference Standard	r	SEE (cm²)	Regression Equation
Centamore (1992) [1]	37 (19 SR, 18 AF)	2-D Planimetry	0.84	-	DOPP = 0.83 x + 0.06
		PHT	0.79	-	DOPP = 0.84 x + 0.09
Rodriguez (1993) [2]	40 (34 SR, 6,AF)	2-D Planimetry	0.91	0.21	DOPP = 1.08 x + 0.13
	40 (34 SR, 6 AF)	PHT	0.89	0.24	DOPP = 1.02 x - 0.14
	26 (24 SR, 2 AF)	Gorlin equation	0.86	0.24	DOPP = 0.89 x + 0.08
Aguilar (1994) [3]	61 (20 SR, 41 AF)	PHT	0.96	0.10	N/A
Deng (1994) [4]	42 (25 SR, 17 AF)	2-D Planimetry	0.98	0.09	2D = 1.11 x +0.12
		PHT	0.89	0.17	PHT = 0.87 x + 0.11
Rifkin (1995) [5]	48 † (22 SR, AF 26)	Gorlin equation	0.78	0.33	CATH = 0.72 x + 0.27
	22 (SR only)		0.75	0.43	CATH = 0.71 x + 0.28
	26 (AF only)		0.79	0.24	CATH = 0.73 x + 0.26
	30 ‡ (11 SR, 17 AF)	Gorlin equation	0.85	0.23	CATH = 0.84 x + 0.18
	11 (SR only)		0.93	0.19	CATH = 0.99 x + 0.01
	17 (AF only)		0.69	0.24	CATH = 0.60 x + 0.41

Abbreviations: 2-D = two-dimensional echocardiography; AF = atrial fibrillation; CATH = catheter-derived valve area; DOPP = Doppler-derived valve area; N/A = not available; PHT = pressure half-time method; SR = sinus rhythm.

† includes all patients with varying degrees of mitral regurgitation: 0-2+ MR (30), 3+ MR (10), 4-5+ MR (8).
‡ includes only patients with 0-2+ MR (30).

Sources: (1) Centamore, G. et al., *G Ital Cardiol 22:1201-1210,1992;* (2) Rodriguez, L. et al., *Circulation 88:1157-1165,1993;* (3) Aguilar, J.A. et al.:, *Arch Inst Cardiol Mex 64:257-263,1994;* (4) Deng, Y-B. et al., *Journal of the American College of Cardiology 24:683-689,1994;* (5) Rifkin, R.D. et al., *Journal of the American College of Cardiology 26:458-465,1995.*

Appendix 9

A. Doppler echocardiographic parameters and values used as indicators of the various grades of severity of mitral regurgitation.

Severity of MR	VTI_s/VTI_d [1]	RJA [2] (cm²)	RJA/LAA [3]	RV [4] (ml)	RF [4] (%)	ERO [4] (mm²)
Mild	> 1.0	≤ 4	< 20	< 30	< 30	< 20
Moderate	0.5 - 1.0	-	20 - 40	30 - 44	30 - 39	20 - 29
Moderately severe	0.0 - 0.5	-	-	45 - 59	40 - 49	30 - 39
Severe	< 0	≥ 8	> 40	≥ 60	≥ 50	≥ 40

Sources:
(1) Seiler, C. et al.: *Journal of the American College of Cardiology 31: 1383-1390, 1998*; (2) Spain, M.G. et al.: *Journal of the American College of Cardiology 13: 585-590, 1989*; (3) Helmcke, F. et al.: *Circulation 75: 175-183, 1987*; (4) Dujardin, K.S. et al.: *Circulation 96: 3409-3415, 1997*.

B. Doppler echocardiographic parameters and values used as indicators of the various grades of severity of aortic regurgitation.

Severity of AR	DS [1] (m/s²)	PHT [2] (ms)	RJH [3] (mm)	RJH/LVOH [3]	RJA/LVOA [4]	RF [5] (%)	ERO [6] (mm²)
Mild	-	-	< 4	< 25	< 4	< 20	-
Moderate	-	-	-	-	4 - 24	20 - 40	-
Moderately severe	-	-	-	-	25 - 59	40 - 60	-
Severe	> 3.5	≤ 200	≥ 8	> 40	≥ 60	≥ 60	≥ 30

Sources:
(1) Labovitz, A. J. et al.: *Journal of the American College of Cardiology 8: 1341-1347, 1986*; (2) Teague, S. M. et al.: Quantification of aortic regurgitation utilising continuous wave Doppler ultrasound. *Journal of the American College of Cardiology. 8:596, 1986*; (3) Dolan, M. S. et al.: *American Heart Journal 129: 1018, 1995*; (4) Perry, G.J et al.: *Journal of the American College of Cardiology. 9: 952-959, 1987*; (5) Nishimura, R.A. et al.: *American Heart Journal 124: 995-1001, 1992*; (6) Tribouilloy, C.M. et al.: *Journal of the American College of Cardiology 32: 1032-1039, 1998*.

Appendix 10

Studies validating the Doppler-derived regurgitant fraction compared with the angiographically-derived regurgitant fraction calculated at cardiac catheterisation, angiographic grade regurgitation (#) or the magnetic resonance imaging-derived regurgitant fraction (*).

First Author (Year)	Pt. No.	Lesion	r	SEE (%)	Regression Equation
Kitabatake (1985) [1]	20	AR	0.96	-	CATH = 1.0 x + 0.08
Touche (1985) [2]	30	AR	0.90	8.8	DOPP = 1.05 x + 0.02
Rokey (1986) [3]	19	MR	0.91	7	CATH = 0.84 x + 1
	6	AR			
Tribouilloy (1991) [4]	27	MR	0.92	-	N/A
Xie (1991) [5] †	20	AR	0.88	9	N/A
Reimold (1996) [6] *	17	AR	0.60	-	DOPP = 0.41 x + 0.33

Abbreviations: AR = aortic regurgitation; **CATH** = catheter-derived regurgitant fraction; **DOPP** = Doppler-derived regurgitant fraction; **MR** = mitral regurgitation; **N/A** = not available; **Pt. No.** = patient number; **r** = correlation coefficient; **SEE** = standard error of the estimate.

Sources: (1) Kitabatake, A., et al., *Circulation 72:523-529,1985*; **(2)** Touche, T. et al., *Circulation 72: 819-824, 1985*; **(3)** Rokey, R., et al., *Journal of the American College of Cardiology 7:1273-1278,1986*; **(4)** Tribouilloy, C., et al., *British Heart Journal 66:290-294,1991*; **(5)** Xie, G-Y., et al., *Journal of the American College of Cardiology 24:1041-1045,1994.* **(6)** Reimold, S.C. et al., *Journal of the American Society of Echocardiography 9: 675-683, 1996.*

† using the simplified regurgitant fraction:

$$RF(\%) = 1 - \left[\frac{1}{0.77} \times \frac{VTI_{MV}}{VTI_{LVOT}} \right] \times 100$$

* using the simplified regurgitant fraction:

$$RF\ (\%) = diastolic\ VTI \div systolic\ VTI$$

Appendix 11

Studies validating the quantitative evaluation of regurgitant severity by the proximal isovelocity surface area (PISA) with other techniques.

First Author (Year)	Pt. No.	Reference Standard	r	SEE	Regression Equation
Recusani (1991) [1]	IV *	Flow rate (Q) - V_N = 54 cm/s	0.96	1.01 L/min	PISA = 0.7355 x + 0.6548
	(n = 9)	- V_N = 41 cm/s	0.96	1.2 L/min	PISA = 0.8759 x + 0.1992
	(n = 9)	- V_N = 27 cm/s	0.98	1.07 L/min	PISA = 0.7226 x + 0.7411
	(n = 11)	Actual area - V_N = 54 cm/s	0.90	13.4 mm²	PISA = 0.5893 x + 4.4311
	IV *	- V_N = 41 cm/s	0.92	11.5 mm²	PISA = 0.5313 x + 10.3905
	(n = 9)	- V_N = 27 cm/s	0.91	15.2 mm²	PISA = 0.8723 x + 9.1971
Utsunomiya (1991) [2]	(n = 9)	Flow rate (Q)	0.99	0.53 L/min	PISA = 1.09 x - 0.41
Bargiggia (1991) [3]	(n = 11)	Left ventriculography vs. Q_{PISA}	0.91	-	N/A
Rivera (1992) [4]	IV *	$RV_D = SV_{MV} - SV_{AV}$	0.93	-	PISA = 0.95 x + 0.55
	45 (MR)	$Q_D = RV_D$ x HR	0.93	-	PISA = 0.95 x + 0.54
	54 (MR)	$RF_D = RV \div SV_{MV}$	0.89	-	PISA = 0.98 x + 0.006
Chen (1993) [5]	42 (MR)	$RV_D = SV_{MV} - SV_{AV}$	0.94	18 ml	DOPP = 1.18 x + 9.5
		Left ventriculography vs. Q_{PISA}	0.89	-	N/A
Vandervoort (1993) [6]	IV	Actual area	0.99	-	PISA = 0.92 x + 1.0
	77 (MR)	$ERO_D = (SV_{MV} - SV_{AV}) \div VTI_{MR}$	0.95	-	PISA = 1.08 x - 1.4
Riveria (1994) [7]	45 **** (TR)	$RV_D = SV_{TV} - SV_{PV}$	0.95	-	PISA = 0.94 x + 0.99
		$Q_D = RV_D$ x HR	0.96	-	PISA = 0.97 x + 0.045
		$RF_D = RV \div SV_{TV}$	0.90	-	PISA = 1.07 x - 2.1
Rivera (1994) [8]	45 **** (TR)	$ERO_D = RV_D \div VTI_{TR}$	0.96	-	PISA = 0.97 x + 0.01
Enriquez-Sarano (1995) [9]	119 (MR)	$ERO_D = (SV_{MV} - SV_{AV}) \div VTI_{MR}$	0.92	15 mm²	N/A
		$ERO_{2-D} = (SV_{LV} - SV_{AV}) \div VTI_{MR}$	0.91	16 mm²	N/A
	112 **	$ERO_D = (SV_{MV} - SV_{AV}) \div VTI_{MR}$	0.97	6 mm²	N/A
		$ERO_{2-D} = (SV_{LV} - SV_{AV}) \div VTI_{MR}$	0.97	7 mm²	N/A
Xie (1995) [10]	20 (MR)	Left ventriculography vs. RV_{PISA}	0.77	-	N/A
		Left ventriculography vs. Q_{PISA}	0.73	-	N/A
Seiler (1998) [11]	100 (MR)	$RF_D = (SV_{LV} - SV_{AV}) \div SV_{LV}$	0.87	10.6%	DOPP = 0.81 x + 5.5
Tribouilloy (1998) [12]	64 (AR)	$ERO_D = (SV_{AV} - SV_{MV}) \div VTI_{AR}$	0.90	8.2 mm²	N/A
		$ERO_{2-D} = ((SV_{LV} - SV_{MV}) \div VTI_{AR}$	0.90	8.0 mm²	N/A
	59 *** (AR)	$ERO_D = (SVAV - SV_{MV}) \div VTI_{AR}$	0.95	5.4 mm²	N/A
		$ERO_{2-D} = ((SV_{LV} - SV_{MV}) \div VTI_{AR}$	0.95	5.8 mm²	N/A

Abbreviations: DOPP = Doppler calculations; **ERO_{2D}** = effective regurgitant orifice by two-dimensional and Doppler echocardiography; **ERO_D** = Doppler effective regurgitant orifice; **HR** = heart rate; **IV** = in vitro; **PISA** = proximal isovelocity surface area; **Q_D** = Doppler regurgitant flow rate; **Q_{PISA}** = regurgitant flow rate by PISA; **RF_D** = Doppler regurgitant fraction; **RJA / LAA** = regurgitant jet area to left atrial area ratio; **RV_D** = Doppler regurgitant volume; **MR** = mitral regurgitation; **N/A** = not available; **PISA** = proximal isovelocity surface area calculations; **RV_{PISA}** = regurgitant volume by PISA; **SV_{AV}** = stroke volume through the aortic valve; **SV_{LV}** = left ventricular stroke volume by Simpson's rule; **SV_{MV}** = stroke volume through the mitral valve; **SV_{TV}** = stroke volume through the tricuspid valve; **TR** = tricuspid regurgitation; **VTI_{MR}** = velocity time integral of mitral regurgitant signal; **VTI_{TR}** = velocity time integral of tricuspid regurgitant signal.

*   in a pulsatile flow model

**   when 7 patients with mitral valve prolapse and eccentric mitral regurgitant jets excluded.

***   flat profile only

****   Using the following equations (where applicable) for calculation of the regurgitant flow rate (Q), regurgitant volume (RV), regurgitant fraction (RF) and effective regurgitant orifice (ERO) from the proximal isovelocity surface area technique as:

$Q = 2\pi r^2 V_N (Vp/Vp - V_N).(\alpha/180)$

$RV = Q (\int V(t)/V_p).dt$

$RF = RV/SV_{TV}$

$ERO = (2\pi r^2 V_N)/(V_p - V_N).(\alpha/180)$

where V_N = aliased velocity; r = radius; $(V_O/V_O - V_N)$ = correction factor for flattening of the isovelocity contour (V_O) measured from the peak orifice velocity from the continuous-wave Doppler; $\alpha/180$ = correction factor for the valve angle; V_p = peak regurgitant velocity; $(\int V(t)dt)$ = regurgitant velocity time integral normalised by the peak regurgitant velocity (V_p).

Sources: (1) Recusani, F., et al., *Circulation 83:594-604,1991*; (2) Utsunomiya, T., et al., *Journal of the American Society of Echocardiography. 4:338-348,1991*; (3) Bargiggia, G.S., et al., *Circulation 84:1481-1489,1991*; (4) Rivera, J.M., et al., *American Heart Journal 124: 1289-1296,1992*; (5) Chen, C., et al., *Journal of the American College of Cardiology 21:374-383,1993*; (6) Vandervoort, P.M. et al., *Circulation 88: 1150-1156, 1993*; (7) Riveria, J.M., et al., *American Heart Journal 127:1354-1362,1994*; (8) Riveria, J.M., et al., *American Heart Journal 128:927-933,1994*; (9) Enriquez-Sarano, M., et al., *Journal of the American College of Cardiology 25:703-709,1995*; (10) Xie, G-Y, et al., *Journal of the American Society of Echocardiography. 8:48-54,1995*; (11) Seiler, C. et al., *Journal of the American College of Cardiology 31: 1383-1390, 1998*; (12) Tribouilloy, C.M. et al., *Journal of the American College of Cardiology 32: 1032-1039, 1998*.

Appendix 12
Studies validating stroke volume and cardiac output calculations by Doppler methods compared with other techniques.

First Author (Year)	Pt. No.	Site (Method)	Reference Standard	r	SEE	Regression Equation
Fisher (1983) [1]	52 *	MV (MVO)	Roller pump	0.974	0.23 L/min	DOPP = 0.982 x + 0.02
Fisher (1983) [2]	95 *	Asc Ao (PW)	Roller pump	0.98-0.99	0.2 L/min	DOPP = 1.001 x + 0.013
Huntsman (1983) [3]	45	Asc Ao (CW)	TD - CO	0.94	0.58 L/min	DOPP = 0.95 x + 0.38
Meijboom (1983) [4]	26 *	RVOT	EM flow - roller pump	0.99	0.134 L/min	DOPP = 0.968 x + 0.073
		MV (MVO)	Roller pump	0.99	0.164 L/min	DOPP = 0.963 x + 0.11
Lewis (1984) [5]	24	MV (circ)	TD - SV	0.96	5.9 ml	TD = 0.91 x + 5.1
			TD - CO	0.87	0.59 L/min	TD = 0.80 x + 0.94
	35	LVOT	TD - SV	0.95	6.4 ml	TD = 0.91 x + 7.8
			TD - CO	0.91	0.63 L/min	TD = 0.85 x + 1.1
Valdes-Cruz (1984) [6]	29 *	Asc Ao (PW)	EM flow	0.96	0.189 L/min	DOPP = 0.889 x + 0.167
	31 *	MPA	EM flow	0.97	0.28 L/min	DOPP = 0.934 x + 0.177
Gillam (1985) [7]	18	LVOT	TD - CO	0.99	-	DOPP = 1.07 x - 0.4
		RVOT		0.97	-	DOPP = 0.99 x - 0.03
		MV (circ)		0.94	-	DOPP = 1.03 x - 0.19
		TV (circ)		0.92	-	DOPP = 0.89 x + 0.4
Nishimura (1984) [8]	54	Asc Ao (CW)	TD - CO	0.94	0.78 L/min	DOPP = 1.0 x - 0.13
Labovitz (1985) [9]	35	Asc Ao (PW)	TD - CO	0.85	0.99 L/min	N/A
	31	LVOT		0.90	0.95 L/min	N/A
	12	RVOT		0.81	0.82 L/min	N/A
Meijboom (1985) [10]	24 *	TV (insp)	EM flow - Roller pump	0.90	0.3 L/min	DOPP = 0.89 x + 0.23
		TV (exp)		0.89	0.35 L/min	DOPP = 0.94 x + 0.12
	10	TV (aver)	TD - CO	0.98	0.43 L/min	DOPP = 1.04 x - 0.29
Stewart (1985) [11]	33 *	LVOT	Roller pump	0.98	0.3 L/min	DOPP = 1.06 x + 0.2
	29 *	MV (MVO)		0.97	0.3 L/min	DOPP = 0.98 x + 0.3
	30 *	RVOT		0.93	0.5 L/min	DOPP = 0.89 x + 0.4
Zhang (1985) [12]	18	MV (MVO)	Fick - SV	0.87	-	DOPP = 0.95 x + 4.83
			Fick - CO	0.98	0.49 L/min	DOPP = 0.97 x + 0.22
Bouchard (1987) [13]	41	LVOT (MM + CW)	TD - SV	0.95	7	DOPP = 0.97 x + 1.7
Dittman (1987) [14]	40	LVOT (MM)	TD - CO	0.93	0.589 l/min	DOPP = 0.94 x + 0.44
		LVOT		0.89	0.695 L/min	DOPP = 0.92 x - 0.18
		MV (circ)		0.86	0.800 L/min	DOPP = 0.88 x + 1.75
		MV (MVO)		091	0.532 L/min	DOPP = 0.79 x + 0.63
De Zuttere (1988) [15]	30	MV (MVO)	TD - SV	0.94	7.3 ml	DOPP = 0.91 x + 5.6
			TD - CO	0.91	0.53 L/min	DOPP = 0.92 x + 0.35
Hoit (1988) [16]	48	MV (MVO)	TD - CO	0.93	0.362 L/min	DOPP = 1.1 x - 0.45
Otto (1988) [17]	52 *	LVOT (AS)	EM flow	0.91	0.25 L/min	DOPP = 1.00 x + 0.03
Dubin (1990) [18]	18	LVOT	TD - SV	0.87	11 ml	TD = 0.92 x + 4.6
		MV (circ)		0.83	10 ml	TD = 0.605 x + 49.4
		MV (MVO)		0.57	19 ml	TD = 0.71 x + 41.5
Rivera (1996) [19]	14	TV (circ)	TD - SV	0.93	-	N/A

* Animal model

Abbreviations: Asc Ao (CW) = ascending aorta using continuous-wave Doppler; **Asc Ao (PW)** = ascending aorta using pulsed-wave Doppler; **DOPP** = Doppler-derived calculation; **EM** = electromagnetic; **L/min** = litres per minute; **LVOT** = left ventricular outflow tract; **LVOT (AS)** = left ventricular outflow tract proximal to aortic stenosis; **LVOT (MM)** = left ventricular outflow tract measured by M-mode; **LVOT (MM + CW)** = left ventricular outflow tract measured by M-mode and using continuous-wave Doppler; **ml** = millilitres; **MPA** = main pulmonary artery; **MV (circ)** = mitral valve assuming circular geometry; **MV (MVO)** = mitral valve orifice method; **N/A** = not available; **Pt. No.** = patient number; **PW** = pulsed-wave Doppler; **r** = correlation coefficient; **RVOT** = right ventricular outflow tract; **SEE** = standard error of the estimate; **TD** = thermodilution-derived calculations; **TD-CO** = thermodilution cardiac output; **TD-SV** = thermodilution stroke volume; **TV (circ)** = tricuspid valve assuming circular orifice; **TV (insp)** = tricuspid valve in inspiration; **TV (exp)** = tricuspid valve in expiration; **TV (aver)** = tricuspid valve averaged over inspiration and expiration.

Sources: (1) Fisher, D.C. et al.: *Circulation 67: 872-877, 1983;* **(2)** Fisher, D.C. et al.: *Circulation 67: 370-376, 1983;* **(3)** Huntsman, L.L. et al.: *Circulation 67: 593-602,1983;* **(4)** Meijboom, E.J. et al.: *Circulation 68: 437-445, 1983;* **(5)** Lewis, J.F. et al.: *Circulation 70: 425-431, 1984;* **(6)** Valdes-Cruz, L.M. et al.: *Circulation 69: 80-86, 1984;* **(7)** Gillam, L.D. et al.: *Circulation 72 (supplement III): III-99, 1985;* **(8)** Nishimura, R.A. et al.: *Mayo Clinic Proceedings 59: 484-489, 1984;* **(9)** Labovitz, A.J. et al.: *American Heart Journal 109: 327-332, 1985;* **(10)** Meijboom, E.J. et al.: *Circulation 71: 551-556, 1985;* **(11)** Stewart, W.J. et al.: *Journal of the American College of Cardiology 6: 653-662, 1985;* **(12)** Zhang, Y. et al.: *British Heart Journal 53: 130-136, 1985;* **(13)** Bouchard, A. et al.: *Journal of the American College of Cardiology 9: 75-83, 1987;* **(14)** Dittmann, H. et al.: *Journal of the American College of Cardiology 10: 818-823, 1987;* **(15)** De Zuttere, D. et al.: *Journal of the American College of Cardiology 11: 343-350, 1988;* **(16)** Hoit, B.D. et al.: *American Journal of Cardiology 62: 131-135, 1988;* **(17)** Otto, C.M. et al.: *Circulation 78: 435-441, 1988;* **(18)** Dubin, J. et al.: *American Heart Journal 120: 116-123, 1990;* **(19)** Rivera, J.M. et al.: *American Heart Journal 131: 742-747, 1996.*

Appendix 13
Studies Validating Doppler-Derived dP/dt by Simultaneous and Nonsimultaneous Cardiac Catheterisation Studies.

First Author (Year)	Pt. No.	Study Type	r	SEE (mm Hg/s)	Regression Equation
Murillo (1988) [1]	16 *	S	0.96	81	N/A
Bargigga (1989) [2]	42	S = 11 NS = 31	0.87	316	DOPP = 1.05 x - 155
Neumann (1989) [3]	14	S	0.84	106	DOPP = 0.55 x + 192
Chung (1990) [4]	9	S	0.95	75	DOPP = 0.93 x + 58
Chen (1991) [5]	28	S	0.94	138	DOPP = 1.18 x - 153
Chung (1992) [6]	14	s	0.98	50	DOPP = 1.1 x + 23
Ge (1993) [7]	53	S	0.93	271	DOPP = 0.862 x + 274.77
Aconina (1993) [8]	8 **	S	0.94	31	DOPP = 0.83 x + 72

*   In patients with tricuspid regurgitation, dP/dt measured between 1 m/s and either 2 m/s or 3 m/s depending on peak tricuspid regurgitant velocity.
**   In patients with tricuspid regurgitation, dP/dt measured between 0 and 2 m/s.

Abbreviations: DOPP = Doppler-derived dP/dt; **N/A** = not available; **NS** = non-simultaneous; **Pt. No.** = patient number; **r** = correlation coefficient; **S** = simultaneous; **SEE** = standard error of the estimate;

Sources: **(1)** Murillo, A. et al.: *Circulation (supplement II) 78: II-650, 1988*; **(2)** Bargiggia, G.S. et al.: *Circulation 80: 1287-1292, 1989*; **(3)** Neumann, A. et al.: *Circulation (supplement II) 80: II-170, 1989*; **(4)** Chung, N. et al.: *Journal of the American College of Cardiology 15: 140A, 1990*; **(5)** Chen, C. et al.: *Circulation 8: 2101-2110, 1991*; **(6)** Chung, N. et al.: *Journal of the American Society of Echocardiography 5: 147-152, 1992*; **(7)** Ge, Z. et al. :*Clinical Cardiology 16: 422-428, 1993*; **(8)** Anconina, J. et al.: *American Journal of Cardiology 71: 1495-1497, 1993*;

Index